Oncology Board Review

Oncology Board Review
Blueprint Study Guide and Q&A

Second Edition

Editors

Francis P. Worden, MD
Clinical Professor of Medicine
Director of Hematology/Oncology Fellowship Program
Division of Hematology/Oncology, Department of Internal Medicine
University of Michigan Medical School
Ann Arbor, Michigan

Rami N. Khoriaty, MD
Assistant Professor
Division of Hematology/Oncology, Department of Internal Medicine
University of Michigan Medical School
Ann Arbor, Michigan

Erin F. Cobain, MD
Clinical Lecturer
Division of Hematology/Oncology, Department of Internal Medicine
University of Michigan Medical School
Ann Arbor, Michigan

Alexander T. Pearson, MD, PhD
Clinical Lecturer
Division of Hematology/Oncology, Department of Internal Medicine
University of Michigan Medical School
Ann Arbor, Michigan

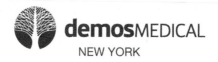

demosMEDICAL

NEW YORK

Visit our website at www.demosmedical.com

ISBN: 9781620701157
e-book ISBN: 9781617052927

Acquisitions Editor: David D'Addona
Compositor: Exeter Premedia Services Private Ltd.

Medicine is an ever-changing science. Research and clinical experience are continually expanding our knowledge, in particular our understanding of proper treatment and drug therapy. The authors, editors, and publisher have made every effort to ensure that all information in this book is in accordance with the state of knowledge at the time of production of the book. Nevertheless, the authors, editors, and publisher are not responsible for errors or omissions or for any consequences from application of the information in this book and make no warranty, expressed or implied, with respect to the contents of the publication. Every reader should examine carefully the package inserts accompanying each drug and should carefully check whether the dosage schedules mentioned therein or the contraindications stated by the manufacturer differ from the statements made in this book. Such examination is particularly important with drugs that are either rarely used or have been newly released on the market.

Library of Congress Cataloging-in-Publication Data

Names: Worden, Francis P., editor. | Khoriaty, Rami N., editor. | Cobain,
    Erin F., editor. | Pearson, Alexander T., editor.
Title: Oncology board review: blueprint study guide and Q&A / [edited by]
    Francis P. Worden, Rami N. Khoriaty, Erin F. Cobain, Alexander T. Pearson.
Other titles: Oncology boards flash review.
Description: Second edition. | New York: Demos, [2017] | Preceded by
    Oncology boards flash review / Francis P. Worden, Rami N. Khoriaty,
    editors. c2013. | Includes index.
Identifiers: LCCN 2016056062 | ISBN 9781620701157 | ISBN 9781617052927 (e-book)
Subjects: | MESH: Neoplasms | Examination Questions | Handbooks
Classification: LCC RC266.5 | NLM QZ 18.2 | DDC 616.99/40076—dc23
LC record available at https://lccn.loc.gov/2016056062

Printed in the United States of America by McNaughton & Gunn.
20 21 22 23 24 / 12 11 10 9

Contents

PART VII. SARCOMA

PART VIII. MELANOMA

PART IX. CENTRAL NERVOUS SYSTEM MALIGNANCIES

PART X. GYNECOLOGIC MALIGNANCIES

PART XI. CANCER OF UNKNOWN PRIMARY

PART XII. GENETICS AND TUMOR BIOLOGY

PART XIII. SUPPORTIVE AND PALLIATIVE CARE

PART XIV. BONE MARROW TRANSPLANTATION

PART XV. BIOSTATISTICS

Contributors

Ajjai Alva, MBBS, Assistant Professor, Division of Hematology/Oncology, Department of Internal Medicine, University of Michigan Medical School, Ann Arbor, Michigan

Dana E. Angelini, MD, Associate Staff, Department of Hematology and Medical Oncology, Cleveland Clinic–Taussig Cancer Center, Cleveland, Ohio

Laurence H. Baker, DO, Collegiate Professor, Cancer Developmental Therapeutics, Professor of Internal Medicine and Pharmacology, Division of Hematology/Oncology, Department of Internal Medicine, University of Michigan Medical School, Ann Arbor, Michigan

Emily Bellile, MS, Statistician, Center for Cancer Biostatistics, Department of Biostatistics, University of Michigan School of Public Health, Ann Arbor, Michigan

Manali Bhave, MD, Hematology and Oncology Fellow, Division of Hematology/Oncology, Department of Internal Medicine, University of Michigan Medical School, Ann Arbor, Michigan

Dale Bixby, MD, PhD, Clinical Associate Professor, Division of Hematology/Oncology, Department of Internal Medicine, University of Michigan Medical School, Ann Arbor, Michigan

Ronald J. Buckanovich, MD, PhD, Associate Professor, Internal Medicine, Division of Medical Oncology, Department of Obstetrics and Gynecology, University of Michigan Medical School, Ann Arbor, Michigan

Monika Burness, MD, Clinical Lecturer, Division of Hematology/Oncology, Department of Internal Medicine, University of Michigan Medical School, Ann Arbor, Michigan

Frank C. Cackowski, MD, PhD, Hematology and Oncology Fellow, Division of Hematology/Oncology, Department of Internal Medicine, University of Michigan Medical School, Ann Arbor, Michigan

Erica Campagnaro, MD, Associate Professor, Division of Hematology/Oncology, Department of Internal Medicine, University of Michigan Medical School, Ann Arbor, Michigan

Megan E. V. Caram, MD, MSc, Clinical Lecturer, Division of Hematology/ Oncology, Department of Internal Medicine, University of Michigan Medical School; Staff Physician, Department of Medicine, Ann Arbor Veterans Affairs, Ann Arbor, Michigan

Rashmi Chugh, MD, Associate Professor, Division of Hematology/Oncology, Department of Internal Medicine, University of Michigan Medical School, Ann Arbor, Michigan

Erin F. Cobain, MD, Clinical Lecturer, Division of Hematology/Oncology, Department of Internal Medicine, University of Michigan Medical School, Ann Arbor, Michigan

Lan G. Coffman, MD, PhD, Clinical Lecturer, Division of Hematology/Oncology, Department of Internal Medicine, University of Michigan Medical School, Ann Arbor, Michigan

Kathleen Ann Cooney, MD, H.A. and Edna Benning Presidential Endowed Chair and Department Chair, Department of Internal Medicine, University of Utah School of Medicine, Salt Lake City, Utah

Paul M. Corsello, MD, Gastroenterology Fellow, Division of Gastroenterology, Department of Internal Medicine, University of Michigan Medical School, Ann Arbor, Michigan

Elizabeth J. Davis, MD, Assistant Professor of Medicine, Division of Hematology/ Oncology, Department of Internal Medicine, Vanderbilt University Medical Center, Nashville, Tennessee

Sumana Devata, MD, Clinical Assistant Professor, Division of Hematology/ Oncology, Department of Internal Medicine, University of Michigan Medical School, Ann Arbor, Michigan

Tobias Else, MD, Assistant Professor, Division of Metabolism, Endocrinology and Diabetes, Department of Internal Medicine, University of Michigan Medical School, Ann Arbor, Michigan

Raymond M. Esper, MD, PhD, Physician, Florida Cancer Specialists and Research Institute, Fort Myers, Florida

Jessica N. Everett, MS, CGC, Clinical Assistant Professor, Department of Internal Medicine, Molecular Medicine and Genetics, University of Michigan Medical School, Ann Arbor, Michigan

Carlos J. Gallego, MD, MS, Assistant Professor, Department of Genetics and Genome Sciences, Case Western Reserve University School of Medicine, Cleveland, Ohio

Kari E. Hacker, MD, PhD, Gynecologic Oncology Fellow, Department of Obstetrics and Gynecology, University of Michigan Medical School, Ann Arbor, Michigan

Khaled A. Hassan, MD, MS, Assistant Professor, Division of Hematology/Oncology, Department of Internal Medicine, University of Michigan Medical School, Ann Arbor, Michigan

James A. Hayman, MD, MBA, Professor, Associate Chair for Clinical Activities, Department of Radiation Oncology, University of Michigan Health System, Ann Arbor, Michigan

Megan R. Haymart, MD, Assistant Professor of Medicine, Division of Metabolism, Endocrinology and Diabetes, University of Michigan Medical School, Ann Arbor, Michigan

Larry Junck, MD, Professor of Neurology, Department of Neurology, University of Michigan; Co-Director, Neuro-Oncology Program, University of Michigan Comprehensive Cancer Center, University of Michigan Medical School, Ann Arbor, Michigan

Kunal C. Kadakia, MD, FACP, Clinical Assistant Professor of Medicine, UNC, Department of Medical Oncology, Levine Cancer Institute, Charlotte, North Carolina

Gregory P. Kalemkerian, MD, Professor of Medicine, Division of Hematology/Oncology, Department of Internal Medicine, University of Michigan Medical School, Ann Arbor, Michigan

Rami N. Khoriaty, MD, Assistant Professor, Division of Hematology/Oncology, Department of Internal Medicine, University of Michigan Medical School, Ann Arbor, Michigan

Darren King, MD, Hematology and Oncology Fellow, Division of Hematology/Oncology, Department of Internal Medicine, University of Michigan Medical School, Ann Arbor, Michigan

Shawna Kraft, PharmD, Clinical Specialist, Division of Hematology/Oncology, Department of Pharmacy; Clinical Assistant Professor, Department of Clinical Pharmacy, University of Michigan College of Pharmacy, Ann Arbor, Michigan

John C. Krauss, MD, Assistant Professor of Internal Medicine, Division of Hematology/Oncology, University of Michigan Medical School, Ann Arbor, Michigan

Christopher Lao, MD, Associate Professor, Division of Hematology/Oncology, Department of Internal Medicine, University of Michigan Medical School, Ann Arbor, Michigan

Aaron Mammoser, MD, MS, Associate Professor, Department of Neurosurgery, Louisiana State University Health Sciences Center, New Orleans, Louisiana

Karen McLean, MD, PhD, Assistant Professor, Gynecologic Oncology, Department of Obstetrics and Gynecology, University of Michigan Medical School, Ann Arbor, Michigan

Neehar D. Parikh, MD, MS, Clinical Lecturer, Medical Director, Liver Tumor Program, Division of Gastroenterology, University of Michigan Medical School, Ann Arbor, Michigan

Alexander T. Pearson, MD, PhD, Clinical Lecturer, Division of Hematology/ Oncology, Department of Internal Medicine, University of Michigan Medical School, Ann Arbor, Michigan

Tycel J. Phillips, MD, Assistant Professor, Division of Hematology/Oncology, Department of Internal Medicine, University of Michigan Medical School, Ann Arbor, Michigan

Angel Qin, MD, Hematology and Oncology Fellow, Division of Hematology/ Oncology, Department of Internal Medicine, University of Michigan Medical School, Ann Arbor, Michigan

Bruce Redman, DO, Professor of Internal Medicine, Division of Hematology/ Oncology, Department of Internal Medicine, University of Michigan Medical School, Ann Arbor, Michigan

Zachery R. Reichert, MD, PhD, Hematology and Oncology Fellow, Division of Hematology/Oncology, Department of Internal Medicine, University of Michigan Medical School, Ann Arbor, Michigan

Mary Mansour Riwes, DO, Clinical Assistant Professor of Medicine, Division of Hematology/Oncology, Department of Internal Medicine, University of Michigan Medical School, Ann Arbor, Michigan

Lyndsey N. Runaas, MD, Hematology and Oncology Fellow, Division of Hematology/Oncology, Department of Internal Medicine, University of Michigan Medical School, Ann Arbor, Michigan

Vaibhav Sahai, MBBS, MS, Assistant Professor of Internal Medicine, Division of Hematology/Oncology, Department of Internal Medicine, University of Michigan Medical School, Ann Arbor, Michigan

Jordan K. Schaefer, MD, Hematology and Oncology Fellow, Division of Hematology/Oncology, Department of Internal Medicine, University of Michigan Medical School, Ann Arbor, Michigan

Benjamin Y. Scheier, MD, Staff Physician, Department of Oncology/Hematology, Kaiser Permanente, Lafayette, Colorado

Erlene K. Seymour, MD, Assistant Professor, Department of Hematology/ Oncology, Karmanos Cancer Institute/Wayne State University, Detroit, Michigan

Maryann Shango, MD, Hematology and Oncology Fellow, Division of Hematology/ Oncology, Department of Internal Medicine, University of Michigan Medical School, Ann Arbor, Michigan

Maria Silveira, MD, Fellow, Division of Geriatric and Palliative Medicine, Department of Internal Medicine, University of Michigan Medical School, Ann Arbor, Michigan

Brittany Siontis, MD, Hematology and Oncology Fellow, Division of Hematology/Oncology, Department of Internal Medicine, University of Michigan Medical School, Ann Arbor, Michigan

David C. Smith, MD, Professor of Medicine and Urology, Associate Chief for Clinical Services, Division of Hematology/Oncology, Department of Internal Medicine, University of Michigan Medical School, Ann Arbor, Michigan

Elena M. Stoffel, MD, MPH, Assistant Professor, Department of Internal Medicine, Director, Cancer Genetics Clinic, University of Michigan Health System, Ann Arbor, Michigan

Paul L. Swiecicki, MD, Hematology/Oncology Fellow, Division of Hematology/Oncology, Department of Internal Medicine, University of Michigan Medical School, Ann Arbor, Michigan

Alon Weizer, MD, Associate Professor of Urology, Associate Chair, Surgical Services, Department of Urology, University of Michigan, Ann Arbor, Michigan

Ryan A. Wilcox, MD, PhD, Assistant Professor, Division of Hematology/Oncology, Department of Internal Medicine, University of Michigan Medical School, Ann Arbor, Michigan

Francis P. Worden, MD, Clinical Professor of Medicine, Director of Hematology/Oncology Fellowship Program, Division of Hematology/Oncology, Department of Internal Medicine, University of Michigan Medical School, Ann Arbor, Michigan

Sarah Yentz, MD, Hematology and Oncology Fellow, Division of Hematology/Oncology, Department of Internal Medicine, University of Michigan Medical School, Ann Arbor, Michigan

Mark M. Zalupski, MD, Professor of Internal Medicine, Division of Hematology/Oncology, Department of Internal Medicine, University of Michigan Medical School, Ann Arbor, Michigan

David B. Zhen, MD, Hematology and Oncology Fellow, Division of Hematology/Oncology, Department of Internal Medicine, University of Michigan Medical School, Ann Arbor, Michigan

Preface

Preparation for board examinations can be a daunting and overwhelming process for many of us. As trainees, we are often busy with research projects, manuscripts, and a large clinical volume, making it difficult to find time to study for board examinations. As practicing physicians, we find it hard to keep up on material needed for board recertification.

Questions on the board examinations are drawn from well-established, validated medical literature and widely accepted clinical guidelines. That said, the University of Michigan Hematology/Oncology Fellowship Program designed this board review book to summarize information that is most pertinent for testing. The *Oncology Board Review: Blueprint Study Guide and Q&A, Second Edition* expands upon the excellent question-based review by providing key updates in all chapters that will be reflected in the medical oncology boards. This book is not intended to be an all-encompassing review. Rather, it is intended to help summarize the important facts that one might need to know for his or her examination, similar to taking notes of pertinent information that one would like to memorize. We created each chapter to cover all of the topics listed in the blueprint provided by the American Board of Internal Medicine as material one should know for the Medical Oncology Board Examination. The authors have endeavored to provide the most accurate and up-to-date information, including well-established chemotherapy regimens for a variety of malignancies. New to this edition, we have also written board review questions to accompany each chapter, providing over 230 multiple choice questions with answers and detailed rationales to those seeking practice questions ahead of their certification or recertification exams.

We hope that fellows and practicing medical oncologists preparing for their certification or recertification will find *Oncology Board Review: Blueprint Study Guide and Q&A, Second Edition* a useful tool. Our goal is to help our readers summarize and solidify many important clinical facts and to help them build confidence in their exam preparation about their knowledge.

As the Hematology/Oncology Fellowship Program director and the chief fellow at the University of Michigan (Ann Arbor, Michigan), we engaged our fellows and faculty to develop *Oncology Board Review: Blueprint Study Guide and Q&A, Second Edition*. Each chapter was written by a fellow and edited by an expert faculty member or an ancillary staff clinician. We gratefully acknowledge the dedication of our fellows, faculty, and medical staff. The successful completion of this project was made possible by the editorial and publishing staff of Demos Medical Publishing, especially David D'Addona, senior editor, and Joseph Stubenrauch, the managing editor who moved the project seamlessly through production.

Finally, we dedicate this book to Michelle Reinhold for her continued devotion and immeasurable service to the University of Michigan Hematology/Oncology Fellowship Program as program coordinator.

Francis P. Worden, MD
Rami N. Khoriaty, MD
Erin F. Cobain, MD
Alexander T. Pearson, MD, PhD

Acknowledgments

The editors would like to acknowledge and thank the contributors from the previous edition for their contributions:

Dawit Aregawi, MD
Grace Chen, MD
Stephanie Daignault-Newton, MS
Irina Dobrosotskaya, MD, PhD
Marwan Fakih, MD
Scott D. Gitlin, MD
Petros D. Grivas, MD, PhD
Maha Hussain, MD
Sadakatsu Ikeda, MD
Mark S. Kaminski, MD
Daniel Lebovic, MD
Binu Malhotra, MD
Jorge Marrero, MD
Kevin McDonnell, MD, PhD
Meaghan W. O'Malley, MD
Phillip Palmbos, MD, PhD
Brian Parkin, MD
Joshua M. Ruch, MD
Igor Rybkin, MD, PhD
Assuntina G. Sacco, MD
Ann W. Silk, MD, MS
Moshe Talpaz, MD
Eduardo Vilar-Sanchez, MD, PhD
Alissa Weber, MD

Acknowledgments

HEMATOLOGIC MALIGNANCIES

I

1

Acute Leukemias and Hairy Cell Leukemia

Lyndsey N. Runaas, Rami N. Khoriaty, and Dale Bixby

Acute Myeloid Leukemia

EPIDEMIOLOGY

1. **What is the median age at diagnosis?**
   - Sixty-seven years

2. **What is the incidence of acute myeloid leukemia (AML)?**
   - Twenty thousand new cases per year in the United States

ETIOLOGY AND RISK FACTORS

1. **What are the common risk factors for AML?**
   - Older age
   - Exposure to chemotherapeutic agents:
     - Topoisomerase II inhibitors: latency of 1 to 3 years, associated with rearrangement of the mixed lineage leukemia (*MLL*) gene (11q23)
     - Alkylating agents: latency period of 3 to 7 years, associated with the del 5q/-5 and/or del 7q/-7 chromosomal abnormalities as well as complex cytogenetic changes
   - Myelodysplastic syndrome (MDS)
   - Myeloproliferative neoplasms
   - Exposure to chemicals: benzene, pesticides, and petroleum products
   - Radiation exposure
   - Congenital disorders: Down syndrome, Bloom syndrome, Fanconi anemia, dyskeratosis congenita (Zinsser–Cole–Engman syndrome), GATA-2 deficiency, Shwachman–Diamond syndrome, Diamond–Blackfan anemia, and others

PATHOLOGY—CLASSIFICATION

1. **Define the subtypes of AML according to the 2016 World Health Organization (WHO) classification.**
   - AML with recurrent genetic abnormalities
     - AML with t(8;21) (q22;q22.1); *RUNX1-RUNX1T1*
     - AML with inv(16) (p13.1;q22) or t(16;16) (p13.1;q22); *CBFB-MYH11*
     - Acute promyelocytic leukemia (APL) with *PML-RARA*

- o AML with t(9;11) (p21.3;q23.3); *MLLT3-KMT2A*
- o AML with t(6;9) (p23;q34.1); *DEK-NUP214*
- o AML with inv(3) (q21.3;q26.2) or t(3;3) (q21.3;q26.2); *GATA2, MECOM*
- o AML (megakaryoloblastic) with t(1;22) (p13.3;q13.3); *RBM15-MKL1*
- o AML with mutated *NPM1*
- o AML with biallelic mutations of *CEBPA*
- o Provisional entities:
  - ■ AML with *BCR-ABL1*
  - ■ AML with mutated *RUNX1*
- • AML with myelodysplasia-related changes
- • Therapy-related myeloid neoplasms
- • AML, not otherwise specified (NOS)
  - o AML with minimal differentiation
  - o AML without maturation
  - o AML with maturation
  - o Acute myelomonocytic leukemia
  - o Acute monoblastic/monocytic leukemia
  - o Pure erythroid leukemia
  - o Acute megakaryoblastic leukemia
  - o Acute basophilic leukemia
  - o Acute panmyelosis with myelofibrosis
- • Myeloid sarcoma
- • Myeloid proliferations related to Down syndrome
  - o Transient abnormal myelopoiesis (TAM)
  - o Myeloid leukemia associated with Down syndrome

SIGNS AND SYMPTOMS

1. **What are the common signs and symptoms of AML?**
   - • Fever and other constitutional symptoms of infections
   - • Bruising or bleeding (due to thrombocytopenia)
   - • Fatigue and other symptoms of anemia
   - • Leukostasis: central nervous system (CNS) manifestations, cardiopulmonary symptoms, retinal hemorrhage, priapism
   - • Disseminated intravascular coagulation (DIC)
   - • Tumor lysis syndrome

DIAGNOSTIC WORKUP

1. **Define the diagnostic criteria for AML.**
   - • Marrow and/or peripheral blood blasts are at least 20%

- The myeloid lineage is established if *any* of the following are identified:
  - Auer rods
  - Blasts are myeloperoxidase positive (by flow cytometry, immunohistochemistry, or cytochemistry)
  - Monocytic differentiation (with at least two of the following: nonspecific esterase, CD11c, CD14, CD64, lysozyme)
- Note: the presence of t(15;17), t(8;21), inv(16), or t(16;16), is diagnostic of AML regardless of the blast percentage, is diagnostic of AML

PROGNOSTIC FACTORS

1. **How are patients with AML stratified into different risk groups?**
   - Age and cytogenetics are independent prognostic factors (older age is a poor prognostic factor).

Risk Status	Cytogenetics/Molecular Abnormalities
Favorable risk	• t(8;21) without c-KIT mutation
	• inv(16) or t(16;16) without c-KIT mutation
	• t(15;17)
	• Normal cytogenetics with *NPM1* mutation in absence of *FLT3*-ITD or with isolated biallelic *CEBPA* mutation
Intermediate risk	• Normal cytogenetics (without better risk or poor risk gene mutations)
	• +8
	• t(9;11)
	• Cytogenetic changes not associated with good or poor risk
Poor risk*	• Complex cytogenetics (at least three chromosomal abnormalities)
	• Monosomal karyotype
	• −5/5q−
	• −7/7q−
	• 11q23 [not t(9;11)]
	• inv(3)/t(3;3)
	• t(6;9)
	• t(9;22)
	• Normal cytogenetics with *FLT3*-ITD mutation
	• *TP53* mutation

*Poor-risk AML: also includes patients with secondary AML—antecedent hematologic disease or treatment-related AML.

2. **How are the patients with APL risk-stratified?**
   - Sanz criteria

Low-risk APL	White blood cell (WBC) <10,000 and platelet >40,000
Intermediate-risk APL	WBC <10,000 and platelet <40,000
High-risk APL	WBC >10,000

TREATMENT

Non-APL AML

1. **What are the induction treatment options for younger patients (<60 years old) with non-APL AML?**
   - Standard-dose cytarabine (100–200 mg/m^2 infusion) over 7 days + idarubicin (12 mg/m^2) or daunorubicin (60–90 mg/m^2) $\times$ 3 days
   - Standard-dose cytarabine (200 mg/m^2 infusion) over 7 days + daunorubicin 60 mg/m^2 $\times$ 3 days and cladribine 5 mg/m^2 $\times$ 5 days
   - High-dose cytarabine 2 g/m^2 every 12 hours $\times$ 6 days or 3 g/m^2 every 12 hours $\times$ 4 days + idarubicin 12 mg/m^2 or daunorubicin 60 mg/m^2 $\times$ 3 days
   - Fludarabine 20 mg/m^2 intravenous (IV) days 2–6, cytarabine 2 g/m^2 over 4 hours starting 4 hours after fludarabine on days 2–6, idarubicin 8 mg/m^2 IV days 4–6, and subcutaneous granulocyte colony-stimulating factor (G-CSF) daily days 1–7
   - Clinical trial (especially for patients with antecedent hematologic disorder or therapy-related AML)

2. **How do we evaluate the efficacy of induction therapy?**
   - Obtain a bone marrow biopsy 7 to 14 days after completion of induction therapy:
     - Aplastic marrow (<5% cellular and <5% blasts): await count recovery and consider growth factor support
     - Significant cytoreduction and a low percentage of blasts: consider repeating the marrow in 7 to 10 days or treat with standard-dose cytarabine (5 days) + idarubicin or daunorubicin (2 days) or a high-dose cytarabine-based regimen
     - Significant residual blasts: high-dose cytarabine (1.5–3 g/m^2)-based regimen or standard-dose cytarabine (7 days) + idarubicin or daunorubicin (3 days)
   - Obtain the next marrow at count recovery (see Question 5)

3. **What are the induction treatment options for older patients (>60 years) with non-APL AML?**
   - Patients with Eastern Cooperative Oncology Group (ECOG) performance status 0 to 2:
     - Standard-dose cytarabine (100–200 mg/m^2) continuous infusion over 7 days with idarubicin (12 mg/m^2) or daunorubicin (60–90 mg/m^2) $\times$ 3 days or mitoxantrone (12 mg/m^2) $\times$ 3 days

- o Decitabine or azacitidine (a special consideration for patients with therapy-related AML or patients with AML with complex cytogenetics)
- o Clinical trial
- Patients with ECOG performance status more than 2 or with significant comorbidities:
  - o Azacitidine or decitabine
  - o Clofarabine +/− cytarabine
  - o Best supportive care—hydroxyurea, transfusion support
  - o Clinical trial

4. **How does the bone marrow result 7 to 10 days after completing induction therapy in patients *older than 60 years* guide therapy?**
   - Aplastic marrow (<5% cellular and <5% blasts): await count recovery and consider growth factor supplementation
   - Significant cytoreduction with low-percentage blasts:
     - o Wait 7 to 10 more days and repeat the marrow
     - o Additional standard-dose cytarabine + anthracycline (5 + 2)
     - o Intermediate-dose cytarabine-based regimen (1–2 g/m^2)
     - o Reduced-intensity allogeneic stem cell transplantation (ASCT)
   - Significant residual blasts:
     - o Additional standard-dose cytarabine + anthracycline (5 + 2)
     - o Intermediate-dose cytarabine-based regimen
     - o Reduced-intensity ASCT
     - o Clinical trial
     - o Supportive care

5. **When is complete remission (CR) evaluated for and how is it defined?**
   - Evaluation of CR requires that a bone marrow biopsy be performed after count recovery—absolute neutrophil count (ANC) ≥1,000, platelets ≥100,000 (independent of transfusions).
     - o *Morphologic CR:* marrow blasts less than 5%, no Auer rods, no persistence of extramedullary disease
     - o *Cytogenetic CR:* normal cytogenetics in patients who had abnormal cytogenetics
     - o *Incomplete CR (CRi):* CR with persistence of cytopenia (usually thrombocytopenia)

6. **What is the postremission treatment of choice for younger patients (*<60 years old*) with non-APL AML in CR?**
   - Favorable-risk AML:
     - o High-dose cytarabine (3 g/m^2) over 3 hours every 12 hours on days 1, 3, and 5 for three to four cycles
     - o Clinical trial

- Intermediate-risk AML:
  - ○ ASCT
  - ○ High-dose cytarabine (2–3 g/m^2) over 3 hours every 12 hours on days 1, 3, 5 for three to four cycles
  - ○ Clinical trial
- Poor-risk AML:
  - ○ ASCT (patients may receive high-dose intermittent ARA-C [HIDAC] consolidation until donor is found)
  - ○ Clinical trial

7. **What is the postremission treatment of choice for older patients (>60 years old) with non-APL AML in CR?**
   - Reduced-intensity ASCT
   - Standard-dose cytarabine (100–200 mg/m^2/day) × 5–7 days ± idarubicin/daunorubicin for one or two cycles
   - Intermediate-dose cytarabine (1–1.5 g/m^2) over 3 hours × 4–6 doses × one or two cycles for patients with favorable- or intermediate-risk AML with good performance status and organ function
   - If patients received hypomethylating agents for AML induction: continue azacitidine or decitabine every 4–6 weeks until toxicity or disease progression
   - Clinical trial
   - Observation

8. **What is the surveillance strategy for patients with AML in CR postconsolidation therapy?**
   - Complete blood count (CBC) every 1 to 3 months for 2 years, then every 3 to 6 months until 5 years
   - Bone marrow aspirate and biopsy only if cytopenias or abnormalities on peripheral smear
   - Donor search at relapse (if not already done)

9. **What is the treatment strategy for relapsed non-APL AML patients?**
   - The only chance for a cure is with ASCT, ideally in the second CR
   - Clinical trial followed by ASCT
   - Salvage chemotherapy followed by ASCT
   - Best supportive care (in some patients >60 years of age who cannot tolerate this therapy)

APL AML

1. **What are the induction and consolidation treatment options for patients with *high-risk* APL?**
   - *Induction:* all-trans retinoic acid (ATRA) 45 mg/m^2 in divided doses until clinical remission + daunorubicin 50 mg/m^2 × 4 days + cytarabine 200 mg/m^2 × 7 days

Consolidation (after CR): arsenic 0.15 mg/kg/day × 5 days for 5 weeks × two cycles, then ATRA 45 mg/m² × 7 days + daunorubicin 50 mg/m² × 3 days for two cycles

Maintenance: ATRA 45 mg/m² in divided doses 7 days on and 7 days off for 1 year

- *Induction:* ATRA 45 mg/m² in divided doses until clinical remission + daunorubicin 60 mg/m² × 3 days + cytarabine 200 mg/m² × 7 days

Consolidation (after CR): daunorubicin 60 mg/m² × 3 days + cytarabine 200 mg/m² × 7 days for one cycle, then cytarabine 1.5 to 2 g/m² (2 g/m² for age <50 or 1.5 g/m² for age 50–60) every 12 hours × 5 days + daunorubicin 45 mg/m² × 3 days for one cycle and 5 doses of intrathecal (IT) chemotherapy

Maintenance: 6-mercaptopurine (50 mg/m² per day), methotrexate (15 mg/m² per week), and intermittent ATRA (45 mg/m² per day) for 15 days every 3 months for 2 years

- *Induction:* ATRA 45 mg/m² in divided doses until clinical remission (may use 25 mg/m²/day in those aged ≤20) + idarubicin 12 mg/m² on days 2, 4, 6, and 8

Consolidation (after CR): ATRA 45 mg/m² × 15 days + idarubicin 5 mg/m² and cytarabine 1 g/m² × 4 days for one cycle, then ATRA × 15 days + mitoxantrone 10 mg/m²/day × 5 days for one cycle, then ATRA × 15 days + idarubicin 12 mg/m² for 1 dose + cytarabine 150 mg/m²/8 h × 4 days for one cycle

Maintenance: mercaptopurine (50 mg/m²/day), intramuscular methotrexate (15 mg/m²/week), and oral ATRA (45 mg/m²/day) for 15 days every 3 months for 2 years

- *Induction:* ATRA 45 mg/m² (days 1–36, divided) + age-adjusted idarubicin 6–12 mg/m² on days 2, 4, 6, and 8 + arsenic trioxide 0.15 mg/kg (days 9–36 as 2 h IV infusion)

Consolidation (after CR): ATRA 45 mg/m² × 28 days + arsenic trioxide 0.15 mg/kg/day × 28 days × one cycle, then ATRA 45 mg/m² × 7 days every 2 weeks × 3 + arsenic trioxide 0.15 mg/kg/day × 5 days for 5 weeks × one cycle.

Maintenance: ATRA (45 mg/m² per day) for days 1 to 14 followed by methotrexate 5 to 15 mg/m²/week on days 15 to 90 and mercaptopurine 50 to 90 mg/m²/day on days 15 to 90. This is repeated every 3 months for 2 years.

- Patients started on an induction regimen according to one treatment protocol should receive consolidation and maintenance following the same protocol. Switching from one protocol to another should not be done.
- All patients with high-risk APL should be considered for CNS prophylaxis with 4 to 6 doses of IT chemotherapy. The first lumbar puncture (LP) is performed at count recovery postinduction therapy.

2. **What is the treatment of choice for patients *with low/intermediate–risk* APL?**

- *Induction:* ATRA 45 mg/m² in divided doses until clinical remission + arsenic trioxide 0.15 mg/kg IV daily until bone marrow remission (preferred)

Consolidation (after CR): Arsenic trioxide 0.15 mg/kg/day IV 5 days/week for 4 weeks every 8 weeks for a total of four cycles, and ATRA 45 mg/m²/day for 2 weeks every 4 weeks for a total of seven cycles

Maintenance: none

- *Induction:* ATRA 45 mg/m² in divided doses until clinical remission + daunorubicin 50 mg/m² × 4 days + cytarabine 200 mg/m² × 7 days

  Consolidation (after CR): arsenic trioxide 0.15 mg/kg/day × 5 days for 5 weeks × two cycles, then ATRA 45 mg/m² × 7 days + daunorubicin 50 mg/m² × 3 days for two cycles

  Maintenance: ATRA 45 mg/m² in divided doses 7 days on and 7 days off for 1 year

- *Induction:* ATRA 45 mg/m² in divided doses until clinical remission + daunorubicin 60 mg/m² × 3 days + cytarabine 200 mg/m² × 7 days

  Consolidation (after CR): daunorubicin 60 mg/m² × 3 days + cytarabine 200 mg/m² × 7 days for one cycle, then cytarabine 1 g/m² every 12 hours × 4 days + daunorubicin 45 mg/m² × 3 days for one cycle

  Maintenance: 6-mercaptopurine (50 mg/m² per day), methotrexate (15 mg/m² per week), and intermittent ATRA (45 mg/m² per day) for 15 days every 3 months for 2 years

- *Induction:* ATRA 45 mg/m² in divided doses until clinical remission + idarubicin 12 mg/m² on days 2, 4, 6, and 8

  Consolidation (after CR): ATRA 45 mg/m² × 15 days + idarubicin 5 mg/m² × 4 days for one cycle, then ATRA × 15 days + mitoxantrone 10 mg/m²/day × 5 days for one cycle, then ATRA × 15 days + idarubicin 12 mg/m² × 1 dose for one cycle

  Maintenance: mercaptopurine (50 mg/m²/day), intramuscular methotrexate (15 mg/m²/week), and oral ATRA (45 mg/m²/day) for 15 days every 3 months for 2 years

- Patients started on an induction regimen according to one treatment protocol, should receive consolidation and maintenance following the same protocol. Switching from one protocol to another should not be done.

3. **How are patients with APL monitored after consolidation and what is the postconsolidation therapy if polymerase chain reaction (PCR) is negative?**
   - Bone marrow biopsy should be performed to document cytogenetic/molecular remission after consolidation.
   - If PCR is negative, patients should receive maintenance therapy as per the initial treatment protocol
   - PCR monitoring should be performed for up to 2 years.

4. **How should patients with PCR-positive disease (after consolidation or if PCR turns positive during postconsolidation therapy) be treated?**
   - PCR should be repeated in 2 to 4 weeks for confirmation and to rule out a false-positive result. If it is confirmed positive, patient are considered in first relapse.
     - No prior exposure to arsenic trioxide or late relapse (≥6 months) after arsenic trioxide containing regimen: arsenic trioxide 0.15 mg/kg IV daily +/− ATRA 45 mg/m² in two divided doses daily until count recovery with marrow confirmation of remission

  ○ Early relapse (<6 months) after ATRA or arsenic trioxide only (no anthra-cycline): consider ATRA 45 mg/m² PO daily + idarubicin 12 mg/m² on days 2, 4, 6, and 8 + arsenic trioxide 0.15 mg/kg IV daily until count recovery with marrow confirmation of remission

  ○ Early relapse (<6 months) after arsenic trioxide/anthracycline containing regimen: arsenic trioxide 0.15 mg/kg IV daily +/− ATRA 45 mg/m² in two divided doses daily until count recovery with marrow confirmation of remission

- Those who achieve second morphologic remission should be strongly considered for CNS prophylaxis.

- If the PCR turns negative, patients should be treated with autologous stem cell transplantation (or with arsenic consolidation for a total of six cycles if not candidates for transplantation).

- If the PCR stays positive, patients should be treated with ASCT (or on a clinical trial if not transplant candidates).

- Patients who do not achieve second morphologic remission are treated on a clinical trial or with ASCT.

Acute Lymphoblastic Leukemia (ALL)

EPIDEMIOLOGY

1. What is the median age at diagnosis?
   - Fifteen years
   - Fifty-seven percent of patients are diagnosed at age less than 20 years, and 27% are diagnosed at age 45 years or older

2. What is the incidence of ALL?
   - Sixty-five hundred new cases per year in the United States

ETIOLOGY AND RISK FACTORS

1. What are the common risk factors for ALL?
   - Hispanics > Whites > African Americans
   - Men > women
   - Intrauterine exposure to radiation
   - Environmental exposure: electromagnetic and nuclear radiation
   - Chemical exposure: insecticides
   - Congenital disorders: Down syndrome, ataxia telangiectasia, Bloom syndrome

PATHOLOGY—CLASSIFICATION

1. What is the WHO classification of ALL?

   B-lymphoblastic leukemia/lymphoma:
   - B-lymphoblastic leukemia/lymphoma, NOS
   - B-lymphoblastic leukemia/lymphoma with recurrent genetic abnormalities
     ○ B-lymphoblastic leukemia/lymphoma with t(9;22)(q34.1;q11.2); *BCR-ABL1*

- B-lymphoblastic leukemia/lymphoma with t(v;11q23.3); *KMT2A* rearranged
- B-lymphoblastic leukemia/lymphoma with t(12;21)(p13.2;q22.1); *ETV6-RUNX1*
- B-lymphoblastic leukemia/lymphoma with hyperdiploidy
- B-lymphoblastic leukemia/lymphoma with hypodiploidy
- B-lymphoblastic leukemia/lymphoma with t(5;14)(q31.1;q32.3); *IL3-IGH*
- B-lymphoblastic leukemia/lymphoma with t(1;19)(q23;p13.3); *TCF3-PBX1*
- Provisional entity: B-lymphoblastic leukemia/lymphoma, *BCR-ABL1*-like
- Provisional entity: B-lymphoblastic leukemia/lymphoma with *iAMP21*

T-lymphoblastic leukemia/lymphoma:

- T-lymphoblastic leukemia/lymphoma, NOS
- Provisional entity: early T-cell precursor lymphoblastic leukemia
- Provisional entity: natural killer (NK) cell lymphoblastic leukemia/lymphoma

2. **What are the different immunophenotypes of ALL?**
- B-precursor ALL
- B-precursor with myeloid features
- Mature B cell
- T-cell

SIGNS AND SYMPTOMS

1. **What are the common signs and symptoms of ALL?**
- Lymphadenopathy and/or hepatosplenomegaly
- Painless testicular swelling
- Fever and other constitutional symptoms of infections
- Bruising or bleeding from thrombocytopenia
- Fatigue and other symptoms of anemia
- Infections (due to neutropenia)
- Leukostasis: CNS manifestations, cardiopulmonary symptoms, retinal hemorrhage, priapism
- Tumor lysis syndrome
- Mediastinal mass
- Musculoskeletal pain

DIAGNOSTIC WORKUP

1. **Define the diagnostic criteria for ALL.**
- Marrow and/or peripheral blood and/or lymph node involvement with lymphoid blasts
  - Typically, there will be $\geq$20% lymphoblasts in the marrow at the time of diagnosis
- Phenotypic and genetic determination of the lymphoblasts to allow for appropriate subclassification as outlined earlier

PROGNOSTIC FACTORS

1. How are patients with ALL stratified into different risk groups?

	Adverse Risk	Standard Risk
Age	<1 y or >35 y	>1 y but <35 y
Immunophenotype	Early T precursor (ETP)	T cell
	Pro-B (especially CD20+)	Pre-B
WBC count	>100,000 for T cell	<100,000 for T cell
	>30,000 for B cell	<30,000 for B cell
Genetic aberrations	Complex (≥5 changes)	Hyperdiploidy (>50 chromosomes)
	Hypodiploidy (<46 chromosomes)	t(1;14)
	t(9;22) or BCR-ABL	t(12;21)
	MLL rearrangement especially t(4;11)	
CNS involvement	Present	Absent
Response to therapy	Time to CR >4 wks	
	Minimal residual disease present after induction	

TREATMENT

1. How are adult patients with Philadelphia chromosome positive (Ph+) ALL treated?

- Patients who are less than 70 years old without major comorbidities: induction chemotherapy + tyrosine kinase inhibitors (TKIs). If CR is achieved, patients should undergo ASCT in first remission followed by consideration for the use of a maintenance TKI for a period of time following the allogeneic transplant. If no donor is available, they should be continued on consolidation multiagent chemotherapy + TKI followed by maintenance therapy + TKI.

  Examples of regimens include:

  ○ TKIs + hyper-CVAD

  ○ TKI + COG AALL-0031

  ○ TKI + EsPhALL

- Patients who are 70 years old or older, or with significant comorbidities: induction therapy with TKI + steroids or TKI + low-dose chemotherapy. If they achieve CR, they should be continued on TKI as consolidation.

  Examples of regimens include:

  ○ LAL1205 protocol—TKI + corticosteroid

  ○ TKI + vincristine + dexamethasone

  ○ EWALL-PH-01 or EWALL-PH-02 protocol

2. **How are adult patients with Ph− ALL treated?**
   - Patients less than 70 years old without major comorbidities: induction with multiagent chemotherapy (multiple regimens available—the backbone of these therapies is steroids + anthracycline + vincristine). For fit patients under age 39, strong consideration should be given for a pediatric-inspired regimen. If CR is achieved, patients should continue multiagent chemotherapy as consolidation followed by maintenance therapy or undergo ASCT if a donor is available (if high risk as outlined in the previous table).

   Examples of regimens include:
   - CALGB 10403
   - COG AALL0232
   - CALGB 8811
   - Linker regimen
   - hyper-CVAD
   - MRC UKALLXII/ECOG2993

   - Patients who are 70 years old or older, or with significant comorbidities: induction with multiagent chemotherapy or steroids. If they achieve CR, they should receive consolidation with chemotherapy followed by maintenance therapy.

3. **How are patients with relapsed/refractory ALL treated?**
   - Ph+ ALL: consider ABL kinase domain mutation testing; treatment options include clinical trial, chemotherapy ± TKI, TKI ± steroids. ASCT is considered if a morphological remission is obtained.
   - Ph− ALL: Treatment options include clinical trial or multiagent chemotherapy. Blinatumomab is considered for B-ALL and nelarabine for T-ALL. ASCT is considered if a morphological remission is obtained.

SPECIAL CONSIDERATIONS IN ACUTE LEUKEMIAS

1. **What are the medical emergencies in leukemias?**
   - *Leukostasis:* needs to be treated aggressively with IV hydration, cytoreduction with hydroxyurea (and steroids in case of lymphoid malignancies) and leukopheresis. Avoid red blood cell transfusions.
   - *DIC:* needs to be treated aggressively with supportive blood and blood product transfusions and disease control. Suspect APL in patients with DIC and start ATRA before diagnosis, especially if morphology is consistent until disease is genetically confirmed.
   - *APL:* need to start ATRA immediately, even before diagnosis is genetically confirmed.
   - *Differentiation syndrome:* develops in APL (ATRA and arsenic are risk factors). The signs and symptoms are fever, weight gain, edema, dyspnea, hypoxia, worsening renal function, opacities on chest imaging, pleural/pericardial effusions, and hypotension. Patients need to be treated with dexamethasone 10 mg every 12 hours. If differentiation syndrome is severe, ATRA (and arsenic) needs to be held and resumed only after it resolves. Starting cytotoxic chemotherapy (if not already done) is recommended. Consider differentiation syndrome

prophylactic therapy with dexamethasone when starting ATRA in patients with WBC greater than 30,000 to 40,000.

- *Tumor lysis syndrome:* could be spontaneous in aggressive hematologic malignancies or induced by therapy. Patients typically have elevated uric acid, potassium and phosphorus, low calcium, and worsening renal function (phosphorus is generally not elevated in spontaneous tumor lysis syndrome). Patients should be treated prophylactically with IV hydration, allopurinol, and monitoring for tumor lysis syndrome through checking potassium, phosphorus, uric acid, and calcium 2 to 3 times a day during therapy. Rasburicase can be used prophylactically in highly proliferative malignancies if the risk of tumor lysis syndrome is elevated and particularly if the renal function is not normal. Treatment of tumor lysis syndrome includes aggressive IV hydration, aggressive measures to correct electrolyte abnormalities, allopurinol, and rasburicase. G6PD deficiency should be ruled out, if suspected, before administration of rasburicase.

Hairy Cell Leukemia (HCL)

EPIDEMIOLOGY

1. What is the median age at diagnosis?
   - Fifty-two years of age

2. What is the incidence of HCL?
   - There are about 600 to 800 new cases per year in the United States (2% of all leukemias)

ETIOLOGY AND RISK FACTORS

1. Is HCL more common in males or females?
   - HCL is more common in males (with male to female ratio of 4:1)

SCREENING

Not applicable

PREVENTION

Not applicable

PATHOLOGY

1. What genetic mutation is seen in virtually all cases of HCL?
   - BRAF V600E

SIGNS AND SYMPTOMS

1. What are the typical clinical manifestations of HCL?
   - Monocytopenia or pancytopenia
   - Fever and other constitutional symptoms
   - Infections
   - Bleeding

- Fatigue and other symptoms of anemia
- Organomegaly (splenomegaly) is common

DIAGNOSIS

1. What is the common microscopic appearance of HCL?

- Hairlike projections from the leukemia cells
- Fried-egg appearance on bone marrow biopsy
- Leukemic cells stain brightly with CD20
- Bone marrow may be hypocellular (need to differentiate from aplastic anemia and hypoplastic MDS)
- Bone marrow fibrosis is often present

2. How is the diagnosis established?

- Typical clinical manifestations with immunophenotype by flow cytometry
- HCL immunophenotype: CD11c+, CD25+, CD103+, CD123+, CD20+, CD22+, CD52+, cyclin D1+, annexin A1+, BRAF V600E+
- Hairy cell variant immunophenotype: CD25−, CD123−, annexin A1−, BRAF V600E−

PROGNOSTIC FACTORS

1. Does the hairy cell variant respond better or worse to treatment?

- The hairy cell variant (immunophenotype CD25−, CD123−) tends not to respond as well to purine nucleoside analog-based therapy. Consideration should be given to treatment with sequential purine nucleoside analog-based therapy followed by rituximab.

TREATMENT

1. When do we initiate therapy in HCL?

- Watch and wait strategy is recommended unless one of the following criteria for starting therapy is met:
  - Symptomatic disease that interferes with daily activities (eg, fatigue with no other reason, symptomatic splenomegaly)
  - Anemia (Hb <12 g/dL)
  - Thrombocytopenia (plt <100,000/mcL)
  - Neutropenia (ANC <1,000)

2. What are the treatment options for HCL?

- Cladribine (7-day continuous infusion, or 1–2 hour bolus IV daily for 5 days, or subcutaneously daily for 5–7 days, or weekly for 5–6 weeks)
- Alternative option: pentostatin IV every 2 weeks until maximal response (every 3 weeks if neutrophil count falls far below the baseline)
- CR is achieved in about 70% to 90% of patients, with a relapse rate of approximately 30% to 40% (at 10–15 years).

3. **How are patients followed after therapy?**
   - Improvement in peripheral blood counts may require weeks to months.
   - Bone marrow to document CR should be done at 3 to 4 months.
   - After CR, CBCs are typically obtained every 1 to 3 months.

4. **How are patients with relapsed HCL treated?**
   - If initial remission was for more than 1 year, consider repeating therapy with the same agent.
   - If the remission was for less than 1 year, consider the alternative purine nucleoside analog, combination of a purine nucleoside analog with rituximab, or vemurafenib.

5. **How are patients with resistant HCL treated?**
   - Consider the alternative purine nucleoside analog, the combination of a purine nucleoside analog with rituximab, or vemurafenib.

QUESTIONS

1. A 45-year-old man presents to his primary care physician (PCP) with symptoms of fatigue and easy bruising. A complete blood count (CBC) reveals a white blood cell (WBC) count of 68, hemoglobin of 9.8, and platelet count of 23. The WBC differential reveals 83% circulating blasts with Auer rods present. Bone marrow biopsy is performed and confirms the diagnosis of acute myeloid leukemia (AML). The patient begins induction chemotherapy with anthracycline and cytarabine in a standard 3 + 7 fashion using daunorubicin 90 mg/m². Human leukocyte antigen (HLA) typing is sent on admission and he is found to have a 10/10 HLA matched sibling. With which of the following findings would you more strongly consider consolidation therapy with high-dose cytarabine in first complete remission (CR1)?
   A. Normal male karyotype, FLT3-ITD mutation positive
   B. Cytogenetics revealing t(6;9)
   C. Cytogenetics revealing t(8;21), c-KIT mutation negative
   D. Monosomal karyotype

2. A 59-year-old woman presents to the emergency department with complaints of fatigue, dyspnea on exertion, vision changes, and headaches. Routine blood work reveals a white blood cell (WBC) count of 120, hemoglobin of 7, and platelet count of 73. Review of the peripheral smear shows 90% blasts with Auer rods. Physical exam confirms the presence of retinal hemorrhages bilaterally. What is the next most important step in management?
   A. Call for an urgent ophthalmology evaluation
   B. Transfuse two units of packed red blood cells (PRBC)
   C. Obtain an echocardiogram
   D. Arrange for urgent leukopheresis, initiate fluids, and begin hydroxyurea

3. A 21-year-old woman completed multiagent chemotherapy including alkylating agents, etoposide, and radiation therapy for Ewing's sarcoma 2 years ago. She has been free of disease since but on routine blood work she was noted to have a white blood cell (WBC) count of 42, hemoglobin of 9, and platelet count of 77. Bone marrow biopsy confirms the diagnosis of acute myeloid leukemia (AML). Which cytogenetic abnormality is she most likely to have?
   A. 11q23 abnormality
   B. t(8;21)
   C. t(15;17)
   D. Monosomy 7

4. A 52-year-old man is 10 days into therapy with all-trans retinoic acid (ATRA) and arsenic trioxide for a diagnosis of low-risk acute promyelocytic leukemia (APL) when he begins to develop hypoxia, dyspnea, and lower extremity edema. Chest x-ray reveals bilateral pulmonary infiltrates. What is the most appropriate step in management?
   A. Obtain a nasopharyngeal swab for presumed viral lower respiratory tract infection
   B. Start dexamethasone 10 mg twice daily for presumed differentiation syndrome
   C. Order a stat CT PE protocol and initiate heparin drip
   D. Perform a stat bedside transthoracic echocardiogram for suspected therapy-induced cardiomyopathy

5. A 39-year-old woman is diagnosed with Philadelphia chromosome positive (Ph+) B-cell acute lymphoblastic leukemia (ALL). After undergoing intensive induction with multiagent chemotherapy and tyrosine kinase inhibitor (TKI), she achieves a complete remission (CR). Minimal residual disease testing is negative. She has a human leukocyte antigen (HLA) matched related sibling. What is the best strategy for additional therapy?
   A. Consolidation with an allogeneic stem cell transplant (ASCT)
   B. Consolidation with maintenance chemotherapy and TKI
   C. Consolidation with maintenance chemotherapy followed by an autologous stem cell transplant
   D. Maintenance therapy with TKI indefinitely

6. A 57-year-old man presents to his primary care physician (PCP) for his annual exam. He is noted to have palpable splenomegaly but is otherwise asymptomatic. A complete blood count (CBC) demonstrates a white blood cell (WBC) count of 2.0 with an absolute neutrophil count (ANC) of 1.5, hemoglobin of 12.5, and platelets of 157. Review of peripheral smear demonstrates presence of hairy cells and diagnosis of hairy cell leukemia is confirmed by flow cytometry. What is the next step in management?
   A. Initiate cladribine, IV daily for 5 days
   B. Initiate pentostatin every 2 weeks until best response
   C. Monitor symptoms and blood counts, no treatment at this time
   D. Referral for bone marrow transplant

ANSWERS

1. **C. Cytogenetics revealing t(8;21), c-KIT mutation negative.** The National Comprehensive Cancer Network (NCCN) recognizes a monosomal karyotype, the t(6;9) (p23;q34); DEK-NUP214 and a normal male karyotype with FLT3-ITD mutation as well validated poor risk prognostic factors in patients with AML. As such, the recommendation for standard postremission therapy would be an ASCT in those patients. Alternatively, the presence of a core binding factor leukemia, t(8;21); is a well validated favorable-risk group. As such, the recommendation for standard postremission therapy is high-dose cytarabine.

2. **D. Arrange for urgent leukopheresis, initiate fluids, and begin hydroxyurea.** This patient is suffering from life-threatening leukostasis as evidenced by complaints of dyspnea, vision changes, and headaches. She needs emergent leukopheresis, fluids, and initiation of a cytoreductive agent. Neither an urgent ophthalmologic exam nor an echocardiogram will alter your initial recommendations. Despite moderate anemia, transfusion of red cells in a patient with active leukostasis would be contraindicated at this time, due to concerns for exacerbating the stasis.

3. **A. 11q23 abnormality.** The multiagent chemotherapy this patient received in treatment for her Ewing's sarcoma has put her at risk for a treatment-related myeloid neoplasm. The latency of 2 years between treatment and onset of AML favors topoisomerase II inhibitor (etoposide) as the culprit. Treatment-related AML caused by topoisomerase II inhibitors is often associated with translocation 11q23 (MLL). Alkylating agents, on the other hand, would be expected to have a longer latency period of 5 to 10 years, tend to be associated with antecedent treatment-related MDS, and are associated with complex cytogenetics as well as monosomy 5 or 7.

4. **B. Start dexamethasone 10 mg twice daily for presumed differentiation syndrome.** Differentiation symptom occurs in 2% to 30% of patients receiving ATRA or arsenic trioxide. Signs and symptoms include leukocytosis, dyspnea, fever, pulmonary edema or infiltrates, effusions, weight gain, and bone pain. Classically, it develops 10 to 12 days after initiation of therapy. Treatment includes prompt initiation of steroids as well as discontinuation of the differentiating agent, depending on the severity of symptoms.

5. **A. Consolidation with an allogeneic stem cell transplant (ASCT).** The National Comprehensive Cancer Network (NCCN) continues to recommend ASCT in the first CR due to lack of data on success of TKI and multiagent chemotherapy alone. Additionally, salvage therapy in the relapsed setting remains challenging and so an ASCT is recommended in the first CR if available.

6. **C. Monitor symptoms and blood counts, no treatment at this time.**
   While cladribine and pentostatin are both considered standard first-line
   options for treatment of hairy cell leukemia, treatment is not indicated at
   this time for this patient. Indications for therapy include systemic symptoms, splenic discomfort, recurrent infection, anemia (hemoglobin <12),
   thrombocytopenia (platelet count <100), or neutropenia (ANC <1). There
   is no indication for upfront bone marrow transplant in this disease.

2

Chronic Lymphocytic Leukemia

Erlene K. Seymour, Rami N. Khoriaty, and Dale Bixby

EPIDEMIOLOGY

1. What is the most common adult leukemia?

- Chronic lymphocytic leukemia (CLL) is the most common adult leukemia in the Western world (about 30% of all leukemias), with approximately 15,000 new cases/year
- Median age at diagnosis: 72 years

2. What is the median overall survival (OS) based on Rai stage?

- Median OS of patients with Rai stages 0, I, II, III, and IV is greater than 150, 101, 71, 19, and 19 months respectively.

ETIOLOGY AND RISK FACTORS

1. What is the etiology of CLL?

- Exact etiology is uncertain. Most cases are acquired; reports of familial CLL do exist, but are rare.

2. What are the common risk factors for CLL?

- Positive family history for CLL or other lymphoid malignancies
- Older age
- Male sex (male to female ratio of 2:1)
- Ethnicity (most common in Whites, rare in Asians)
- CLL is **not associated** with radiation exposure, solvents, or chemicals.

STAGING

1. Define the staging for CLL.

Rai Stage	Modified Rai Stage	Definition
0	Low risk	Lymphocytosis only
I	Intermediate risk	Lymphocytosis and lymphadenopathy
II	Intermediate risk	Lymphocytosis with hepatomegaly or splenomegaly
III	High risk	Lymphocytosis and anemia (hemoglobin <11 g/dL)
IV	High risk	Lymphocytosis and thrombocytopenia (platelets <100,000/mcL)

Binet Stage	Definition
A	Less than three nodal sites*
B	Three or more nodal sites*
C	Anemia (hemoglobin <10 g/dL) and/or thrombocytopenia (platelets <100,000/mcL)

*The five nodal sites for Binet staging are cervical (including Waldeyer ring), axillary, inguinal, spleen, and liver.

- CT scans are not needed to stage CLL. Serial CT scans are not indicated in CLL. CT scans should only be obtained to follow and monitor disease progression in patients with new symptoms when peripheral adenopathy is not present.

SIGNS AND SYMPTOMS

1. What is the most common presentation of CLL?

- Incidental lymphocytosis
- Asymptomatic lymphadenopathy

2. What are the common signs and symptoms of CLL?

- Fatigue and malaise associated with anemia
- Early satiety or abdominal discomfort secondary to splenomegaly
- B symptoms: fevers, night sweats, and weight loss
- Recurrent infections due to neutropenia

3. What are the characteristic peripheral blood smear findings of CLL?

- Typical CLL smear: small mature lymphocytes with clumped chromatin and a narrow rim of cytoplasm
- Smudge cells: characteristic of CLL

DIAGNOSTIC CRITERIA

1. Define the three diagnostic criteria for CLL.

- Peripheral blood monoclonal B-lymphocyte count ≥5,000/mcL
- Characteristic peripheral blood lymphocyte flow cytometric immunophenotype: CD5+/CD23+
- Percentage of prolymphocytes <55% of the lymphocytes
  - A bone marrow biopsy is not needed to make the diagnosis of CLL.

2. Define monoclonal B-cell lymphocytosis?

- If the monoclonal B-lymphocyte count is <5,000/mcL in the setting of a characteristic flow cytometry pattern and absence of lymphadenopathy or hepatosplenomegaly, then the patient's diagnosis is a monoclonal B-cell lymphocytosis.

3. What is prolymphocytic leukemia?

- If monoclonal B-lymphocyte count is ≥5,000/mcL and the percentage of prolymphocytes is ≥55% of the lymphocytes, then the patient's diagnosis is prolymphocytic leukemia.

4. What is small lymphocytic lymphoma (SLL)?

- If the clonal B-cells seen within an enlarged lymph node (LN), liver, or spleen have a CLL immunophenotype, but the patient does not have a peripheral monoclonal B-lymphocyte count ≥5,000/mcL, then the patient has a diagnosis of SLL. CLL and SLL are for all clinical purposes treated the same.

5. What do you see in flow cytometry in CLL?

- Restriction to either kappa or lambda immunoglobulin light chains (monoclonal disease).
- CD5+, CD19+, CD23+, monoclonal B-cell population that also typically expresses CD20 dim, CD79b dim, surface immunoglobulins (sIg) dim.
- Differs from mantle cell lymphoma, which is CD5+, CD19+, CD23−. In mantle cell lymphoma, cytogenetics (or fluorescence in situ hybridization [FISH]) demonstrates t(11;14), and cyclin D1 is positive immunohistochemically.
- CD23 can be negative in CLL (atypical CLL). Cyclin D1 differentiates atypical CLL from mantle cell lymphoma.

INDICATIONS FOR TREATMENT

1. How do you treat asymptomatic CLL?

- Careful monitoring without therapy, typically with follow-up visits every 3 to 6 months without surveillance imaging unless indicated for symptoms. The average time to first therapy is 4 to 5 years from diagnosis.

2. What are the indications for therapy?

- New or worsening anemia (Rai stage III disease) (not associated with autoimmune hemolytic anemia [AIHA])
- New or worsening thrombocytopenia (Rai stage IV disease) (not due to immune thrombocytopenic purpura [ITP])
- Threatened end organ function due to adenopathy
- Progressive bulky disease (spleen >6 cm below the left costal margin, or LN >10 cm in longest diameter)
- Lymphocyte doubling time <6 months or an increase in absolute lymphocyte count (ALC) of >50% over a period of 2 months (use this criterion only in patients with ALC >30,000)
- B symptoms: fevers (>100.5°F or >38.0°C for more than 2 weeks with no evidence of infection), night sweats (for >1 month with no evidence of infection), unintentional weight loss (≥10% in the last 6 months)
- Severe fatigue resulting in an Eastern Cooperative Oncology Group (ECOG) performance status of ≥2 (rule out other causes of fatigue)
- AIHA or autoimmune thrombocytopenia ineffectively responding to steroids or other standard therapy

3. When is therapy for CLL not indicated?

- Do not treat CLL in the absence of the criteria listed in the prior question even if the patient has:
  - Significantly elevated white blood cell (WBC) count

○ Hypogammaglobulinemia

○ Paraproteinemia

○ High-risk cytogenetic features without indications to treat

PROGNOSTIC FACTORS

1. **What are the important FISH testing abnormalities in CLL?**
   - Eighty percent of patients with CLL have FISH abnormalities, including:
     ○ Deletion 13q (~50%)
     ○ Trisomy 12 (~20%)
     ○ Deletion 11q (~15%)
     ○ Deletion 17p (~7%–10%)

2. **What are the poor risk factors on FISH testing?**
   - Deletion 17p (median OS: 2–3 years)
   - Deletion 11q (median OS: 6–7 years)

3. **What are the intermediate prognosis risk factors on FISH testing?**
   - Trisomy 12 (median OS ~9 years)
   - Normal karyotype on FISH (median OS ~9 years)

4. **What generates a favorable prognosis on FISH testing?**
   - Deletion 13q (median OS ~11 years)

5. **What are other prognostic factors in CLL?**
   - Mutated *IgVH* (>2% mutation) portends an excellent OS (~22.8 years) (exception: patients expressing the *VH3-21* gene have a poor survival). Patients with unmutated *IgVH* (≤2% mutation) have shorter OS (~6.6 years).
   - Positive ZAP-70 expression (≥20%), measured by flow cytometry in CD19+/CD5+ cells, predicts short time to treatment (TTT)—2.9 years for those who are ZAP-70 positive versus 9.2 years for those that are ZAP-70 negative.
   - Positive CD38 (≥30%): predicts for short TTT.
   - Complex karyotype (≥3 chromosome abnormalities in more than one cell on conventional cytogenetics)
   - Elevated beta-2 microglobulin level

TREATMENT

First-Line Therapy

1. **What factors are important to consider when choosing a therapeutic regimen for CLL?**
   - Age
   - Functional status and comorbidities
   - Results of the FISH study

2. **What are treatment options for young patients (<65 years) with good performance status, no significant comorbidities, and no del 17p?**

- Fludarabine, cyclophosphamide, and rituximab (FCR); fludarabine and rituximab (FR; Note that FR is not an appropriate treatment option for patients with del11q.); pentostatin, cyclophosphamide and rituximab (PCR); and bendamustine and rituximab (BR), ibrutinib. Chemoimmunotherapy is preferred first.

3. **What are treatment options for "physically fit" elderly patients (>65 years of age) without significant comorbidities?**
   - Obinutuzumab and chlorambucil; ibrutinib; ofatumumab and chlorambucil; rituximab and chlorambucil; BR; obinutuzumab single agent; chlorambucil single agent; and rituximab single agent

4. **What are treatment options for younger CLL patients (≤65 years of age) with significant comorbid conditions?**
   - Same as physically fit elderly patients (see the previous question)

5. **What are treatment options for frail patients with poor performance status without del(17p) (not able to tolerate purine analogs)?**
   - Obinutuzumab and chlorambucil; ibrutinib; ofatumumab and chlorambucil; rituximab and chlorambucil; obinutuzumab; rituximab; chlorambucil

6. **What are initial treatment options for patients with CLL and del 17p/p53 mutation?**
   - Ibrutinib; high-dose methylprednisolone and rituximab; obinutuzumab and chlorambucil; and alemtuzumab (+/− rituximab)
   - Patients with del 17p CLL should be considered for allogeneic stem cell transplant (ASCT) after the first response, particularly if patients have complex cytogenetics.

7. **What type of transplant is preferred in CLL if transplant is indicated?**
   - Reduced intensity ASCT is preferred.
   - Myeloablative ASCT is acceptable in young and fit patients without comorbidities if they have a poorly controlled disease.
   - Matched sibling is preferred over matched unrelated donor.

Response Criteria

1. **How are complete response and partial response defined? How are progressive disease and stable disease defined?**
   - Complete response: peripheral blood lymphocytes $<4 \times 10^9$/L, normalization of peripheral blood counts without growth factor support (ANC $>1.5 \times 10^9$/L, Hb >11 g/dL, platelets $>100,000 \times 10^6$/L), absence of lymphadenopathy (≤ 1.5 cm palpable LNs), absence of hepatomegaly, absence of splenomegaly, and absence of constitutional symptoms.
   - Partial response: At least two of the following criteria should be achieved: $\geq 50\%$ decrease in peripheral blood lymphocytes, lymphadenopathy, hepatomegaly, and/or splenomegaly. Additionally, at least one of the peripheral blood counts should be normalized or increased by $\geq 50\%$ from baseline.
   - Progressive disease is defined by any of the following: $\geq 50\%$ increase in lymphocyte count, lymphadenopathy, hepatomegaly, or splenomegaly. Progressive

disease can also be defined if there is appearance of a new lesion or cytopenias due to disease (>2 g/dL drop in hemoglobin or ≥50% drop in platelet count).

- Stable disease: defined as patients without progressive disease not meeting criteria for complete response or partial response.
- Exceptions: lenalidomide causes tumor flare reaction (increase in size of LNs and worsening lymphocytosis), which actually correlates with response to this drug. Ibrutinib and idelalisib are known to result in transient lymphocytosis, which results from mobilization of lymphocytes from LNs to the peripheral blood.

Second-Line Therapy

1. **How are CLL patients treated following failure of first-line therapy?**
   - Asymptomatic patients at relapse: monitor closely, and start therapy if one of the previously noted treatment criteria is met.
   - Repeat FISH testing prior to treatment initiation.
   - If duration of first remission is >12 months: consider repeating the first-line treatment regimen.
   - If refractory to nucleoside analogs (response duration <1 year or no response): enroll into a well-designed clinical trial if possible. ASCT is recommended for patients who are candidates for this approach.
     - Physically fit patients with del 17p: the preferred options are ibrutinib; venetoclax, idelalisib (+/− rituximab); high-dose methylprednisolone and rituximab; lenalidomide (+/− rituximab), alemtuzumab (+/− rituximab); ofatumumab; and oxaliplatin, fludarabine, cytarabine, and rituximab (OFAR). All patients should be referred for ASCT, if eligible.
     - Physically fit patients without del 17p: ibrutinib and idelalisib (+/− rituximab); venetoclax; BR; FCR; PCR; fludarabine and alemtuzumab; rituximab, cyclophosphamide, doxorubicin, vincristine, and prednisone (R-CHOP); OFAR; BR and ibrutinib; BR and idelalisib; ofatumumab; obinutuzumab; lenalidomide (+/− rituximab); alemtuzumab (+/− rituximab); and high-dose methylprednisolone and rituximab. Therapy should be followed by ASCT in transplant-eligible patients.

SPECIAL CONSIDERATIONS

1. **What are the causes of anemia in patients with CLL?**
   - The differential diagnosis includes: progressive marrow failure from CLL, splenomegaly, autoimmune process, and pure red cell aplasia in cases of isolated anemia.
   - Cytopenia(s) from marrow failure secondary to CLL should be documented by a bone marrow biopsy.
   - **Pure red cell aplasia** (diagnosis suspected by lack of reticulocyte response and confirmed by absence of erythroid precursors in the bone marrow): rule out viral infections including Epstein–Barr virus, cytomegalovirus (CMV), and parvovirus before presuming an autoimmune etiology.
   - **AIHA** diagnosis is based on exclusion of other causes of anemia, and the presence of elevated lactate dehydrogenase (LDH), high unconjugated bilirubin, elevated reticulocyte count, low haptoglobin, and positive direct antiglobulin test (DAT).

2. **How is AIHA in patients with CLL treated?**
   - If indication for CLL therapy exists independent of the anemia: treat CLL (purine analogs may potentially worsen AIHA. Therefore, it is prudent to avoid fludarabine in patients with active AIHA and in patients with a history of AIHA, particularly if purine analog induced).
   - If no independent indication for CLL therapy: prednisone 1 mg/kg/day for 4 weeks + folic acid, followed by a *slow* steroid taper (fast tapers can result in relapse). If no response or if relapse after steroid withdrawal, options include: rituximab, intravenous immunoglobulins, cyclosporine A, mycophenolate mofetil, azathioprine, daily low-dose oral cyclophosphamide, rituximab, or alemtuzumab. A trial of rituximab and at least one immunosuppressive agent is generally recommended prior to consideration of splenectomy.
   - Treatment refractory AIHA: treat CLL with chemoimmunotherapy.

3. **What are the common side effects of ibrutinib?**
   - Diarrhea, peripheral lymphocytosis, rash, atrial fibrillation, and antiplatelet effect (resulting in increased tendency to bleeding). Therefore ibrutinib should be avoided in patients receiving anticoagulants. It is otherwise relatively well tolerated.

4. **Is prolonged peripheral lymphocytosis on ibrutinib or idelalisib indicative of disease progression?**
   - No, the peripheral lymphocytosis that occurs after initiation of ibrutinib or idelalisib may vary among patients, can last for months up to a year, and is not indicative of progression of disease.

5. **What is the treatment of patients with CLL and recurrent sinopulmonary infections?**
   - Check serum IgG levels. If <500 mg/dL: administer monthly IVIG. Adjust dose/interval to maintain nadir IgG of approximately 500 mg/dL.

6. **What anti-infective prophylaxis is indicated in patients receiving purine analog or alemtuzumab?**
   - Purine analog:
     o Herpes prophylaxis with acyclovir
     o PCP prophylaxis with sulfamethoxazole/trimethoprim or equivalent
   - Alemtuzumab:
     o Herpes prophylaxis with acyclovir
     o PCP prophylaxis with sulfamethoxazole/trimethoprim or equivalent
     o Monitor for CMV viremia by polymerase chain reaction every 2 to 3 weeks while on therapy. If present or if viral load is rising, use ganciclovir and consult with infectious disease

7. **When is Richter's transformation suspected in CLL and how is it treated?**
   - Richter's transformation (transformation to diffuse large B-cell lymphoma [DLBCL] or Hodgkin lymphoma) is suspected in:

- ○ Patients with prominent B symptoms (fevers, night sweats, weight loss)
- ○ Rapidly enlarging LNs
- ○ If LDH is significantly elevated (in the absence of hemolysis)
- ○ Pancytopenia is common
- ○ Hypercalcemia +/− lytic bone lesions can be seen
- Patients with DLBCL transformation should be treated with regimens developed for DLBCL. Patients should be considered for ASCT after complete response or partial response to initial therapy. High-dose therapy with autologous stem cell rescue should be considered after response to first-line therapy in patients who are not candidates for ASCT.
- Patients with Hodgkin lymphoma transformation should be treated with a standard regimen used to treat Hodgkin lymphoma.

QUESTIONS

1. A 57-year-old woman presents with an elevated white blood cell (WBC) count of 55,000/mcL, hemoglobin of 13.5 g/dL, and platelet count of 160,000/mcL. A peripheral flow cytometry is sent and reveals a monoclonal population of cells expressing CD5, CD20 (dim), CD19, and CD23. The cells were negative immunohistochemically for cyclin D1. Which of the following is not associated with a poorer prognosis in this diagnosis?
   A. Deletion 17p
   B. Deletion 11q
   C. ZAP-70 expression greater than 20%
   D. Mutated *IgVH* status
   E. CD38 expression

2. A 55-year-old gentleman with chronic lymphocytic leukemia (CLL) presents with fevers, severe fatigue, weight loss, and increased lymphadenopathy. His complete blood counts are significant for a white blood cell (WBC) count of 80,000/mcL, absolute lymphocyte count (ALC) of 70,000/mcL, hemoglobin of 10 g/dL, and platelet count of 102,000/mcL. His CLL fluorescence in situ hybridization (FISH) reveals a del(17p). He is initiated on ibrutinib 420 mg PO daily and has mild diarrhea but otherwise tolerates therapy in his first week. On his subsequent labs in 2 weeks, his WBC has increased to 180,000/mcL, ALC 160,0000/mcL, and hemoglobin and platelet counts are stable. In 1 month, his WBC has increased to 225,000/mcL, ALC 200,000/mcL, hemoglobin and platelet counts remain stable. His palpable lymphadenopathy has resolved.
   What is the next appropriate step in management of his CLL?
   A. Perform CT of chest/abdomen/pelvis to evaluate for bulky disease in areas that are not palpable by exam
   B. Switch therapy to idelalisib
   C. Continue ibrutinib 420 mg PO daily

D. Increase ibrutinib to 560 mg PO daily
E. Refer him for a reduced intensity allogeneic bone marrow transplantation

3. A 45-year-old gentleman presents to clinic for the first time with a new diagnosis of chronic lymphocytic leukemia (CLL). He feels well and denies any fevers, chills, night sweats, or weight loss. He was noted to have an elevated white blood cell (WBC) count of 40,000/mcL, and absolute lymphocyte count (ALC) of 35,000/mcL on routine bloodwork that was obtained during a routine physical exam 6 months ago. His WBC in clinic today is now 65,000/mcL with an absolute lymphocyte count of 59,000/mcL.
Which of the following diagnostic tests would be appropriate to obtain for both prognostic and future therapeutic management?
A. *IgVH* mutation status
B. ZAP-70 expression
C. CLL fluorescence in situ hybridization (FISH)
D. CD38 expression by flow cytometry
E. PET scan

4. An 85-year-old gentleman with a history of congestive heart failure, chronic kidney disease, and uncontrolled diabetes presents for a follow-up appointment in regard to his chronic lymphocytic leukemia (CLL). He has been noticing enlargement of his lymph nodes in his neck and also developed severe fatigue and night sweats over the last 4 weeks. His Eastern Cooperative Oncology Group (ECOG) performance status is 2. On laboratory studies that day, he has a white blood cell (WBC) count of 90,000/mcL, hemoglobin of 9 g/dL, and platelet count of 80,000/mcL. His hemoglobin was 11 g/dL at his appointment 3 months earlier. His CLL fluorescence in situ hybridization (FISH) was remarkable for del13q only. There is no evidence of an autoimmune hemolytic anemia on laboratory testing.
Which of the following would be an appropriate first therapeutic option?
A. Fludarabine and rituximab (FR)
B. Obinutuzumab and chlorambucil
C. Fludarabine, cyclophosphamide, and rituximab (FCR)
D. Rituximab and idelalisib
E. Alemtuzumab

5. A 47-year-old woman with known chronic lymphocytic leukemia (CLL) presents to clinic with worsening lymphadenopathy, night sweats, and shortness of breath. Her white blood cell (WBC) count is 102,000/mcL, hemoglobin 8 g/dL, and platelet count 90,000/mcL. A CT scan of the chest/abdomen/pelvis demonstrates bulky lymphadenopathy in her cervical, axillary, retroperitoneal, and mesenteric lymph nodes. Her CLL fluorescence in situ hybridization (FISH) demonstrates a deletion 17p. She has not been previously treated for her CLL.

Which of the following would be the most appropriate frontline therapy option?

A. Fludarabine, cyclophosphamide, and rituximab (FCR)
B. Rituximab, cyclophosphamide, doxorubicin, vincristine, and prednisone (R-CHOP)
C. Ibrutinib
D. Bendamustine and rituximab (BR)
E. Fludarabine and rituximab (FR)

6. A 67-year-old woman presents to clinic with a new diagnosis of chronic lymphocytic leukemia (CLL). She was incidentally found to have an elevated white blood cell (WBC) count of 23,000/mcL, absolute lymphocyte count (ALC) of 20,000/mcL, hemoglobin 13 g/dL, and platelet count of 175,000/mcL. She continues to work full time and is at her baseline state of health. On physical exam there are no appreciable palpable lymph nodes and no hepatosplenomegaly.
Which of the following is the most appropriate next step in the management of her disease?

A. Baseline CT scan of the chest, abdomen, and pelvis
B. Baseline PET scan
C. Bone marrow biopsy
D. No additional studies, follow up in 3 months with labs only
E. No additional studies, follow up as needed when symptomatic

ANSWERS

1. **D. Mutated *IgVH* status.** This is associated with a better prognosis in chronic lymphocytic leukemia (CLL) than unmutated *IgVH* status, which is associated with unfavorable prognosis. (A), (B), (C), and (E) have all been associated with unfavorable prognosis in CLL.

2. **C. Continue ibrutinib 420 mg PO daily.** Increased peripheral lymphocytosis after initiating treatment with ibrutinib therapy is common and may last for several months. The development of peripheral lymphocytosis secondary to ibrutinib has not been shown to be detrimental to long-term clinical outcomes.

3. **C. CLL fluorescence in-situ hybridization (FISH).** This is needed to help with treatment management, which would help evaluate for deletion 17p, deletion 11q, trisomy 12, or deletion 13q. For example, in a young patient with deletion11q we would consider regimens with alkylating agents. In patients with deletion 17p, we could consider ibrutinib therapy as a possible first-line therapy. The other answer options would not necessarily determine specific therapies.

4. **B. Obinutuzumab and chlorambucil.** These have been shown to have improved clinical outcomes in patients with CLL with multiple comorbid conditions compared to chlorambucil alone. Given its more tolerable toxicity profile, it is one of the preferred regimens to use in frail elderly patients and patients with comorbid conditions.

5. **C. Ibrutinib.** This has been shown to have high overall response rates in deletion 17p patients and is currently a preferred first-line therapy. Deletion 17p and patients with TP53 mutations have poor outcomes with conventional chemoimmunotherapy regimens.

6. **D. No additional studies, follow up in 3 months with labs only.** For an early stage asymptomatic CLL patient, there is no indication for baseline CT scans or baseline bone marrow biopsy. Avoidance of baseline and serial CT scans in early stage asymptomatic CLL patients was recently encouraged as a part of the American Society of Hematology Choosing Wisely Campaign. General follow-up every 3 to 6 months is the current standard of care.

Chronic Myeloid Leukemia and Myeloproliferative Neoplasms

3

Brittany Siontis and Rami N. Khoriaty

Chronic Myelogenous Leukemia (CML)

EPIDEMIOLOGY

1. What is the median age at diagnosis of CML?
   - Sixty-seven years; incidence increases with age

ETIOLOGY AND RISK FACTORS

1. What is the one known causative factor?
   - Ionizing radiation

2. What two genes are involved in the hallmark Philadelphia (Ph) chromosomal translocation of CML and what chromosomes are they on?
   - *Breakpoint cluster region* (*BCR*) on chromosome 22 and *ABL1* proto-oncogene on chromosome 9

3. What is the protein product of balanced translocation between the long arms of chromosomes 9 and 22?
   - The BCR-ABL1 oncoprotein

DIAGNOSTIC CRITERIA

1. What is required to make a diagnosis of CML?
   - Identification of t(9;22) in cytogenetic analysis of bone marrow (BM), or
   - Identification of the *BCR-ABL1* fusion gene by fluorescence in situ hybridization (FISH), or
   - Identification of the BCR-ABL1 transcript with quantitative reverse transcription polymerase chain reaction (RT-PCR)

2. Name two other hematologic malignancies that can harbor t(9;22).
   - Ph+ acute lymphoblastic leukemia
   - Ph+ acute myeloid leukemia (AML)

STAGING

1. **What are the three phases of CML, and what characterizes each phase by World Health Organization (WHO) criteria?**

Chronic Phase (CP)	Accelerated Phase (AP)	Blast Phase (BP)
No features of accelerated or blast phase	Peripheral or marrow blasts 10%–19%, peripheral blood basophils ≥20%, platelets <100,000 unrelated to therapy, platelets >1,000,000 unresponsive to therapy, clonal evolution by cytogenetics, increasing spleen size and white blood cell (WBC) count unresponsive to therapy	Peripheral or marrow blasts ≥20%, extramedullary blasts, large clusters or foci of blasts in bone marrow (BM)

SIGNS AND SYMPTOMS

1. **What is the classic presentation of CML?**
   - Asymptomatic neutrophilia (+/− left shift) on routine complete blood count (CBC), gradual onset of fatigue, weight loss, night sweats, splenomegaly, early satiety, gout, and leukocytosis

2. **Are infections rare or common at presentation?**
   - Rare, because neutrophil function is preserved

3. **What is a typical CBC on presentation?**
   - Leukocytosis (20,000 to as high as 700,000) with left shift and circulating myeloblasts, myelocytes, metamyelocytes, and band forms
   - Basophilia (+/− eosinophilia): a hallmark feature of CML
   - Mild normochromic, normocytic anemia
   - Normal or elevated platelet count

PROGNOSTIC FACTORS

1. **What are two important poor prognostic factors?**
   - Disease status at diagnosis
   - Failure to achieve (or loss of) hematologic, cytogenetic, and molecular responses (see the table in Question 7 found on page 34)

2. **What prognostic factors are associated with worse outcomes in CML?**
   - Age, spleen size, platelet count, and blast percentage on the peripheral blood (all included in the Sokal risk assessment score). Additionally, peripheral blood basophil and eosinophil percentages have prognostic values in the Hasford scoring system.

TREATMENT

1. **How is newly diagnosed CML in chronic phase treated?**
   - Tyrosine kinase inhibitor (TKI) therapy: nilotinib (300 mg BID) dasatinib (100 mg daily), and imatinib (400 mg daily) are the three Food and Drug Administration (FDA)-approved TKIs for first-line treatment of chronic phase CML
   - Consider hydroxyurea for patients with white blood cell (WBC) count greater than 100,000 (only temporarily until WBC goes down)
   - Addition of allopurinol 300 mg daily until blood counts normalize

2. **What should be taken into consideration when selecting one of the three TKIs (dasatinib, nilotinib, imatinib) in the first-line treatment of chronic phase CML?**
   - Side effects of the different TKIs (see following Questions 3–6)
   - Patient comorbidities
   - Sokal and Hasford prognostic scores: consider nilotinib or dasatinib, rather than imatinib, in patients with intermediate or high risk scores
   - Patient preference and cost/insurance coverage

3. **What are some characteristic toxicities associated with nilotinib?**
   - QT prolongation, gastrointestinal (GI) upset, pancreatitis, hyperglycemia, hypercholesterolemia, liver toxicity. Nilotinib is the only TKI that needs to be taken twice a day. Patients cannot have PO intake for 2 hours before or 1 hour after each dose of nilotinib.

4. **What are some characteristic toxicities associated with dasatinib?**
   - QT prolongation, thrombocytopenia, gastroesophageal reflux disease (GERD), pleural effusion, bleeding from platelet dysfunction, pulmonary hypertension

5. **What are some characteristic toxicities associated with imatinib?**
   - Skin rash, muscle cramps, diarrhea, periorbital swelling, edema, liver function test abnormalities, hypophosphatemia, QT prolongation

6. **Based on the toxicities of the different TKIs, which TKI of the three TKIs approved in the first-line treatment setting (imatinib, dasatinib, nilotinib) should be avoided in the following conditions?**
   - History of pancreatitis: avoid nilotinib
   - History of pericardial/pleural disease: avoid dasatinib
   - History of (or significant risk factors for) arterial thrombotic events: avoid nilotinib
   - Patients on anticoagulants: avoid dasatinib
   - Patient with pulmonary hypertension: avoid dasatinib
   - Patients who are not able to fast for 3 hours (2 hours before and 1 hour after each dose of medication) twice a day: avoid nilotinib

7. What are the treatment response goals and criteria for CML patients treated with first-line TKIs?

Goal	Definition	Optimal Response	Treatment Failure*	Recommended Monitoring
Hematologic response	**Complete hematologic response (CHR):** Platelet count <450,000, white blood cell (WBC) <10,000, no peripheral blood immature granulocytes, basophils <5%, no palpable spleen	CHR by 3 months	No CHR by 3 months	Complete blood count (CBC): every week for first 6 weeks, then every 2 weeks until CHR, then every 3 months
Cytogenetic response (CyR)	**Minor (MCyR):** Ph+ cells 36%–65% **Partial (PCyR):** Ph+ cells 1%–35% **Complete (CCyR):** Ph+ cells 0%	At least PCyR at 3 months, and CCyR at 6 months	No PCyR at 6 months, no CCyR at 12 months	Bone marrow (BM) cytogenetics: at diagnosis; at 3 and 6 months if quantitative polymerase chain reaction (qPCR) is not available; at 12 months if no CCyR documented prior or no MMR; if there is a 1 log increase in BCR-ABL transcript with loss of MMR
Molecular response (MR)	**Major (MMR):** BCR-ABL1:control gene ratio <0.1 **Complete:** BCR-ABL1 transcripts undetectable in a lab where PCR sensitivity of at least 4.5 logs below standardized baseline	BCR-ABL ≤10% at 3 months, <1% at 6 months, and ≤0.1% at 12 months	BCR-ABL >10% at 6 months, BCR-ABL >1% at 12 months. 1 log increase in BCR-ABL transcript with loss of MMR is an indication for BM biopsy	qPCR: every 3 months until 2 years after CCyR, then every 3–6 months; perform mutational analysis only if response is suboptimal or if failure

*Treatment failure also includes: loss of CHR or CCyR, and clonal chromosomal abnormalities.

8. What is a practical approach to monitor chronic phase CML after first-line TKI therapy?

- CBC every 1 to 2 weeks until complete hematologic response (CHR) then every 3 months. At 3 months: if no CHR, then this is treatment failure, and patients need to be treated as such (see Question 10). For patients in CHR by 3 months, further monitoring is as follows:

- At 3 months: perform quantitative polymerase chain reaction (qPCR) (or BM cytogenetics if qPCR is not available):
  - If BCR-ABL transcripts ≤10% (or if partial cytogenetic response [PCyR] is achieved): this is optimal response. Continue the same treatment and monitor qPCR every 3 months.
  - If BCR-ABL transcripts >10% (or if no PCyR): this is suboptimal response, but not treatment failure. Evaluate for compliance, drug interactions, and check for ABL kinase mutation.
    - If patient was on imatinib, consider switching to nilotinib or dasatinib (recommended) or increasing the imatinib dose to a maximum of 800 mg a day if not a candidate for the second-generation TKIs. Evaluate for allogeneic stem cell transplant (ASCT).
    - If patient was on dasatinib or nilotinib: consider switching to the other second-generation TKI or keeping the same course. Do not switch from second-generation TKI to imatinib. Evaluate for ASCT.
- At 6 months: perform qPCR (or BM cytogenetics if qPCR is not available):
  - BCR-ABL transcripts <1% constitutes optimal response.
  - If BCR-ABL transcripts ≤10% (or if PCyR is achieved): continue the same treatment and monitor qPCR in 3 months if available (or BM biopsy).
  - If BCR-ABL transcripts >10% (or if no PCyR): this is treatment failure.
- At 12 months: perform qPCR (or BM cytogenetics if qPCR is not available):
  - If BCR-ABL transcripts ≤1% (or if complete cytogenetic response [CCyR] is achieved): continue same treatment. Monitor qPCR every 3 months for 2 years post-CCyR then every 3 to 6 months.
  - If BCR-ABL transcripts >1%: This is treatment failure. Switch to an alternate TKI (see Question 10) and evaluate for ASCT.
- Despite the ease of PCR monitoring, BM biopsy is typically still recommended at diagnosis, to document CCyR, and if there is suspicion of loss of response.

9. **What are the management options for patients with TKI intolerance?**
   - Patients with intolerance to one TKI can be switched to one of the other three TKIs approved in first-line treatment. An additional option is bosutinib, a second-generation TKI, FDA-approved for patients with intolerance or resistance to imatinib or other second-generation TKIs (dasatinib and nilotinib).

10. **What are the management options for patients with failure to first-line TKI therapy?**
    - Evaluate for compliance and drug interactions.
    - Test for ABL kinase mutations to help guide the choice of the second-line TKI (see the following): approximately 50% of patients with treatment failure have mutation in the ABL kinase.
    - For most patients, switching to a/another second-generation TKI is appropriate: patients who fail first-line imatinib, dasatinib, or nilotinib can be treated with one of the (other) second-generation TKIs (dasatinib, nilotinib, or bosutinib) in the second-line setting (patients who fail dasatinib or nilotinib

should not be switched to imatinib). Third-line treatment options include any of the remaining second-generation TKIs, ponatinib, and ASCT. Further options for patients not eligible for ASCT include ponatinib, omacetaxine, and clinical trials.

- Evaluate for ASCT (indications for ASCT are included in a Question 15.
- Other possibilities include: clinical trials, interferon alpha.

11. **What ABL kinase mutation confers resistance to all first- and second-generation TKIs: imatinib, nilotinib, dasatinib, and bosutinib?**
    - T315I mutation
    - Patients with treatment failure due to T315I mutation should be considered for early ASCT, and could be treated with the third-generation TKI ponatinib (or with omacetaxine as a less favorable alternative) while a donor is identified.

12. **What ABL kinase mutations help decide the choice of the second-line TKI therapy?**
    - Patients without the T315I can be switched to a second-generation TKI (dasatinib, nilotinib, or bosutinib).
    - The V299L mutations predict a better response to nilotinib than dasatinib or bosutinib.
    - The T315A, F317L/V/I/C mutations are more sensitive to nilotinib or bosutinib than to dasatinib.
    - The Y253H, E255K/V, F359V/C/I mutations predict a better response to dasatinib or bosutinib than nilotinib.

13. **What are some characteristic toxicities associated with ponatinib?**
    - Arterial thrombotic events, heart failure, hepatotoxicity, QT prolongation, pancreatitis, fluid retention.

14. **What are some characteristic toxicities associated with bosutinib?**
    - Diarrhea, nausea/vomiting, hepatotoxicity, rash, low incidence of pleural effusion, vascular events, and cardiac toxicity. In contrast to other TKIs, bosutinib has minimal QT prolongation.

15. **What is the role of ASCT in CML?**
    - Reserved for fourth (or third)-line treatment after TKI failure in chronic phase CML patients
    - ASCT should be prioritized in patients with low probability of response to second-generation TKIs (patients with no cytogenetic response to imatinib or other second-generation TKIs or with mutations predicting low sensitivity to second-generation TKIs)
    - Indicated for accelerated phase (AP) or blast phase (BP) after best response to TKI is achieved (regardless of the depth of response)
    - Should be considered for patients younger than 30 years of age, given that it is the only curative option for CML

16. **How successful is ASCT for CML?**
    - Long-term cure rate of approximately 65% for patients transplanted in chronic phase
    - Transplant-related mortality and relapse are higher in patients transplanted for AP or BP

17. **How should accelerated phase chronic myelogenous leukemia (AP CML) be treated?**
    - Patients in AP CML should be treated with dasatinib 140 mg daily, nilotinib 400 mg BID, or bosutinib 500 mg daily (and less favorably imatinib 600 mg PO daily), followed by ASCT (if eligible) after best response is achieved with the TKI. Patients with optimal/deep response to the TKI might choose to be monitored very carefully with deferring ASCT until the first sign of disease progression. This relapse requires another TKI followed by ASCT.

18. **How are patients with blast phase chronic myelogenous leukemia (BP CML) treated?**
    - Patients with BP CML should undergo ABL kinase mutation analysis to help select the best TKI. All patients should be evaluated for ASCT.
    - Patients with lymphoid blast crisis are treated with combination chemotherapy with second-generation TKI, followed by ASCT.
    - Myeloid blast crisis does not typically respond well to AML induction regimens. Patients in de novo myeloid blast crisis CML are treated with a second-generation TKI without chemotherapy until best response, followed by ASCT. Patients with blast crisis CML that develops on TKI therapy are treated with combination chemotherapy + more potent TKI, followed by ASCT.

Myeloproliferative Neoplasms (General)

1. **What characterizes a myeloproliferative neoplasm (MPN)?**
   - Clonal hematopoietic stem cell disease with overproduction of one or more blood cell lines
   - Normal maturation with effective hematopoiesis and extramedullary hematopoiesis
   - Risk for leukemic transformation

2. **What are the eight MPNs recognized by the WHO in 2016?**
   - BCR-ABL1-positive CML
   - Polycythemia vera (PV)
   - Essential thrombocythemia (ET)
   - Primary myelofibrosis (PMF)
   - Chronic neutrophilic leukemia
   - Chronic eosinophilic leukemia, not otherwise specified
   - Mast cell disease
   - MPNs, unclassifiable

3. **What is the most common gene mutated in PV, ET, and PMF?**
   - *JAK2*

4. **What is *JAK2*'s normal function?**
   - Tyrosine kinase, which is critical in intracellular signaling for the erythropoietin, thrombopoietin, interleukin-3, granulocyte colony-stimulating factor (G-CSF), and granulocyte macrophage colony-stimulating factor (GM-CSF) receptors

5. **What *JAK2* mutations are tested for in MPN?**
   - *JAK2* V617F (most common) and *JAK2* exon 12 mutations
   - *JAK2* V617F mutation causes constitutive activation of downstream messengers through the JAK–STAT, PI3K, and AKT pathways

6. **In which MPN is *JAK2* mutation most prevalent?**
   - PV (98%–99%), ET (~60%), PMF (~55%)

7. **Name two additional mutations implicated in ET and PMF?**
   - *MPL* (mutation in the transmembrane domain of the thrombopoietin receptor)
   - *CALR*

8. **What thrombophilic condition should raise the suspicion of a *JAK2* mutation?**
   - Budd–Chiari syndrome

Polycythemia Vera

EPIDEMIOLOGY

1. **What is the median age at diagnosis of PV?**
   - Approximately 60 years old, but occurs in all age groups

2. **What is the median survival of PV patients?**
   - Median survival is approximately 14 years (and ~24 years in patients <60 years)

3. **What are prognostic factors for worse survival in PV?**
   - Risk factors predicting worsening survival in PV are: age >57 (with age >67 being even higher risk), leucocytosis (WBC >15,000), venous thrombosis, and abnormal karyotype

4. **What are the risks of transformation to myelofibrosis and risk of leukemic transformation in PV?**
   - Risk of transformation to myelofibrosis: 5% to 6% at 10 years, and 6% to 14% at 15 years. Risk factor: JAK2V617F allele burden of >50%.
   - Risk of transformation to AML: <10% at 20 years. Risk factors: advanced age, leucocytosis, and abnormal karyotype.

5. **What characterizes PV pathophysiologically?**
   - Growth factor (epo)-independent proliferation of erythroid cells, producing an elevated red cell mass

DIAGNOSTIC CRITERIA

1. What are the WHO diagnostic criteria for PV?

	2008 WHO Criteria*	Proposed 2016 WHO Criteria**
Major	1. Hgb >18.5 g/dL (men) or Hgb >16.5 g/dL (women), OR Hgb or Hct >99th percentile of reference for age, sex, and altitude of residence	A1. Hgb >16.5 g/dL(men) or Hgb >16 g/dL (women) OR Hct >49% (men) or Hct >48% (women)
	2. Presence of *JAK2* mutation	A2. Hypercellular bone marrow (age-adjusted) with panmyelosis and pleomorphic mature megakaryocytes
		A3. Presence of *JAK2* mutation
Minor	1. Bone marrow trilineage myeloproliferation	B. Subnormal epo level
	2. Subnormal serum epo level	
	3. endogenous erythroid colony (EEC) growth	

*2008 WHO criteria: diagnosis requires meeting either both major criteria and one minor criterion, or first major criterion and two minor criteria.

**PV diagnosis in the proposed 2016 revisions requires meeting criteria A1 to A3, or meeting criteria A1 and A2 and B.

Hgb, hemoglobin.

2. What are the features that help distinguish PV from secondary polycythemia?

- Splenomegaly
- Leukocytosis
- Thrombocytosis
- Low epo level
- Panhyperplasia in BM
- Normal arterial oxygen saturation
- Increased vitamin B12 level

SIGNS AND SYMPTOMS

1. What are the common presenting signs/symptoms in patients with PV?

- Incidental polycythemia (+/− thrombocytosis +/− leucocytosis) on CBC, hypertension, pruritus aggravated by hot shower, erythromelalgia, gout, kidney stones, palpable splenomegaly (50%–70%), early satiety, joint pain, thrombosis symptoms (arterial or venous), and neurologic symptoms such as headache and confusion

TREATMENT

1. **Which patients should be treated with aspirin?**
   - All patients with PV who do not have a contraindication should be treated with aspirin 81 mg daily

2. **In addition to aspirin, what are the treatment options for patients with PV, in the first-line setting?**
   - Phlebotomy and cytoreduction with hydrea

3. **What is the goal hematocrit when the patient is getting phlebotomies or hydrea?**
   - Hematocrit less than 45% with either treatment

4. **What are the indications for cytoreductive therapy with hydrea?**
   - Hydrea should be used in these situations:
     - Patients older than 60 years
     - Patients with history of thromboembolism (consider in patients with risk factors for thromboembolic disease)
     - Platelets greater than 1.5 million or acquired von Willebrand disease (VWD). Always check von Willebrand factor (VWF) activity if platelets are >1 million before administering aspirin (see the section on Essential Thrombocythemia).
   - Patients who do not have any of these criteria should be treated with aspirin and PRN phlebotomies

5. **In addition to aspirin, which therapy in PV has demonstrated the greatest reduction in thrombotic events?**
   - Hydroxyurea

6. **What are second-line treatment options for PV?**
   - Interferon alpha
   - Busulfan
   - Ruxolitinib (particularly if significant splenomegaly or constitutional symptoms)
   - Anagrelide (will only control the platelet count)
   - ASCT is the only curative option, but is almost never needed in PV (for treatment of post-PCR myelofibrosis, refer to the section on Primary Myelofibrosis)

Essential Thrombocythemia

EPIDEMIOLOGY

1. **What is the typical age at presentation for ET?**
   - Bimodal: One peak around age 30 with a second (larger) peak at age 50 to 60
   - Women to men ratio is 1.5 to 2:1 in the early peak

2. **What is the median survival in ET patients?**
   - Median survival is approximately 20 years (and ~33 years in patients <60 years of age); in some reports survival is comparable to that of the age-matched population

3. **What is the prevalence of the *JAK2* mutation in ET? What other genes are mutated in ET?**
   - *JAK2* is mutated in approximately 60% of patients
   - *CALR* is mutated in approximately 22% of patients
   - *MPL* is mutated in approximately 3% of patients

4. **What are prognostic factors for worse survival in ET?**
   - Risk factors predicting worse survival in ET are: age >60 years, leucocytosis (WBC >11,000), and history of thrombosis

5. **What are the risk of transformation to myelofibrosis and risk of leukemic transformation in ET?**
   - Risk of transformation to myelofibrosis: 1% to 5% at 10 years, and 4% to 11% at 15 years (risk factors: advanced age and anemia. Presence of *JAK2* V617F mutation appears to be associated with lower risk of fibrotic transformation).
   - Risk of transformation to AML: approximately 5% at 20 years. Risk factors: thrombosis and extreme thrombocytosis (platelets >1 million).

DIAGNOSTIC CRITERIA

1. **What are the WHO diagnostic criteria for ET?**

	2008 WHO Criteria*	Proposed 2016 WHO Criteria**
Major criteria	1. Platelet count >450,000	A1. Platelet count >450,000
	2. Megakaryocyte proliferation with large and mature morphology, with no or little granulocyte or erythroid proliferation	A2. Megakaryocyte proliferation with large and mature morphology, with no or little granulocyte or erythroid proliferation, and very rarely minor (grade 1) reticulin fibrosis
	3. Not meeting WHO criteria for chronic myelogenous leukemia (CML), polycythemia vera (PV), primary myelofibrosis (PMF), myelodysplastic syndrome (MDS), or other myeloid neoplasms	A3. Not meeting WHO criteria for CML, PV, PMF, MDS, or other myeloid neoplasms
	4. Demonstration of *JAK2* V617F or another clonal marker or no evidence of reactive thrombocytosis	A4. Presence of *JAK2*, *CALR*, or *MPL* mutation
Minor criteria		B. Presence of a clonal marker or absence or evidence of reactive thrombocytosis

*2008 WHO criteria: ET diagnosis requires meeting all four major criteria.

** ET diagnosis in the proposed 2016 WHO revisions requires meeting criteria A1 to A4, or meeting criteria A1 to A3 and the B criterion.

SIGNS AND SYMPTOMS

1. **What are the most common presenting symptoms in ET?**
   - Asymptomatic (50%)
   - Vasomotor symptoms: visual changes, lightheadedness, headaches, palpitations, typical/atypical chest pain, erythromelalgia, livedo reticularis, acral paresthesias
   - Palpable splenomegaly and early satiety
   - Thrombosis (15% at presentation)

2. **In addition to the thrombosis risk and the risk of transformation to myelofibrosis and AML, what are the other complications of this disease?**
   - Major hemorrhage (5%–10%) from acquired VWD
   - Recurrent first trimester abortions

TREATMENT

1. **Who should receive aspirin therapy?**
   - All patients without contraindication for aspirin
   - In patients with platelets ≥1 million/µL, check VWD ristocetin cofactor activity before starting aspirin. Patients with VWD ristocetin activity ≤30% are at high risk of bleeding and should undergo platelet cytoreduction to result in VWD ristocetin activity ≥30% prior to starting aspirin.

2. **What are the indications for cytoreductive treatment?**
   - Age greater than 60, or
   - History of thrombosis (consider in patients with risk factors for thrombosis), or
   - Platelets greater than 1 million/µL
   - Patients without any of these indications for cytoreductive therapy should receive aspirin only

3. **What is the preferred first-line cytoreductive agent in treating high-risk ET?**
   - Hydroxyurea

4. **What second-line agents are used in treating high-risk ET?**
   - Anagrelide
   - Interferon alpha
   - Busulfan

5. **What is the mechanism of action of anagrelide?**
   - Interferes with terminal differentiation of megakaryocytes

6. **In what group of patients should anagrelide therapy be avoided and why?**
   - In those with cardiovascular comorbidities because it can cause fluid retention, palpitations, and pulmonary hypertension

Primary Myelofibrosis

EPIDEMIOLOGY

1. **In addition to PMF, which two hematologic disorders most commonly lead to secondary myelofibrosis?**
   - Myelofibrosis could be a primary disease (PMF) or secondary to ET or PV.
   - Fibrosis in the BM could result from other etiologies such as hairy cell leukemia, metastatic solid tumor to the BM, and so on.

2. **What is the median survival of patients with PMF?**
   - Median survival of approximately 6 years (~15 years in patients <60 years of age)

DIAGNOSTIC CRITERIA

1. **What are the WHO 2008 diagnostic criteria for PMF?**

		2008 WHO Criteria*	Proposed 2016 WHO Criteria**
Major*	1.	Megakaryocyte proliferation and atypia accompanied by either reticulin and/or collagen fibrosis. In prefibrotic/early PMF, the megakaryocytic changes are accompanied by increased cellularity with granulocytic proliferation and often decreased erythropoiesis	A1. Megakaryocyte proliferation and atypia accompanied by either reticulin and/or collagen fibrosis (grades 2–3 on 0–3 scale). In prefibrotic/early PMF, the megakaryocytic changes are not accompanied by fibrosis, and the bone marrow shows increased cellularity with granulocytic proliferation and often decreased erythropoiesis
	2.	Not meeting WHO criteria for chronic myelogenous leukemia (CML), polycythemia vera (PV), myelodysplastic syndrome (MDS), or other myeloid neoplasms	A2. Not meeting WHO criteria for CML, PV, essential thrombocythemia (ET), MDS, or other myeloid neoplasms
	3.	Demonstration of *JAK2* V617F or another clonal marker or no evidence of reactive marrow fibrosis	A3. Demonstration of *JAK2*, *CALR*, or *MPL* mutation or another clonal marker or no evidence of reactive marrow fibrosis
Minor	1.	Leukoerythroblastosis	B1. Leukoerythroblastosis (absent in prefibrotic PMF)
	2.	Increased serum lactate dehydrogenase (LDH)	B2. Increased serum LDH
	3.	Anemia	B3. Anemia

(continued)

(continued)

2008 WHO Criteria*	Proposed 2016 WHO Criteria**
4. Palpable splenomegaly	B4. Palpable splenomegaly
	B5. Leukocytosis (white blood cell [WBC] >11,000)

*2008 WHO criteria: PMF diagnosis requires meeting all three major criteria and two minor criteria.

** PMF diagnosis in the proposed 2016 WHO revisions requires meeting criteria A1 to A3 and at least one B criterion.

2. **What are the three most commonly mutated genes in PMF?**
   - *JAK2* (~55% of patients)
   - *CALR* (27%)
   - *MPL* W515L (7% of patients)
   - Approximately 10% of patients with PMF do not have any of the above mutations

3. **What are the diagnostic criteria of post-PV and post-ET myelofibrosis?**

		Post-PV Myelofibrosis*	Post-ET Myelofibrosis**
Major*	1.	Documentation of a prior diagnosis of PV	1. Documentation of a prior diagnosis of ET
	2.	Bone marrow fibrosis (grade 2–3 on 0–3 scale)	2. Bone marrow fibrosis (grade 2–3 on 0–3 scale)
Minor	1.	Anemia or lack of requirement of phlebotomies in absence of cytoreductive therapy	1. Anemia and ≥ 2 g/dL decrease from baseline Hgb
	2.	Leukoerythroblastosis	2. Leukoerythroblastosis
	3.	New splenomegaly or increase in palpable splenomegaly of ≥5 cm	3. New splenomegaly or increase in palpable splenomegaly of ≥5 cm
	4.	One or more of these constitutional symptoms: unexplained fever (>37.5°C, night sweats, or >10% weight loss in 6 months)	4. One or more of these constitutional symptoms: unexplained fever (>37.5°C, night sweats, or >10% weight loss in 6 months)
	5.		5. Increased lactate dehydrogenase (LDH)

*For diagnosis of post-PV myelofibrosis: two major and two minor criteria are required.

**For diagnosis of post-ET myelofibrosis: two major and two minor criteria are required.

SIGNS AND SYMPTOMS

1. **Name several common presenting symptoms of PMF?**
   - Fatigue, anemia, abdominal discomfort and early satiety (from splenomegaly), fever, night sweats, weight loss, bone pain, pruritus, complications of portal hypertension (such as variceal bleed, ascites)

2. **What are the two most common physical exam findings in patients with PMF?**
   - Palpable splenomegaly and hepatomegaly.

3. **What does the classic peripheral blood smear of PMF show?**
   - Leukoerythroblastosis (immature cells of the granulocytic series and nucleated red blood cells) and teardrop-shaped red blood cells (seen in fibrotic PMF).

PROGNOSTIC FACTORS

1. **What are the factors associated with decreased survival in PMF based on the Dynamic International Prognostic Scoring System-plus (DIPSS-plus)?**
   - Age >65 years
   - Presence of constitutional symptoms
   - Anemia, Hgb ≤10 g/dL
   - Leukocytosis, WBC greater than $25,000 \times 10^6$/L
   - Presence of ≥1% circulating peripheral blasts
   - Presence of unfavorable karyotype (complex karyotype, +8, −7/7q−, i(17q), inv(3), −5/5q, 12p−, or 11q23 rearrangement)
   - Platelet count <100,000/μL
   - Red blood cell transfusion need (patients with red blood cell transfusion need will automatically get 2 points because their Hgb would be <10 g/dL)

2. **How are patients with PMF divided into risk groups? What is the median survival in each risk group?**
   - High risk: at least four of the aforementioned risk factors; median survival is approximately 1.3 years
   - Intermediate-2 risk: two or three risk factors; median survival is approximately 2.9 years
   - Intermediate-1 risk: one risk factor; median survival is approximately 6.5 years
   - Low risk: zero risk factors; median survival is approximately 15.4 years

TREATMENT

1. **What is the goal of treatment in PMF?**
   - Palliation in most cases, except in patients who are candidates for BM transplantation, where cure might be attained (see the following)

2. **How do you treat patients with low and intermediate-1 risk PMF?**
   - The mainstay of therapy is supportive care and symptom control
     - Asymptomatic: observation is reasonable
     - MF-associated anemia: options include danazol, talidomine +/− prednisone, lenalidomine +/− prednisone (use lenalidomine particularly in presence of del 5q), and erythropoiesis stimulating agents (an option if epo level is inadequate). Avoid erythropoiesis stimulating agents in patients with significant splenomegaly, because they are not very effective in transfusion-dependent patients and might worsen splenomegaly. Splenectomy can be

considered in refractory cases; however, this decision should not be taken lightly because of the associated morbidity and mortality (~10% perisurgical mortality) and because a subset of patients develop compensatory hepatomegaly, some of whom might die of liver failure.

o Symptomatic splenomegaly: hydroxyurea or ruxolitinib are reasonable as first-line therapies for symptomatic splenomegaly. Other less favorable options include splenectomy and splenic irradiation. The response of splenomegaly to ruxolitinib is superior to the response to hydroxyurea. Ruxolitinib should be considered as first-line therapy in cases of significantly symptomatic splenomegaly, while hydroxyurea could be used as the first-line option in the other cases. Splenectomy is associated with significant risks, and the decision to proceed with splenectomy should be individualized (see the previous item). The risks of splenic irradiation include profound cytopenias and the benefit of this modality is only transient.

3. **How do you treat patients with intermediate-2 and high-risk PMF?**
   - These patients should be considered for BM transplantation, which is the only curative modality in myelofibrosis. Patients who are not candidates for BM transplantation should be treated on a clinical trial (if available) or should undergo symptom-adjusted therapy.
   - Patients with symptomatic splenomegaly or constitutional symptoms: use ruxolitinib.

4. **How is myelofibrosis associated pulmonary hypertension diagnosed and treated?**
   - Diagnosis is confirmed by a technetium 99m sulfur colloid scintigraphy.
   - Single fraction whole lung radiation (100 cGy) has been shown to be effective.

QUESTIONS

1. A 70-year-old woman with a past medical history notable for hypertension, diabetes, and stroke is found to have leukocytosis (white blood cell [WBC] count of 25,000) on routine labs. Hemoglobin is mildly reduced at 11.5 g/dL and platelet count is mildly elevated at 500,000. She notes some mild fatigue but is otherwise asymptomatic. Examination is notable for a spleen tip palpable 3 cm below the left costal margin. Further testing reveals BCR-ABL by fluorescence in situ hybridization (FISH) to be positive. You calculate her Sokal score, and she is found to be high risk. What is the next best step in management?
   A. Initiation of hydrea
   B. Initiation of imatinib
   C. Initiation of nilotinib
   D. Initiation of dasatinib

2. A 63-year-old gentleman with a history of chronic myelogenous leukemia (CML) on imatinib presents to clinic for routine follow-up. Labs are notable for a white blood cell (WBC) count of 50,000 (10,000 6 months ago) and platelet count of 650,000 (normal 6 months ago). Quantitative polymerase chain reaction (PCR) for BCR-ABL returns

elevated at 5% (previously undetected), and this result was confirmed by repeat testing. The patient confirms that he is taking imatinib religiously and has not missed any dose. What is the next best step in management?

A. Continue imatinib and repeat PCR again in 1 month
B. Transition to nilotinib or dasatinib
C. Perform a molecular mutation analysis
D. Switch to ponatinib

3. A 67-year-old woman with a past medical history notable for hypertension, glaucoma, and diabetes presents to clinic for evaluation of 2 months of progressive fatigue, early satiety, and weight loss. Labs are obtained and complete blood count (CBC) shows a white blood cell (WBC) count of 95,000 with basophilia (22%). Hemoglobin is 9.5 and platelets are 650,000. Differential reveals 12% blasts. Fluorescence in situ hybridization (FISH) for BCR-ABL is positive. Bone marrow biopsy shows 15% blasts, with cytogenetics revealing the Philadelphia chromosome in 20 out of 20 cells examined. What is the next best step in management?

A. Admit to hospital for cytotoxic chemotherapy
B. Initiate second-generation tyrosine kinase inhibitor (TKI)
C. Refer for consideration of allogeneic stem cell transplant (ASCT)
D. B and C

4. A 55-year-old woman is referred to hematology for evaluation of a hemoglobin of 16.8/hematocrit of 51% found on routine labs. White blood cell (WBC) and platelet counts are normal. Upon further questioning she reports minimal pruritus following a hot bath but denies burning and erythema of her hands. Her past medical history is otherwise notable for mild hypertension and tobacco dependency. She denies any family history of hematologic disorders. There is no personal or family history of thrombosis. Physical examination is unremarkable. What is the next best step in management?

A. Initiate JAK2 inhibitor therapy and evaluate for etiology
B. Immediately phlebotomize and evaluate for etiology
C. Evaluate for etiology
D. Initiate hydrea and evaluate for etiology

5. A 46-year-old man presents with polycythemia (hemoglobin 18.7, hematocrit 56%). He does not have a history of prior thromboembolic events. Workup demonstrated negative JAK2 V617F mutation. Bone marrow biopsy demonstrated increased cellularity with panmyelosis and pleomorphic mature megakaryocytes. Epo level is low. How should this patient be managed?

A. Initiate JAK2 inhibitor therapy
B. Aspirin and phlebotomy
C. Aspirin only
D. Observation and optimizing risk factors for thrombosis

6. A 68-year-old woman is found to have a platelet count of 800,000 on routine labs. She is asymptomatic. She has no history of arterial or venous thrombotic events. Physical examination is notable for a palpable spleen tip 2 cm below the costal margin. Testing for *JAK2* V617F is positive. Bone marrow biopsy demonstrates findings consistent with essential thrombocythemia (ET) and rules out other possible disorders. What is the next best step in management?
   A. Hydrea and aspirin
   B. Interferon alpha and aspirin
   C. Aspirin monotherapy
   D. Check von Willebrand factor (VWF) activity. No therapy is needed because she is asymptomatic

7. A 78-year-old man with a past medical history of diabetes, coronary artery disease, heart failure, and hypertension presents for evaluation of fatigue, night sweats, unintentional weight loss, left upper quadrant abdominal pain, and early satiety. The patient developed these symptoms gradually over the past 6 months. Physical exam is notable for splenomegaly (spleen tip palpated about 15 cm below the left costal margin). Labs are obtained: a white blood cell (WBC) count of 14,000 (2% circulating blasts), hemoglobin 11 g/dL, and platelet count of 160,000. Peripheral smear is notable for teardrop cells. *JAK2* V617F and exon 12 mutations are negative, as is *MPL* mutation. The patient has a *CALR* mutation identified. Infections are ruled out. What is the best management option for this patient?
   A. Supportive care with transfusions as needed
   B. Hydroxyurea
   C. Ruxolitinib
   D. Cytotoxic chemotherapy followed by bone marrow transplantation

ANSWERS

1. **D. Initiation of dasatinib.** The patient is high risk based on her Sokal score; therefore, outcomes are improved with nilotinib or dasatinib compared to imatinib. She has a history of arterial events (as well as multiple risk factors for arterial thrombosis), making nilotinib a less desirable option. Therefore, the best option for this patient is dasatinib. Hydrea is typically considered briefly for patients with WBC >100,000 who need immediate leukoreduction.

2. **C. Perform a molecular mutation analysis.** Patients who show resistance to imatinib should be evaluated for mutations in the *ABL* kinase domain. Certain mutations may guide therapy and therefore this test should be done before transitioning to a second-generation tyrosine kinase inhibitor (TKI). Continuing current therapy would not be a good choice given the loss of response to the current therapy. Ponatinib should be limited to specific clinical situations given its high risk of arterial thrombosis.

3. **D. B and C.** This patient is in an accelerated phase of chronic myelogenous leukemia (CML). Cytotoxic chemotherapy is not indicated. Patients in accelerated phase CML should be treated with a second-generation TKI followed by ASCT after best response is obtained.

4. **C. Evaluate for etiology.** Patients who present with elevated hematocrit should be evaluated for the etiology prior to initiation of therapy directed at the etiology. If the patient has polycythemia secondary to hypoxemia, for example, dropping the hemoglobin/hematocrit might result in respiratory compromise.

5. **B. Aspirin and phlebotomy.** Patients who present with polycythemia and exhibit typical bone marrow abnormalities for polycythemia vera (PV), as well as low epo level, have a diagnosis of PV. *JAK2* V617F mutation is present in most patients with PV, but approximately 5% to 7% of patients with PV have the *JAK2* exon 12 mutation instead, while approximately 1% to 2% of patients with PV do not have either *JAK2* V617F or *JAK2* exon 12 mutations. In these patients, the typical bone marrow findings coupled with a low epo level clinch the diagnosis. This patient is <60 years of age, and has no prior history of thromboembolic events; therefore, he should be treated with aspirin and PRN phlebotomy (goal hematocrit <45%).

6. **A. Hydrea and aspirin.** This is a patient with high-risk ET given her age >60 years. She needs to be treated with aspirin and hydrea. Hydrea is teratogenic but this not a problem in this patient. Patients of childbearing age who desire to become pregnant should be counseled about pregnancy while on hydrea, and should employ safe contraception methods that do not increase risk of thrombosis, and hydrea should be stopped before pregnancy. Interferon therapy is not first line for ET. VWF activity should be checked in patients with a very high platelet count (>1 million) prior to aspirin administration.

7. **C. Ruxolitinib.** This patient meets criteria for higher risk (intermediate-2/ high risk) primary myelofibrosis. He is not a candidate for allogeneic stem cell transplantation given his age and comorbidities. He has symptomatic splenomegaly and constitutional symptoms; therefore, he would benefit from ruxolitinib therapy as opposed to supportive care alone or hydrea.

Myelodysplastic Syndromes

Rami N. Khoriaty and Dale Bixby

EPIDEMIOLOGY

1. **What is the median age at diagnosis for myelodysplastic syndrome (MDS)?**
   - Sixty-eight years

2. **What is the incidence of MDS?**
   - Ten thousand to 15,000 new cases per year in the United States (likely an underestimation)

Etiology and Risk Factors

1. **What is the etiology of MDS?**
   - Exact etiology is uncertain

2. **What are the common risk factors for MDS?**
   - Older age (incidence rises exponentially with age)
   - Male sex
   - Exposure to chemotherapeutic agents (alkylating agents, anthracyclines, and other topoisomerase II inhibitors)
   - Radiation exposure
   - Exposure to benzene and other organic solvents
   - Congenital disorders: Down syndrome, neurofibromatosis type 1, Fanconi anemia, congenital neutropenic disorders, dyskeratosis congenita, GATA-2 mutations, and others

CLASSIFICATION

1. **What are the subtypes of MDS according to World Health Organization (WHO) classification?**

MDS Subtype	Blood	Bone Marrow
Refractory cytopenia with unilineage dysplasia (RCUD)	Single or bicytopenia, <1% blasts	<5% blasts, dysplasia in one cell line
Refractory anemia with ringed sideroblasts (RARS)	Anemia, no blasts	<5% blasts, erythroid dysplasia only, ≥15% ringed sideroblasts

(continued)

1. **What are the subtypes of MDS according to World Health Organization (WHO) classification?** (*continued*)

MDS Subtype	Blood	Bone Marrow
MDS associated with isolated del(5q)	Anemia, normal or elevated platelets, <1% blasts	<5% blasts, erythroid dysplasia only, isolated del(5q), hypolobated megakaryocytes
Refractory cytopenia with multilineage dysplasia (RCMD)	Cytopenia(s), <1% blasts, no Auer rods	<5% blasts, dysplasia in ≥2 lineages, no Auer rods, ± ringed sideroblasts
Refractory anemia with excess blasts-1 (RAEB-1)	<5% blasts, no Auer rods	5%–9% blasts, no Auer rods, dysplasia in ≥1 lineage
Refractory anemia with excess blasts-2 (RAEB-2)	Blasts 5%–19%	10%–19% blasts or presence of Auer rods, dysplasia in ≥1 lineage
Myelodysplastic syndrome, unclassified (MDS-U)*	Cytopenias	<5% blasts, dysplasia or no dysplasia with MDS characteristic cytogenetics

Notes: Dysplasia is considered present if it involves at least 10% of a lineage.
Monocyte count is less than 1,000/mcL in all subtypes of MDS.
*Pancytopenia with dysplasia in one lineage is classified as MDS-U.

SIGNS AND SYMPTOMS

1. **What are the common signs and symptoms of MDS?**
   - Incidental cytopenias
   - Infections (due to neutropenia)
   - Bleeding (due to thrombocytopenia)
   - Fatigue and other signs/symptoms of anemia

DIAGNOSTIC CRITERIA

1. **What are the diagnostic criteria for MDS?**
   - The diagnosis relies on bone marrow examination showing dysplasia in one or more lineages (increased blasts are a sign of dysplasia) in addition to cytopenias.
   - In the absence of dysplasia, a diagnosis of MDS could be made in the correct clinical setting if MDS-specific karyotypic abnormalities are present (and if other bone marrow disorders are ruled out).

PROGNOSTIC FACTORS

1. **How are patients with MDS stratified into different risk groups?**
   - The International Prognostic Scoring System (IPSS) stratifies MDS into four risk groups: low risk (IPSS score 0), intermediate-1 risk (IPSS score

0.5–1), intermediate-2 risk (IPSS score 1.5–2), and high risk (IPSS score 2.5–3.5). Patients with low, intermediate-1, intermediate-2, and high-risk MDS by IPSS have median overall survivals of 5.7, 3.5, 1.2, and 0.4 years, respectively.

IPSS Scores

	0	0.5	1	1.5	2
Percentage of bone marrow blasts	<5	5–10	—	11–20	>20
Karyotype*		Good	Intermediate	Poor	—	—
Number of cytopenias**	0–1	2–3		—	—

*Good karyotype risk: normal, −Y, del(5q), del(20q); poor karyotype risk: complex karyotype (≥ 3 abnormalities), chromosome 7 abnormalities; intermediate karyotype risk: all others.

**Neutropenia: absolute neutrophil count <1,800; anemia: Hgb <10; thrombocytopenia: platelets <100,000.

- The IPSS scoring system should only be used at diagnosis in nontherapy-related MDS.
- WHO classification–based Prognostic Scoring System (WPSS) for MDS can be used throughout the MDS disease course. It stratifies patients into very low (WPSS score 0), low (WPSS score 1), intermediate (WPSS score 2), high (WPSS score 3–4), and very high (WPSS score 5–6) risk groups, with median overall survival of 103, 72, 40, 21, and 12 months, respectively, and cumulative 5-year probability of acute myeloid leukemia (AML) progression of 0.06, 0.24, 0.48, 0.63, and 1.0, respectively.

WPSS Score

	0	1	2	3
WHO subtype	RA, RARS, 5q−	RCMD, RCMD-RS	RAEB-1	RAEB-2
Transfusion requirement	None	≥1 red blood cell (RBC) unit every 8 weeks	—	—
IPSS cytogenetic risk	Good	Intermediate	Poor	—

- More recently, the IPSS has been refined (revised IPSS or IPSS-R) utilizing a larger patient cohort and has added additional risk groups of cytogenetic changes and has added the degree of anemia and thrombocytopenia into the model system. However, this still applies only to treatment naïve patients with de novo disease. This has allowed a further refinement of outcomes of patients, especially those with low-risk disease per IPSS.

Revised IPSS

	0	0.5	1	1.5	2		3	4
Bone marrow blasts	≤2		>2 to <5		5–10		>10	
Cytogenetics*	Very good		Good		Intermediate		Poor	Very poor
Hemoglobin	≥10		8 to <10	<8				
Platelets	≥100	50–100	<50					
Absolute neutrophil count	≥0.8	<0.8						

*Very good karyotype includes –Y or del(11q); good karyotype includes normal karyotype, del(5q), del(12p), del(20q), or a double abnormality including del(5q); intermediate karyotype includes del(7q), +8, +19, i(17q), and any other single or double independent clones; poor karyotype includes −7, inv(3)/t(3q)/del(3q), double abnormalities including −7/del(7q), or three abnormalities; very poor karyotype includes complex karyotype (≥3 abnormalities).

INDICATIONS FOR TREATMENT

1. **What are the indications of therapy in MDS?**
   - Transfusion dependence or symptoms related to cytopenias
   - Intermediate-2 or high-risk MDS

TREATMENT

1. **What is the treatment of choice for patients with low or intermediate-1 risk MDS with symptomatic/transfusion-dependent anemia and del(5q) as the sole cytogenetic abnormality?**
   - Lenalidomide (10 mg a day) is the treatment of choice for these patients. Transfusion-dependent patients with low/intermediate-1 risk MDS and del(5q) have an approximately 67% chance of becoming transfusion-independent (for medial duration of ~2–2.5 years) and approximately 62% chance of achieving complete cytogenetic response with lenalidomide.

2. **Is lenalidomide indicated for patients with low/intermediate-1 risk MDS with symptomatic or transfusion-dependent anemia but lacking del(5q)?**
   - Lenalidomide results in an overall response rate of 26% in patients with low/intermediate-1 risk MDS without del(5q). This response rate is lower than that achieved with DNA methyltransferase inhibitors. Lenalidomide, as a single agent, is therefore not generally recommended as frontline therapy for MDS patients without del(5q).

3. **What is the treatment of choice for patients with low or intermediate-1 risk MDS with symptomatic/transfusion-dependent anemia but lacking del(5q)?**

- The treatment of these patients is based on the erythropoietin level and the number of red blood cell (RBC) transfusions per month, as shown by the Hellström-Lindberg model.

Hellström-Lindberg Score

	Level	Score
Erythropoietin level	<100	+2
	100–500	+1
	>500	−3
Number of RBC units transfused per month	<2	+2
	≥2	−2

- Patients with a total Hellström-Lindberg score of greater than +1, −1 to +1, and less than −1 have a 74%, 23%, and 7% chance of achieving an erythroid response with erythropoietin-stimulating agents (ESAs), respectively. Most responses occur within 8 weeks of treatment, though some patients might respond after 12 weeks of treatment. The median time of response is ~2 years.

- ESAs represent a good treatment option for patients with a high chance of achieving an erythroid response with these agents (low epo levels and less than 2 units of transfusion a month). Occasionally, the addition of filgrastim may lead to erythroid responses in patients failing an ESA alone.

- Patients predicted to have a low chance of responding to ESAs could be treated with RBC transfusions. DNA methyltransferase inhibitors (azacitidine or decitabine) could also be considered.

- Iron chelation may be required depending on the ferritin levels (which should be monitored) and if the patient is undergoing curative intent therapy. Currently, no iron chelation therapy is Food and Drug Administration (FDA) approved for patients with myeloid neoplasms.

4. **What is the treatment of choice for patients with low/intermediate-1 risk MDS with thrombocytopenia and/or neutropenia?**

- Observation, if the thrombocytopenia and/or neutropenia are not severe
- Azacitidine or decitabine, if the thrombocytopenia and/or neutropenia are significant
- Patients with low/intermediate-1 risk MDS have better overall survival (according to retrospective data review) if allogeneic stem cell transplant (ASCT) is delayed until progression.

5. **When is immunosuppressive therapy (antithymocyte globulin and cyclosporine) considered in MDS?**

- Antithymocyte globulin and cyclosporine could be considered in a specific subgroup of younger patients (<60 years of age) with low/intermediate-1 risk MDS with the following characteristics: hypocellular bone marrow, <5% blasts, presence of a paroxysmal nocturnal hemoglobinuria clone, presence of an HLA-DR15 haplotype, or the presence of STAT-3 mutated T cell clones.

6. **What are the treatment options for patients with intermediate-2/high-risk MDS?**

   - ASCT is the only curative modality in MDS and should be strongly considered in patients with intermediate-2/high-risk MDS. A retrospective analysis showed that patients with intermediate-2/high-risk MDS have better overall survivals if they undergo ASCT. Administration of azacitidine or decitabine prior to ASCT is not routinely recommended because it has not been shown to add value in patients planning to proceed with ASCT; however, this should be considered in patients whose ASCT is expected to be delayed.

   - Patients who are not candidates for or who decline ASCT should be treated with azacitidine or decitabine. Azacitidine is the only one of these two drugs that was shown in a randomized control trial to confer a survival benefit compared to best supportive care. However, this is felt to be due to the different designs of the azacitidine and decitabine trials, and both drugs are considered to have equal value in MDS.

7. **For how many cycles should azacitidine or decitabine be given?**

   - Patients receiving azacitidine or decitabine who are not candidates for ASCT should continue receiving these drugs unless their MDS progresses or they develop side effects prohibiting their use if they are responding to therapy. Patients should receive a minimum or four to six cycles of azacitidine or decitabine before declaring the patient nonresponsive to therapy.

SPECIAL CONSIDERATIONS

1. **What is chronic myelomonocytic leukemia (CMML)?**

   - CMML is an overlap syndrome between MDS and myeloproliferative neoplasms, and has features of both (MDS features: dysplasia, anemia, and/or thrombocytopenia; myeloproliferative features: leucocytosis, monocytosis, and splenomegaly). CMML is characterized by absolute monocytosis (≥ 1000), persistent for more than 3 months and with no other etiologies identified. CMML can only be diagnosed after ruling out other myeloid neoplasms (such as myelogenous [CML]), and secondary causes of monocytosis. PDGFRA, PDGFRB, and FGFR rearrangements should be ruled out, particularly in cases with concomitant eosinophilia. Cytogenetic abnormalities are found in ~30% of patients with CMML. In patients without cytogenetic abnormalities and without significant dysplasia on the bone marrow, other causes of monocytosis need to be carefully ruled out before a diagnosis of CMML can be made.

   - CMML can be subdivided into CMML-1 (<5% peripheral blood blasts and <10% bone marrow blasts) and CMML-2 (5%–19% peripheral blood blasts or 10%–19% bone marrow blasts).

2. **How is CMML treated?**

   - Asymptomatic patients with no significant anemia or thrombocytosis could be observed. Hydrea could be utilized in these patients if they have a significantly increased leukocyte count or symptomatic splenomegaly.

   - The only curative option for CMML is ASCT. Patients who require therapy should be directed toward ASCT if clinically appropriate.

(•) Patients who require therapy but are not candidates for ASCT, or in whom ASCT has to be significantly delayed, should be treated with hypomethylating agents, azacitidine or decitabine

QUESTIONS

1. A 65-year-old woman had a complete blood count (CBC) performed for fatigue, which showed: white blood cell (WBC) count 5.0 (absolute neutrophil count [ANC] 2.5), hemoglobin 8.5 g/dL (mean corpuscular volume [MCV] 104), and platelets 505. Iron, vitamin B12, and folic acid levels were normal. The patient had a bone marrow biopsy, which showed a hypercellular marrow, with dysplasia in the erythroid lineage but normal myeloid and megakaryocytic lineages. There were 1.5% blasts seen in the aspirate smear. Cytogenetics showed del(5q) as the sole abnormality. Which of the following is the best treatment option for the patient at this point?
   A. Azacitidine or decitabine
   B. Allogeneic bone marrow transplantation
   C. Lenalidomide single agent
   D. Lenalidomide + a hypomethylating agent
   E. Red blood cell transfusions only

2. A 64-year-old man presents with a transfusion-dependent anemia (two units of red cells every 6 weeks). Otherwise, he has a normal white blood cell (WBC) count (6) and absolute neutrophil count (ANC) (4) as well as a normal platelet count (250). A bone marrow aspirate and biopsy demonstrated myelodysplastic syndrome (MDS) with dysplasia in the erythroid lineage only. There were 1.8% blasts seen in the aspi-rate smear and no increased ringed sideroblasts. Cytogenetics showed del 20q. A serum erythropoietin level is 90. Which of the following is the best treatment option for this patient?
   A. Red blood cell (RBC) transfusions only
   B. Allogeneic stem cell transplantation
   C. Lenalidomide single agent
   D. Erythropoietin-stimulating agent
   E. Hypomethylating agent

3. A 62-year-old man with no other comorbidities and a good perfor-mance status was diagnosed with myelodysplastic syndrome (MDS) 2 years ago. He was on observation because he had mild cytopenias initially and he was asymptomatic. Over the recent few months, his counts started to drop, and his most recent complete blood count (CBC) showed white blood cell (WBC) count 1, absolute neutrophil count (ANC) 0.5, hemoglobin 8.5, and platelets 40. A bone marrow biopsy was repeated and demonstrated a hypercellular marrow with dysplasia in all lineages, 12% blasts on the aspirate smear, and a com-plex karyotype. Which of the following is the best treatment option for this patient?
   A. Red blood cell transfusions only
   B. Allogeneic stem cell transplant (ASCT)

   C. Lenalidomide
   D. Erythropoietin-stimulating agent in combination with thrombopoietin-stimulating agent
   E. Hypomethylating agent

4. A 78-year-old man with a history of coronary artery disease, chronic obstructive pulmonary disease (COPD), and hypertension has high-risk myelodysplastic syndrome (MDS) with pancytopenia (white blood cell [WBC] count 0.8, absolute neutrophil count [ANC] 0.3, hemoglobin 8.5, platelets 35). Bone marrow showed 11% blasts and cytogenetics demonstrated a complex karyotype. Which of the following is the best treatment option for this patient?
   A. Red blood cell transfusions only
   B. Allogeneic stem cell transplant (ASCT)
   C. Lenalidomide
   D. Erythropoietin-stimulating agent in combination with thrombopoietin-stimulating agent
   E. Hypomethylating agent

5. A 59-year-woman has a diagnosis of chronic myelomonocytic leukemia (CMML) with a most recent complete blood count (CBC) showing a white blood cell (WBC) count 40,000 (absolute neutrophil count [ANC] 25, absolute monocyte count [AMC] 10), hemoglobin 7.5, and platelets of 200. Her spleen is palpated 6 cm below the left costal margin. A recent bone marrow aspiration and biopsy showed 5% blasts. She has fatigue and shortness of breath on moderate exertion. The patient has no other comorbidities. Which of the following is the best treatment option for this patient?
   A. Allogeneic stem cell transplant (ASCT)
   B. Lenalidomide
   C. Erythropoietin-stimulating agent in combination with thrombopoietin-stimulating agent
   D. Hypomethylating agent

ANSWERS

1. **C. Lenalidomide single agent.** This patient has low-risk myelodysplastic syndrome (MDS) with symptomatic anemia and del(5q) as the sole cytogenetic abnormality (5q syndrome). Lenalidomide 10 mg a day is the treatment of choice for this patient. Prior studies have shown that 67% of patients with the 5q syndrome treated with lenalidomide no longer needed transfusions and 45% had a complete cytogenetic response.

2. **D. Erythropoietin-stimulating agent.** This patient has low-risk MDS with transfusion-dependent anemia, no del (5q), and no other cytopenias. Because his erythropoietin level is low and he gets less than two units of RBC transfusions a month, his chance of responding to erythropoietin-stimulating agents is ~74%.

3. **B. Allogeneic stem cell transplant (ASCT).** This is a patient with high-risk MDS. ASCT is the only curative modality. A retrospective analysis showed that patients with high-risk MDS have better overall survival if they undergo ASCT. Hypomethylating agents prior to ASCT are not routinely recommended and have not been shown to add value in patients planning to proceed with ASCT; therefore, hypomethylating agents should be considered in patients whose ASCT is expected to be delayed. This patient has a good performance status and does not have other comorbidities and would be a candidate for ASCT.

4. **E. Hypomethylating agent.** This is a patient with high-risk MDS. Though ASCT is the only curative modality, this patient is not a candidate for ASCT. Hypomethylating agents are the agents of choice. Studies have demonstrated that a hypomethylating agent (azacitidine) given to intermediate-2 or high-risk MDS patients delayed progression to acute myeloid leukemia (AML) and improved overall survival compared to supportive care alone.

5. **A. Allogeneic stem cell transplant (ASCT).** The patient has CMML-1 with symptomatic anemia. The only curative option is ASCT. This patient requires therapy for CMML given the symptomatic anemia and should be directed toward ASCT. If ASCT has to be delayed, then a hypomethylating agent should be strongly considered as a bridge to curative intent therapy.

5

Hodgkin Lymphoma

Darren King and Ryan A. Wilcox

EPIDEMIOLOGY

1. **How common is Hodgkin lymphoma?**
   - Hodgkin lymphoma accounts for approximately 12% of all lymphomas in the United States (about 9,060 cases annually).

2. **How is Hodgkin lymphoma classified?**
   - Classical Hodgkin lymphoma (cHL) makes up 95% of cases. Its subtypes are: nodular sclerosis (70%), mixed cellularity (25%), lymphocyte rich (5%), and lymphocyte depleted (<1%).
   - Nodular lymphocyte predominant Hodgkin lymphoma (NLPHL) makes up 5% of "Hodgkin lymphoma" cases. It is characterized by an indolent course, late relapses, and is clinically managed like an indolent non-Hodgkin lymphoma (NHL).

3. **What are the demographics of Hodgkin lymphoma?**
   - Bimodal age distribution with the first peak around age 20 and the second near age 65
   - In cHL there is a slight male predominance, whereas 75% of patients with NLPHL are male

ETIOLOGY AND RISK FACTORS

1. **What are risk factors for Hodgkin lymphoma?**
   - Socioeconomic status is directly associated with the nodular sclerosing subtype and inversely associated with the mixed cellularity variant
   - Immunosuppression (eg, solid organ or hematopoietic transplants)
   - Autoimmune diseases (eg, rheumatoid arthritis)
   - HIV/AIDS is associated with Epstein–Barr virus (EBV) positive, lymphocyte-depleted subtype
   - There is an increased incidence in patients with affected family members, but no known genetic predisposition

STAGING

1. Define the staging for Hodgkin lymphoma.

Ann Arbor Staging

Stage	Description
I	Involvement of single lymph node region or structure (eg, spleen, thymus, Waldeyer's ring) or a single extranodal site
II	Involvement of two or more lymph nodes or lymphoid structures on the same side of the diaphragm
III	Involvement of lymph nodes or lymphoid structures on both sides of the diaphragm
IV	Diffuse or disseminated involvement of one or more extranodal organs beyond I_E* including any liver or bone marrow involvement, with or without associated lymph node involvement

*Contiguous extranodal extension indicated by "E."

Note: B symptoms (significant unexplained fever, night sweats, or unexplained weight loss exceeding 10% of body weight during the 6 months prior to diagnosis) indicated by "A" (absence) or "B" (presence); bulky disease (mediastinal mass >1/3 diameter of thorax or any mass >10 cm) indicated by "X."

SIGNS AND SYMPTOMS

1. What are the common signs and symptoms of Hodgkin lymphoma?
   - Most patients present with asymptomatic lymphadenopathy or an incidentally discovered mediastinal mass.
   - B symptoms include fevers (unexplained, persistent/recurring temperature >38°C), drenching night sweats, and weight loss (>10% over preceding 6 months), seen in 20% of early- and 50% of advanced-stage disease.

2. What is the pattern of disease involvement in Hodgkin lymphoma?
   - Cervical nodes are most commonly affected followed by mediastinal nodes
   - Spread is generally to adjacent lymph nodes.
   - Bone marrow involvement is observed in fewer than 5% of cases.

DIAGNOSTIC CRITERIA

1. What is the optimal approach to the diagnosis of Hodgkin lymphoma?
   - Excisional lymph node biopsy. Tumor in Hodgkin lymphoma has a very small component of malignant cells, with a surrounding reactive milieu of lymphocytes, eosinophils, and fibrosis (sclerosis). Excisional lymph node biopsy is far better at documenting this architecture than core biopsy.
   - Clinical staging done using CT and PET/CT scans.
   - Bone marrow biopsy is no longer required for staging if PET/CT is consistent with marrow involvement. Bone marrow biopsy should be performed in the presence of cytopenias and a negative PET/CT.

FIGURE 5.1 ■ Reed–Sternberg cell surrounded by inflammatory infiltrate.

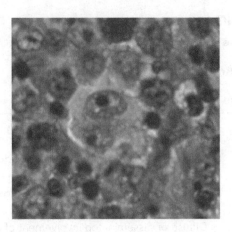

2. **How is the diagnosis of cHL made?**

   ● Presence of multinucleate Reed–Sternberg (RS) cells in an inflammatory background (see Figure 5.1).

   ● Typical immunophenotype of cHL is CD15 and CD30 positive with absence of the usual B-cell markers CD20, CD79a, and the common leukocyte antigen CD45. PD-L1 is often expressed.

3. **How is NLPHL diagnosed?**

   ● Presence of lymphocytic and histiocytic cells with "popcorn" appearance

   ● Typical immunophenotype CD15 and CD30 negative with positivity for the B-cell markers CD20, CD79a, and the common leukocyte antigen CD45

4. **What is the cell of origin of Hodgkin lymphoma?**

   ● Despite their unique immunophenotype, cHL cells have been shown to derive from germinal center B-cells.

INDICATIONS FOR TREATMENT

1. **Who requires treatment for Hodgkin lymphoma?**

   ● All patients with cHL should be considered for initial treatment with curative intent.

   ● Likewise, all patients with NLPHL should be considered for therapy at the time of diagnosis (eg, radiation with nonbulky stage IA/IIA disease, immunochemotherapy—eg, rituximab, cyclophosphamide, doxorubicin, vincristine, and prednisone [R-CHOP]—in bulky limited-stage or advanced-stage disease; however, observation alone may be considered for some patients—eg, excised stage I disease).

PROGNOSTIC FACTORS

1. **What are unfavorable factors in early-stage (I–IIA) cHL?**

   ● Large mediastinal mass (greater than 1/3 of mediastinal diameter), extranodal disease, erythrocyte sedimentation rate (ESR) ≥50 mm/hour without or ≥30 mm/hour with B symptoms, greater than or equal to three nodal sites, and/or bulky disease

2. **What are unfavorable prognostic factors in advanced-stage (IIB–IV) cHL? How does this International Prognostic Factor score impact outcome?**
   - Factors include: age >45, male sex, stage IV, albumin <4 g/dL, hemoglobin <10.5 g/dL, white blood cell count >15,000/mm^3, lymphopenia (one point for each).

Score	5-Year FFP (%)	5-Year OS (%)
0	84	89
1	77	90
2	67	81
3	60	78
4	51	61
5–7	42	56

FFP, freedom from progression; OS, overall survival.

3. **What are other poor prognostic factors on Hodgkin lymphoma?**
   - Positive PET scan after two cycles of Adriamycin, bleomycin, vinblastine, dacarbazine (ABVD) strongly associated with inferior 2-year progression-free survival (PFS)
   - Increased density of lymphoma-associated macrophages (CD68 positive cells)

4. **What is the prognosis for Hodgkin lymphoma?**
   - Cure is obtained in over 80% of all patients.
   - Five-year survival is >90% in early and >75% in advanced-stage disease.

TREATMENT

1. **What is the initial treatment for early-stage (I–IIA) cHL?**
   - In limited-stage favorable-risk disease, a standard approach is combined modality therapy with two cycles of ABVD (doxorubicin/bleomycin/vinblastine/dacarbazine) with restaging PET/CT followed by 20 Gy of involved site radiation therapy (ISRT). Limited-stage, unfavorable-risk disease may be treated with four cycles of ABVD followed by 30 Gy of ISRT. An alternative approach, sparing radiation therapy and its potential risks, is 3 to 6 cycles of ABVD alone, in a risk-adapted fashion (ie, depending upon the quality of response observed on interim PET/CT).
   - The Stanford V regimen (doxorubicin, vinblastine, mechlorethamine, etoposide, vincristine, bleomycin, prednisone) is an alternative to ABVD.

2. **How is advanced-stage (IIB–IV) cHL managed?**
   - Chemotherapy alone with ABVD for six cycles. Outcome appears to be optimized if treatment delays and dose reductions are avoided.
   - Bleomycin, etoposide, Adriamycin, cyclophosphamide, vincristine (Oncovin), procarbazine, prednisone (BEACOPP) and Stanford V are alternative regimens.
   - Consolidative radiation therapy is an option for patients with bulky disease.

3. **What are treatment options for relapsed/refractory Hodgkin lymphoma?**
   - First relapse or progression following initial standard treatment (eg, ABVD +/− radiation) can be treated with brentuximab vedotin or salvage chemotherapy, such as ifosfamide/carboplatin/etoposide (ICE) or a gemcitabine-containing regimen. Those patients who achieve a remission are candidates for high-dose chemotherapy followed by autologous stem cell transplant (auto-SCT), with consideration of posttransplant brentuximab.
   - Patients who relapse or progress following these salvage regimens can be considered for therapy with brentuximab, a checkpoint inhibitor, or further chemotherapy (eg, bendamustine). Those achieving a response are candidates for allogeneic stem cell transplant.
   - Relapse or progression following allogeneic stem cell transplant may be treated with observation alone, a clinical trial, single-agent therapy (eg, mTOR inhibitor, HDAC inhibitor), or radiation therapy, depending on the patient's disease and performance status.

4. **What is brentuximab vedotin? What are its usual toxicities?**
   - Brentuximab vedotin is an anti-CD30 monoclonal antibody conjugated to a mitotic spindle inhibitor. Its use has been approved in patients who relapse following auto-SCT or who are not deemed candidates for transplant. Its main toxicity as a single agent is peripheral neuropathy. Its use in combination with bleomycin is contraindicated, given the risk for potentiating pulmonary toxicity.

5. **How is nodular lymphocyte predominant disease managed?**
   - Radiation therapy alone for stages IA and IIA
   - Chemotherapy ± radiation for stages IB and IIB
   - Observation may be appropriate for asymptomatic patients with advanced-stage disease that is nonbulky and slowly progressive
   - Immunochemotherapy (eg, R-CHOP) for symptomatic advanced disease

SPECIAL CONSIDERATIONS

1. **What are the significant toxicities from treatment?**
   - Pulmonary toxicity from bleomycin. Bleomycin can be safely omitted from cycles #3 to 6 of ABVD in patients with advanced-stage disease.
   - Myelosuppression with ABVD. Less than 10% of patients develop febrile neutropenia. It is important (and safe) to maintain dose intensity through cytopenias.
   - Infertility (much more common with BEACOPP regimen than ABVD).
   - Cardiac dysfunction from radiation (eg, pericarditis, coronary artery disease, and valvular disease) or chemotherapy (eg, heart failure due to anthracyclines).
   - Secondary malignancies (eg, breast cancer in females who have received thoracic radiation). Therapy-related myelodysplastic syndrome (MDS) and acute myeloid leukemia (AML) are less common in patients receiving ABVD than in patients who received mechlorethamine/vincristine/procarbazine/prednisone (MOPP) or BEACOPP regimens.

QUESTIONS

1. A 30-year-old female smoker has begun treatment for stage IIIA Hodgkin lymphoma. She is receiving Adriamycin, bleomycin, vinblastine, dacarbazine (ABVD). She has read about bleomycin-induced pulmonary toxicity, and is very anxious about this potential side effect. Which of the following does *not* increase the risk of bleomycin-induced pulmonary toxicity?
   A. Renal insufficiency
   B. Concomitant use of brentuximab
   C. Smoking
   D. Younger age

2. An otherwise healthy 45-year-old male completed six cycles of Adriamycin, bleomycin, vinblastine, dacarbazine (ABVD) for stage IV classical Hodgkin lymphoma (cHL). Six months following completion of treatment, he noticed an enlarging cervical lymph node. Biopsy was performed, which confirmed relapse. PET/CT shows diffuse disease. Which of the following is the most appropriate next step in management?
   A. Initiate bleomycin, etoposide, Adriamycin, cyclophosphamide, vincristine (Oncovin), procarbazine, prednisone (BEACOPP)
   B. Initiate brentuximab
   C. Initiate salvage chemotherapy with ifosfamide/carboplatin/etoposide (ICE) and plan for autologous stem cell transplant (auto-SCT)
   D. Proceed to nonmyeloablative allogeneic stem cell transplant

3. A 35-year-old female is receiving treatment for stage IIA classical Hodgkin lymphoma (cHL) with Adriamycin, bleomycin, vinblastine, dacarbazine (ABVD). Following her first two cycles of ABVD, which of the following is most predictive of a worse progression-free survival (PFS)?
   A. Unchanged size of mediastinal mass per interim CT
   B. No change in fluorodeoxyglucose (FDG) avidity of mediastinal mass per interim PET
   C. Elevation of lactate dehydrogenase (LDH)
   D. Persistence of B symptoms

4. A 24-year-old female was diagnosed with stage IIIB classical Hodgkin lymphoma (cHL) with a bulky mediastinal mass. Her treatment comprised six cycles of Adriamycin, bleomycin, vinblastine, dacarbazine (ABVD) and radiation to the mediastinum. She completed treatment 4 years ago. Long-term surveillance does *not* include which of the following:
   A. Breast MRI or early mammogram
   B. Thyroid function testing
   C. Yearly history and physical exam
   D. Annual PET scan

5. A 20-year-old male undergoes biopsy of an enlarged left cervical lymph node, and is diagnosed with classical Hodgkin lymphoma (cHL), nodular sclerosing subtype. PET/CT is performed, which shows fluoro-deoxyglucose (FDG) uptake in the left cervical lymph node region, but no other areas of pathologic uptake. Complete blood count (CBC) and lactate dehydrogenase (LDH) are normal. The patient has no B symptoms. The patient is very hesitant about undergoing bone marrow biopsy as part of his staging workup. Which of these staging steps/results can best reassure his hematologist that a bone marrow biopsy is not essential?
   A. Normal CBC
   B. Normal lactate dehydrogenase (LDH)
   C. Lack of B symptoms
   D. PET/CT

6. A 75-year-old male was diagnosed with stage IA nodular lympho-cyte predominant Hodgkin lymphoma (NLPHL) of the mediastinum. He underwent radiation therapy to the mediastinum and did well for 5 years. Now, at age 80, he has a biopsy-proven recurrence in the right cervical lymph node chain, outside his prior radiation field. He is asymptomatic. PET/CT staging is consistent with stage III disease. The patient has an Eastern Cooperative Oncology Group (ECOG) performance status of 1–2, but desires further treatment. Which of the following would *not* be a reasonable treatment strategy?
   A. Observation
   B. Single agent rituximab
   C. Rituximab, cyclophosphamide, doxorubicin, vincristine, and prednisone (R-CHOP)
   D. Bleomycin, etoposide, Adriamycin, cyclophosphamide, vincristine (Oncovin), procarbazine, prednisone (BEACOPP)

ANSWERS

1. **D. Younger age.** Older age is associated with increased risk of bleomycin-induced pulmonary toxicity, and as a result this drug is usually removed from treatment in elderly patients. Renal insufficiency, concomitant use of brentuximab, and smoking have all been associated with increased risk of bleomycin-induced pulmonary toxicity. It remains unclear whether granulocyte colony-stimulating factor (G-CSF) may potentiate bleomycin-induced pulmonary toxicity; however, many clinicians avoid its use.

2. **C. Initiate salvage chemotherapy with ifosfamide/carboplatin/ etoposide (ICE) and plan for autologous stem cell transplant (auto-SCT).** Standard initial treatment for relapsed cHL is salvage chemo-therapy (such as ICE) followed by auto-SCT. Re-treating with a combina-tion chemotherapy regimen without auto-SCT would not be indicated with a relapse this early. Brentuximab and allogeneic stem cell transplant are indicated in patients relapsing following auto-SCT.

3. **B. No change in fluorodeoxyglucose (FDG) avidity of mediastinal mass per interim PET.** Interim PET scan following two cycles of ABVD has been shown to be the most powerful predictor of PFS. Its prognostic signifi-cance is superior to the International Prognostic Score (IPS).

4. **D. Annual PET scan.** Because of its high cure rates, long-term follow-up for cHL requires monitoring of a number of possible late complications. Women who received radiation therapy to the chest are at higher risk of developing (often bilateral) breast cancer, and require close monitoring with breast MRI or early mammogram. Thyroid function should be moni-tored, as the gland may be affected by mediastinal radiation. After com-pletion of treatment, National Comprehensive Cancer Network (NCCN) guidelines recommend that a history and physical should be performed every 3 to 6 months for the first 1 to 2 years, then every 6 to 12 months until year 3, and then yearly. Surveillance with PET scan is **not** indicated in the absence of clinical concern for relapse.

5. **D. PET/CT.** Bone marrow biopsy is no longer always considered an essen-tial part of the staging workup for Hodgkin lymphoma, given the sensitiv-ity/specificity of PET scan for marrow involvement.

6. **D. Bleomycin, etoposide, Adriamycin, cyclophosphamide, vincristine (Oncovin), procarbazine, prednisone (BEACOPP).** NLPHL typically fol-lows an indolent course, but often with late relapses. Given its distinct clinical course and immunophenotype, the decision to treat should be approached in a way similar to the indolent non-Hodgkin lymphomas. Observation in an asymptomatic patient, single agent rituximab, and combination therapy with R-CHOP are reasonable options in a patient with advanced age and borderline performance status. BEACOPP would not be appropriate.

Non-Hodgkin Lymphoma— Low Grade

Erlene K. Seymour and Tycel J. Phillips

EPIDEMIOLOGY

1. **Classify lymphomas into indolent or aggressive categories.**

Indolent	Aggressive
Follicular lymphoma	Diffuse large B-cell lymphoma
Marginal zone lymphoma	Burkitt lymphoma
Small lymphocytic lymphoma/ Chronic lymphocytic leukemia	Lymphoblastic lymphoma
	Mantle cell lymphoma*
Lymphoplasmacytic lymphoma/ Waldenström macroglobulinemia	Primary mediastinal large B-cell lymphoma
Cutaneous T-cell lymphoma (mycosis fungoides and Sézary syndrome)	Anaplastic large cell lymphoma
	Angioimmunoblastic T-cell lymphoma
Mantle cell lymphoma*	Extranodal NK/T-cell lymphoma
	Peripheral T-cell lymphoma not otherwise specified

*Can have indolent and aggressive presentations and is discussed in Chapter 7.

ETIOLOGY AND RISK FACTORS

1. **What risk factors are associated with the development of non-Hodgkin lymphoma (NHL)?**
   - Farming (exposure to herbicides and pesticides, such as organochlorine, organophosphate, and phenoxyacid compounds)
   - Infections (see the next question)
   - Immunosuppressive drug use
   - Autoimmune diseases
   - Post solid organ transplantation

2. **What infections are associated with lymphoma, and what is the associated subtype of lymphoma?**
   - HIV: AIDS-associated lymphoma
   - *Epstein–Barr virus* (EBV): Burkitt lymphoma in Africa, posttransplant lymphoproliferative disorders, NK/T-cell lymphoma, diffuse large B-cell lymphoma (DLBCL) of the elderly

- HTLV-I: adult T-cell leukemia/lymphoma
- *Helicobacter pylori:* mucosa-associated lymphoid tissue (MALT) lymphoma
- Human herpesvirus-8: body cavity lymphoma
- Hepatitis C: splenic marginal zone lymphoma
- *Chlamydia psittaci:* orbital adnexal lymphoma
- *Campylobacter jejuni:* intestinal lymphoma
- *Borrelia burgdorferi:* cutaneous MALT lymphoma

STAGING

1. How is NHL staged?

- Ann Arbor Staging System: refer to Chapter 5

SIGNS AND SYMPTOMS

1. What are the common presenting signs and symptoms of NHLs?

- Lymphadenopathy
- B symptoms
  - Fever (T $>100.5°F$)
  - Drenching night sweats
  - Unintentional weight loss ($>10\%$ loss within a 6-month period of time)
  - Anorexia
  - Fatigue
- Splenomegaly

DIAGNOSTIC FEATURES

1. What are the immumophenotypic markers of the indolent NHLs?

Non-Hodgkin Lymphoma Subtype	sIg	CD5	CD10	CD20	Other	Cyclin D1
CLL/SLL	Weak	+	−	Dim	CD23 + FMC−	−
Follicular lymphoma	++	−	+	+	BCL−2+	−
Mantle cell lymphoma	++	+	−	+	CD23− FMC+	+
Marginal zone lymphoma/extranodal marginal zone lymphoma	+	−/+	−	+	MUM−1+ IRTA1+	−
Lymphoplasmacytic lymphoma	++	−	−	+	CD25+/− CD38+/−	−

CLL, chronic lymphocytic leukemia; SLL, small lymphocytic lymphoma.

2. What are the chromosomal translocations and their oncogene (and function) associated with indolent NHLs?

Non-Hodgkin Lymphoma Subtype	Cytogenetics	Oncogene	Function
Follicular lymphoma	t(14;18)	BCL2	Antiapoptosis
Mantle cell lymphoma	t(11:14)	Cyclin D1	Cell cycle regulator
Marginal zone lymphoma/extranodal marginal zone lymphoma	t(11;18)	API2-MALT	Resistance to H. pylori treatment
Lymphoplasmacytic lymphoma	t(9;14)	PAX-5	Deregulation of PAX-5 gene

Follicular Lymphoma

GRADE AND PROGNOSTIC FACTORS

1. How do we determine the grade of follicular lymphoma (FL)?
   - Grade 1 to grade 2: less than 15 centroblasts per high-power field
   - Grade 3: more than 15 centroblasts per high-power field

2. What are the components of the Follicular Lymphoma International Prognostic Index (FLIPI)?

Criteria (one point for each)	Risk Group
Age >60	Low (0–1 points)
Number of nodal sites >4	Intermediate (2 points)
Elevated lactate dehydrogenase (LDH)	High (3–5 points)
Hemoglobin level <12 g/dL	
Ann Arbor Stage III or IV	

3. What is the 5-year and 10-year overall survival (OS) rate of low-, intermediate-, and high-risk FL by FLIPI?

Risk	5-Year OS (%)	10-Year OS (%)
Low	86	71
Intermediate	71	40
High	51	37

4. **What are the poor prognostic factors associated with FL?**
   - According to the Groupe d'Etude des Lymphomes Folliculaires (GELF) criteria, the poor prognostic factors are:
     - Involvement of three or more nodal sites, each with a diameter of at least 3 cm
     - Any nodal/extranodal mass with a diameter of at least 7 cm
     - Presence of B symptoms
     - Splenomegaly
     - Pleural effusion or ascites
     - Cytopenia(s)
     - Circulating tumor cells ($>$5,000 malignant cells/mm^3)

TREATMENT

1. **What are the indications for treatment of FL?**
   - Symptomatic (B symptoms present)
   - Threatened end-organ function
   - Cytopenia secondary to lymphoma marrow involvement
   - Bulky disease
   - Steady progression

2. **How do you treat asymptomatic advanced-stage FL?**
   - Observation

3. **How do you treat grade 3 FL or an aggressive presentation of FL?**
   - Same management as DLBCL; treat with rituximab, cyclophosphamide, doxorubicin, vincristine, and prednisone (R-CHOP)

4. **What are the treatment options for limited-stage (I–II) grade 1/2 FL?**
   - Potentially curative local radiotherapy for stage I or contiguous stage II
   - Rituxan monotherapy
   - Observation

5. **What are some first-line treatment regimens for stage III/IV grade 1/2 FL?**
   - Bendamustine and rituximab (BR)
   - Rituximab, cyclophosphamide, vincristine, prednisone (R-CVP)
   - R-CHOP
   - Rituximab monotherapy

6. **What is the role of maintenance rituximab?**
   - The role for maintenance is controversial. It has been demonstrated to improve progression-free survival but has not demonstrated any survival benefit in any of the studies conducted to date. As currently indicated, this can be considered in all patients with FL after initial therapy.

7. **What are some second-line treatment regimens for relapsed/refractory low-grade FL?**
   - First-line chemoimmunotherapy regimen that has not been used can be utilized for second-line therapy
   - Radioactive monoclonal antibody (radioimmunotherapy)
   - Idelalisib
   - Lenalidomide and rituximab

8. **How should we treat histological transformation of FL to aggressive lymphoma (such as DLBCL)?**
   - Transformed FL should be treated the same way as a DLBCL (see details in Chapter 7)

Marginal Zone Lymphoma

SIGNS AND SYMPTOMS

1. **What is the clinical presentation of extranodal marginal zone (MALT) lymphoma?**
   - Signs and symptoms from involvement of the gastrointestinal (GI) tract, respiratory tract, salivary gland, kidney, prostate, lung, eye (conjunctiva), and other organs
   - Associated with autoimmune disease, such as Sjögren syndrome or Hashimoto thyroiditis

2. **What is the clinical presentation of splenic marginal zone lymphoma?**
   - Splenomegaly, circulating lymphocytosis, cytopenias
   - Peripheral circulating malignant lymphocytes may display villous cytoplasmic projections

TREATMENT

1. **What is the initial treatment for stage I or II, gastric MALT lymphoma with positive *H. pylori*?**
   - Treatment of *H. pylori* with antibiotics

2. **What are the initial treatment options for stage I or II, gastric MALT lymphoma without *H. pylori* infection?**
   - Local radiation
   - Single agent rituximab (if radiation is contraindicated)

3. **What is the treatment of stage III/IV MALT lymphoma that involves the stomach?**
   - Rare. Should confirm diagnosis. If confirmed, can consider rituximab + focal radiation to stomach or systemic chemoimmunotherapy.

4. **What is the treatment for nodal marginal zone lymphoma?**
   - Same as that for FL

5. **What is the initial treatment for symptomatic, splenic marginal zone lymphoma without hepatitis C infection?**
   - Splenectomy or single agent rituximab

6. **What is the treatment for symptomatic, splenic marginal zone lymphoma with hepatitis C infection?**
   - Treat hepatitis C infection first. If resolution of the lymphoma does not occur, then treat similar to splenic marginal zone without hepatitis C.

7. **What is the treatment for asymptomatic, splenic marginal zone lymphoma?**
   - Observation
   - Treat hepatitis C

Lymphoplasmacytic Lymphoma/Waldenström Macroglobulinemia

SIGNS AND SYMPTOMS

1. **What is the clinical presentation of lymphoplasmacytic lymphomas?**
   - Monoclonal gammopathy, hyperviscosity syndrome (30%), neuropathy, amyloidosis, cryoglobulinemia, cold agglutinin disease
   - Associated with hepatitis C infection

TREATMENT

1. **What are the indications for treatment of lymphoplasmacytic lymphoma?**
   - Hyperviscosity syndrome
   - Organomegaly
   - Cryoglobulinemia
   - Cold agglutinin disease
   - Cytopenia
   - Other disease-related symptoms

2. **What are some treatment regimens for lymphoplasmacytic lymphoma?**
   - Proteasome inhibitor based regimens (bortezomib/rituximab, bortezomib/dexamethasone [VD], bortezomib/dexamethasone/rituximab [RVD], carfilzomib/rituximab/dexamethasone [CRD])
   - Chemoimmunotherapy (rituximab monotherapy, rituximab/cyclophosphamide/prednisone, rituximab/cyclophosphamide/dexamethasone, R-CHOP), BR
   - Ibrutinib
   - Avoid single agent rituximab in patients with a markedly elevated serum IgM/serum viscosity without prior plasmapheresis due to concern for IgM flare, which can temporarily cause marked elevation in IgM and subsequent hyperviscosity.

3. **What is the treatment for hyperviscosity syndrome as related to Waldenström macroglobulinemia?**
   - Plasmapheresis in emergent situations, then proceed with definitive therapy

Small Lymphocytic Lymphoma

For details about small lymphocytic lymphoma, see Chapter 2.

QUESTIONS

1. A 47-year-old male presents with raised, erythematous nodular rash on his arm. He just came back from a hiking trip in the Rocky Mountains a few weeks ago. He unfortunately got sick with fevers and joint pain during his trip, but was treated with antibiotics, although he does not remember the name of the antibiotic. He notices that this rash has not resolved and underwent a biopsy, which revealed a cutaneous mucosa-associated lymphoid tissue (MALT) lymphoma.
   What infection is associated with his cutaneous MALT lymphoma?
   A. *Rickettsia rickettsii*
   B. *Bartonella henselae*
   C. *Trypanosoma brucei*
   D. *Borrelia burgdorferi*
   E. *Neisseria gonorrhoeae*

2. The following clinical vignette is a two-part question:
   A 65-year-old female presents with enlarged lymph nodes in her axillary and inguinal regions. She undergoes an excisional lymph node biopsy, which is consistent with follicular lymphoma, grade 2. She denies any fevers, night sweats, or weight loss. She has no other symptoms associated with her enlarged lymph nodes. She otherwise continues to work full time, with an Eastern Cooperative Oncology Group (ECOG) performance score of 0. A PET scan reveals uptake in her cervical, axillary, and inguinal lymph nodes, and all nodes are less than 3 cm. She does not demonstrate any splenomegaly. Her lactate dehydrogenase (LDH) is 180 U/L. Her complete blood counts reveal a white blood cell (WBC) of 7.7/mcL, hemoglobin of 13.5 g/dL, and platelet count of 165/mcL. Her bone marrow biopsy is negative for involvement of her follicular lymphoma.

   I. What is her Follicular Lymphoma International Prognostic Index (FLIPI) risk?
      A. Low risk
      B. Intermediate risk
      C. High risk
      D. Very high risk

II. What is the appropriate initial step in management?
   A. Treatment with rituximab and bendamustine
   B. Treatment with rituximab, cyclophosphamide, doxorubicin, vincristine, and prednisone (R-CHOP)
   C. Watch and wait
   D. Treatment with rituximab monotherapy × four doses

3. A 60-year-old female was treated with six cycles of rituximab, cyclophosphamide, doxorubicin, vincristine, and prednisone (R-CHOP) for symptomatic follicular lymphoma. Her follow-up PET scan reveals a complete remission. She has come to your clinic today and asks about the role of maintenance rituximab after chemotherapy.
   What is the benefit of maintenance rituximab in follicular lymphoma patients treated with chemotherapy?
   A. Decreased risk of infection
   B. Increased overall survival
   C. Increased progression-free survival
   D. Increased quality of life
   E. Decreased risk of transformation

4. A 66-year-old female is evaluated for palpable lymph nodes, which she noted in her axillary regions. She undergoes a CT scan of her chest, abdomen, and pelvis, which demonstrates axillary, retroperitoneal, and mesenteric lymphadenopathy. An excisional lymph node biopsy is performed of an axillary node. The flow cytometry is positive for CD20, CD5, surface immunoglobulin, and cyclin D1; and negative for CD10 and CD23.
   What is the associated chromosomal translocation with her lymphoma?
   A. (14;18)
   B. t(11;18)
   C. t(11;14)
   D. t(9;14)
   E. t(9;22)

5. A 56-year-old female presents with worsening abdominal discomfort and weight loss. She was evaluated by her gastroenterologist and underwent an upper endoscopy, which revealed a gastric ulcer and mild mucosal erythema of her gastric wall. Her ulcer is biopsied and is remarkable for gastric mucosa-associated lymphoid tissue (MALT) lymphoma. Her *Helicobacter pylori* testing is positive. Her complete blood counts and comprehensive metabolic panel are all within normal range. She does not exhibit any lymphadenopathy on physical exam or on her recent CT scan of the abdomen and pelvis.
   What is the next appropriate step in treatment?
   A. Referral for radiation therapy
   B. Start proton pump inhibitor therapy and repeat an endoscopy in 3 months
   C. Treat her *H. pylori* with antibiotics and a proton pump inhibitor
   D. Treat with rituximab monotherapy
   E. Treat her *H. pylori* with antibiotics and a proton pump inhibitor with concurrent radiation therapy

ANSWERS

1. **D. *Borrelia burgdorferi*.** This is associated with Lyme disease and also with cutaneous B-cell lymphomas. A, B, C, and E are not associated with cutaneous B-cell lymphoma.

2. **I. B. Intermediate risk.** Her FLIPI score is 2 because she has one point for age >60, and one point for stage III disease.

   II. C. Watch and wait. She has asymptomatic grade 2 follicular lymphoma; observation is appropriate at this time.

3. **C. Increased progression-free survival.** The PRIMA trial demonstrated increased progression-free survival after using maintenance rituximab for 2 years after the completion of chemotherapy for follicular lymphoma. It did not demonstrate increased overall survival, decreased risk of transformation, or improved quality of life. It demonstrated an increased risk of infection in the maintenance rituximab arm.

4. **C. t(11;14).** This is associated with cyclin D1, which is associated with mantle cell lymphoma. t(14;18) is associated with BCL2 and follicular lymphoma. t(11;18) is associated with marginal zone lymphoma. t(9;14) is associated with lymphoplasmacytic lymphoma. t(9;22) is associated with the BCR/ABL and chronic myeloid leukemia.

5. **C. Treat her *H. pylori* with antibiotics and a proton pump inhibitor.** After therapy is complete, a repeat endoscopy should confirm eradication of her gastric MALT lymphoma and *H. pylori*. If eradicated, she can be observed. If her disease is still persistent, other treatment modalities could be considered.

Non-Hodgkin Lymphoma— High Grade

7

Erlene K. Seymour and Tycel J. Phillips

EPIDEMIOLOGY

1. **What is the most common subtype of non-Hodgkin lymphoma (NHL)?**
   - Diffuse large B-cell lymphoma (DLBCL) comprises approximately one third of all NHLs and is the most common aggressive NHL.

STAGING

1. **How are aggressive NHLs staged?**
   - Same as Hodgkin lymphoma using the Ann Arbor staging system (see Chapter 5)

DIAGNOSTIC CRITERIA

1. **How is the diagnosis of high-grade NHL made?**
   - Excisional biopsy preferred, except for nodes that are inaccessible, in which case a core needle biopsy is acceptable. Fine needle aspiration should be avoided since nodal architecture is difficult to fully assess.

2. **What are the immumophenotypic markers of the aggressive NHLs?**

NHL Subtype	sIg	CD5	CD10	CD20	Other	Cyclin D1
DLBCL	+	Rare	+/−	+	MUM-1 +/−	−
					Bcl-6 +/−	
					C-Myc +/−	
					BCL-2 +/−	
Mantle cell lymphoma	++	+	−	+	CD23−FMC+	+
PMBCL*	+	−	+/−	+	CD30 +/−	−
Burkitt lymphoma	+	−	+	+	TdT-	−

*PMBCL, primary mediastinal B-cell lymphoma.

3. **What are the chromosomal translocations and their associated oncogene (and function) associated with aggressive non-Hodgkin lymphomas?**

Non-Hodgkin Lymphoma Subtype	Cytogenetics	Oncogene	Function
DLBCL	t(14;18), t(3;14)	*BCL2*	Antiapoptosis
	t(3;v)	*BCL6*	Transcription factor
	t(2;8), t(8;14), t(8;22)	*c-Myc*	
Mantle cell lymphoma	t(11;14)	Cyclin D1	Cell cycle regulator
PMBCL	t(16;X)	*CIITA*	MHC class II transactivator
Burkitt lymphoma	t(8;14) most common t(2;8), t(8;22)	*cMYC*	Transcription factor

Diffuse Large B-Cell Lymphoma

EPIDEMIOLOGY

1. **What is the median age of DLBCL patients?**
   - Median age is 65 years

ETIOLOGY

1. **What is the cell of origin of DLBCL?**
   - Mature B-lymphocyte
     - GCB: germinal center B-cell, better survival
     - ABC: activated B-cell, inferior survival
   - DLBCL may arise de novo or as a result of Richter's, only called Richter's when CLL transforms from a more indolent lymphoproliferative condition.

PATHOLOGY AND STAGING

1. **What are the pathological characteristics of DLBCL?**
   - Hematoxylin and eosin (H&E) appearance
     - There is effacement of the normal, follicular architecture of the lymph node.
     - Tumor cells are large with abundant cytoplasm and often multiple nucleoli.
     - The tumor cells are surrounded by nonmalignant cells.

2. **What studies are important in staging and workup of DLBCL?**
   - PET/CT
   - Complete blood count (CBC)
   - Liver function test (LFT), serum creatinine
   - Lactate dehydrogenase (LDH), uric acid, potassium, phosphorus, calcium (to evaluate for tumor lysis syndrome [TLS])

- Bilateral bone marrow biopsy and aspirate if PET/CT scan was not performed or if there is concern for bone marrow involvement or other underlying bone marrow disorder based on presenting labs.
- HIV testing
- Multigated acquisition scan (MUGA) scan or two-dimensional transthoracic echocardiography (TTE) prior to anthracycline-containing regimen (ie, R-CHOP)
- Hepatitis B surface antigen (Hep B S Ag) and core antibody (Hep B C Ab) testing
- Fertility counseling

PROGNOSTIC FACTORS

1. How is DLBCL risk-stratified?

- There are two currently utilized prognostic scores, which stratify patients based on several presenting factors, the IPI score and the age-adjusted IPI score.

Risk Factors (1 Point Each)	IPI Score	IPI Risk Category	5-Year Overall Survival (%)
Age >60 years	0–1	Low	73
Serum LDH >upper limit of normal	2	Low intermediate	51
ECOG performance status 2–4	3	High intermediate	43
Stages III–IV	4–5	High	26
>2 Extranodal sites			

Risk Factors (1 point each)	Age-Adjusted IPI Score (Age ≤60)	IPI Risk Category	5-Year Overall Survival (%)
Serum LDH >upper limit of normal	0	Low	83
	1	Low intermediate	69
ECOG performance status 2–4	2	High intermediate	46
Stages III–IV	3	High	32

2. What are the risk factors for central nervous system (CNS) recurrence?

- Clinical risk factors: elevated LDH, multiple extranodal sites, and particular extranodal sites (eg, paranasal sinuses, orbit, bone marrow, breast, testes, kidney, adrenal gland)
- Molecular/cytogenetic risk factors: c-Myc+ and double-hit lymphomas
- Presence of multiple risk factors confers increased risk compared with a single risk factor alone
- Check cell counts, protein, glucose, cytology, and flow cytometry on cerebrospinal fluid (CSF) examination

- CNS prophylaxis in these patients includes intrathecal treatments with methotrexate or ara-C. If very high risk (such as testicular or double-hit), consider high-dose systemic methotrexate

TREATMENT

1. **What is the most commonly used chemotherapy regimen in DLBCL?**
   - R-CHOP (rituximab, cyclophosphamide, doxorubicin, vincristine, and prednisone) is the most commonly used regimen. R-CHOP should be given in 21-day cycles (R-CHOP-21). Monitor for signs of congestive heart failure (CHF), neuropathy, myelosuppression, and liver or renal dysfunction.
   - Frontline treatment currently is not dependent on the DLBCL subtype (GC versus ABC), although clinical trials currently are being designed to determine if improvements to R-CHOP can be obtained.
     - ○ Response rate to R-CHOP is inferior in the ABC subtype compared to GC based on historical data.

     In the relapse/refractory setting, knowledge of subtype is important as several treatments have demonstrated differing response rates based on the subtype.
   - If an anthracycline is contraindicated, regimens without doxorubicin such as R-CEOP (etoposide substituted for doxorubicin) can be used.

2. **What is the first-line treatment for different stages of DLBCL?**
   - Stages I–II, nonbulky: R-CHOP × three cycles, followed by involved field radiation therapy (IFRT), or R-CHOP × six cycles with or without IFRT
   - Stages I–II, bulky: R-CHOP × six cycles followed by radiation to the "bulky" area
   - Stages III–IV: R-CHOP × six cycles, consider IFRT to the "bulky" areas
   - If presentation includes systemic and parenchymal CNS disease, incorporate high-dose systemic methotrexate
   - If presentation includes concurrent leptomeningeal disease, then use R-CHOP plus high-dose systemic methotrexate or intrathecal methotrexate
   - There is no definitive role for high-dose chemotherapy/autologous stem cell rescue (HDT/ASCR) in the first-line setting
   - There is no role for maintenance rituximab

3. **What is the treatment of relapsed or refractory DLBCL?**
   - High-dose chemotherapy followed by HDT/autologous stem cell transplant after achieving CR or PR. The high-dose chemotherapy could be: R-ICE (rituximab, ifosfamide, carboplatin, etoposide), gemcitabine-based regimen (GDP [gemcitabine, dexamethasone, cisplatin], or GemOx [Rituxan, gemcitabine, oxaliplatin]), or R-DHAP (rituximab, dexamethasone, cisplatin, cytarabine).
   - Repeat biopsy if contemplating changing the course of treatment in patients with relapsed disease, or if there is a concern regarding the original subtyping of DLBCL in the biopsy obtained at diagnosis.
   - If the patient is not eligible for transplant, options include: R-ICE, R-GemOx/R-GDP, R-DHAP, or a less intensive regimen such as single-agent Rituxan, lenalidomide with Rituxan, or a clinical trial.

4. **How should TLS be monitored and prevented?**
   - Risk factors include stage III/IV disease, bulky disease, elevated LDH at baseline, evidence of spontaneous TLS, and decreased renal function at baseline.
   - Monitor uric acid, potassium, phosphorus, creatinine, calcium, and LDH.
   - Consider allopurinol in cases with evidence of TLS.

5. **How are response to therapy and ongoing remission monitored (role of PET scan)?**
   - Repeat PET-CT after 3 to 4 cycles to determine interval response to initial therapy, then after completion of chemotherapy but before planned RT.
   - After completion of all treatment, obtain posttreatment PET/CT in 6 to 8 weeks.
   - Frequent false positive PET scans in this setting have been described. Therefore, a change in treatment plan should be backed up by a repeat biopsy of the PET-positive areas.
   - Imaging can be considered for surveillance for up to 2 years from completion of treatment in a patient with a sustained remission, but surveillance imaging has not been shown to have any direct impact on patient outcomes in retrospective studies.

6. **What is the role of hepatitis B prophylaxis in patients infected with hepatitis B during treatment with rituximab?**
   - Treatment with rituximab may cause hepatitis B reactivation.
   - Antiviral prophylaxis should be instituted in hepatitis B infected patients who are planned to receive rituximab to prevent flares and related deaths.
   - Obtain baseline viral load before therapy; monitor viral loads monthly while on treatment and 3 months afterward.

SPECIAL CONSIDERATIONS

1. **What are the clinical features and management of primary mediastinal B-cell lymphoma (PMBCL)?**
   - Arises from thymic B-cells
   - Young (30s–40s) females with mediastinal (stage I/II) disease
   - Often presents with superior vena cava (SVC) syndrome, pleural or pericardial effusion
   - Widespread extranodal involvement is uncommon on initial presentation
   - First-line treatment with DA-R-EPOCH (dose-adjusted rituximab, etoposide, prednisone, vincristine, cyclophosphamide, and Adriamycin)

2. **What are special features of transformation of follicular lymphoma to DLBCL?**
   - Transformation happens at a rate of approximately 3% per year in the first 10 years, less afterward.
   - Prognosis is better in previously untreated patients with a localized area of transformation.

- Transformation should be considered if there is a disproportionately rapid growth of a lymph node group with elevated LDH (biopsy that lymph node group) or if an isolated area on a PET scan demonstrates higher fluorodeoxyglucose (FDG) avidity than the rest of the disease areas (biopsy the more intensely PET avid lymph node).
- Treat initially with R-CHOP. If the patient has previously received chemotherapy then consolidation with autologous stem cell transplant should be performed in patients that obtain a complete remission or substantial partial remission. If the patient has previously received R-CHOP then treatment should be given with salvage regimens such as RICE, RDHAP, R-GemOX/R-GDP followed by autologous stem cell transplant.

Burkitt Lymphoma (BL)

EPIDEMIOLOGY

1. How common is BL?
   - BL is rare
   - There are three variants:
     - Endemic—most common childhood malignancy in equatorial Africa, associated with Epstein–Barr virus (EBV) infection.
     - Sporadic—1% to 2% of all lymphomas in American adults.
     - Immunodeficiency-associated—seen in patients with HIV, postorgan transplant, congenital immunodeficiency.

STAGING

1. What studies are important in workup/staging of BL?
   - Same as DLBCL (see the section on Diffuse Large B-Cell Lymphoma), with the addition of CSF exam in all patients

PATHOLOGY

1. What is the classic pathologic description of BL?
   - Described as a classic "starry sky" appearance

SIGNS AND SYMPTOMS

1. What are the frequent clinical features of BL?
   - Constitutional symptoms
   - Spontaneous TLS
   - Bone marrow involvement in up to 70% of patients at presentation
   - Leptomeningeal involvement in up to 40% of patients at presentation
   - Bulky abdominal (in adults) adenopathy (see Figure 7.1).

TREATMENT

1. What is the preferred initial treatment for BL?

FIGURE 7.1 ■ PET scan of a patient with Burkitt lymphoma. Image courtesy of Dr. Ryan Wilcox.

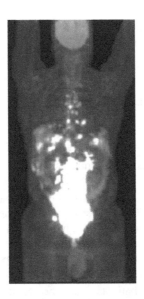

- One of the intensive, multiagent chemo regimens with CSF prophylaxis, two of which are listed in the following. CNS prophylaxis is essential in BL. R-CHOP is not adequate therapy.
- CODOX-M (cyclophosphamide, vincristine, doxorubicin, high-dose methotrexate) alternating with IVAC (ifosfamide, etoposide, high-dose cytarabine), with intrathecal methotrexate or ara-C. Addition of rituximab may further improve outcomes in these patients.
- R-Hyper-CVAD (rituximab, hyperfractionated cyclophosphamide, vincristine, doxorubicin, dexamethasone, alternating with methotrexate and cytarabine) with intrathecal methotrexate gives similar outcomes.

SPECIAL CONSIDERATIONS

1. **What is a "double-hit" lymphoma?**
   - Defined by *MYC* translocation with an additional translocation, usually *BCL2* or less commonly *BCL6*. Rarely, triple-hit lymphomas (*MYC*, *BCL2*, and *BCL6*) also exist.
   - Histologic features are intermediate between DLBCL and BL: presence of "starry sky" pattern, some large cells, Ki-67 >90%.
   - Poor prognosis.
   - There is some evidence to consider DA-R-EPOCH as a first-line therapy in double-hit lymphomas since they historically do not respond well to R-CHOP.

Mantle Cell Lymphoma (MCL)

DIAGNOSTIC CRITERIA

1. **How should a patient with MCL be worked up and staged?**
   - Same as described earlier for DLBCL

- Lumbar puncture (LP) in patients with blastic variant even if no other risk factors for CNS involvement

2. Is MCL an aggressive lymphoma?
- 85% to 90% of cases are clinically aggressive; however, approximately 10% to 15% of cases behave as indolent lymphomas.

TREATMENT
1. What is the typical first-line treatment for MCL?
- Although rare, patients with limited-stage (stages I–II) disease should be treated with IFRT and combination chemotherapy.
- For bulky stage II and for stages III/IV, optimal treatment is debatable. Patients who are candidates for autologous stem cell transplant should undergo induction chemotherapy, followed by high-dose therapy with autologous stem cell rescue. Regimens that include high dose Ara-c appear to be important in this setting (eg, Nordic regimen, consisting of rituximab, cyclophosphamide, vincristine, doxorubicin, and prednisone, alternating with rituximab + high dose Ara-c).
- Transplant ineligible patients can be treated with R-bendamustine, R-HyperCVAD, or R-CHOP. R-CHOP is the least optimal of these three options; therefore, patients treated with R-CHOP should receive rituximab maintenance, typically every 2 months for 2 years. The addition of R-maintenance to frontline R-CHOP has been shown to extend progression free survival in elderly patients with MCL. Current evidence does not indicate a benefit of rituximab maintenance after R-bendamustine. R-CHOP + rituximab maintenance has similar outcomes to R-bendamustine without maintenance.
- About 15% of patients have indolent disease and can be observed until symptomatic. Most asymptomatic patients should be observed until symptoms arise that warrant therapy.

Lymphomas in HIV/AIDS Patients

SPECIAL CONSIDERATIONS
1. What are AIDS-defining malignancies?
- Invasive cervical cancer
- Kaposi sarcoma
- BL
- Immunoblastic lymphoma (B- or T-cell)
- Primary CNS lymphoma

2. What other lymphomas are also seen more frequently in HIV/AIDS patients?
- Primary effusion lymphoma (associated with HHV8, often coinfected with EBV)
- Plasmablastic lymphoma
- Multicentric Castleman disease (associated with HHV8)

3. **What are special considerations in working up an HIV/AIDS patient with lymphoma?**
   - Monitor CD4+ counts.

4. **What are special considerations in treating an HIV/AIDS patient with lymphoma?**
   - Early initiation of highly active antiretroviral therapy (HAART) improves the outcomes of these patients.
   - There is increased risk of infectious complications of chemotherapy with CD4 count <50.
   - Use granulocyte colony stimulating factor support aggressively.
   - Use prophylactic antimicrobials.
   - Given the aggressive nature of these lymphomas, CNS prophylaxis is generally recommended.

Posttransplant Lymphoproliferative Disorder

EPIDEMIOLOGY

1. **Which transplants are associated with a higher incidence of posttransplant lymphoproliferative disorder?**
   - Solid organ tumor transplants, particularly those that require higher degrees of immunosuppression such as heart and lung (10%–25%) transplants.

TREATMENT

1. **How is posttransplant lymphoproliferative disorder treated?**
   - Treatment depends on the subtype of lymphoma.
   - If Hodgkin lymphoma, treat as Hodgkin lymphoma (see Chapter 5).
   - If diagnosed with non-Hodgkin and patient noted to have low burden disease, reduction of immunosuppressives may be enough. If there is a complete response to reduction of immunosuppressives alone, then monitoring after this is appropriate. If there is persistent/progressive disease despite reduction of immunosuppression, then treat with rituximab alone. In patients with more advanced stage disease, treatment with single-agent Rituxan can be considered versus treatment with rituximab + chemotherapy.
   - If monomorphic B-cell lymphoma—reduce immunosuppressives followed by rituximab alone or chemoimmunotherapy.
   - If polymorphic B-cell lymphoma with extensive disease—reduce immunosuppressives followed by rituximab alone or chemoimmunotherapy.
   - If polymorphic B-cell lymphoma with localized disease—reduce immunosuppressive therapy followed by rituximab alone. Local treatment such as radiation therapy or surgery along with rituximab can also be considered.

QUESTIONS

1. A 59-year-old female presents with night sweats, weight loss, and palpable lymphadenopathy. On laboratory studies, she has a white blood cell (WBC) count of 12/mcL, hemoglobin of 12 g/dL, and platelet count of 120/mcL. Lactate dehydrogenase (LDH) is 450 U/L. A PET scan is performed, which demonstrates fluorodeoxyglucose (FDG) avid lymphadenopathy in cervical, axillary, mesenteric, and inguinal lymph nodes. An excisional lymph node biopsy is performed. Morphology reveals sheets of large atypical lymphocytes. Flow cytometry is positive for CD20, CD10, and surface immunoglobulin, negative for CD5 and cyclin D1. Fluorescence in situ hybridization (FISH) is performed, which is negative for BCL6 and MYC but positive for BCL2.
   What is the function of the BCL2 in her lymphoma?
   A. Overexpression of a transcription factor
   B. Overexpression of an antiapoptotic gene
   C. Overexpression of a cell cycle regulator
   D. Loss of function of a transcription factor
   E. Loss of function of an antiapoptotic gene

2. A 30-year-old female presents with shortness of breath and swelling in her neck. A CT of the thorax reveals a large mediastinal mass as well as axillary and cervical lymphadenopathy. PET scan redemonstrates activity in these areas. A lymph node biopsy is performed, which is consistent with a primary B-cell mediastinal lymphoma. A bone marrow biopsy is performed, which is unremarkable for involvement with lymphoma.
   Which of the following is the appropriate treatment regimen?
   A. Treatment with rituximab, cyclophosphamide, and fludarabine
   B. Treatment with R-HyperCVAD
   C. Treatment with dose-adjusted EPOCH with rituximab
   D. Radiation therapy first to the mediastinum because of impending superior vena cava syndrome
   E. Treatment with rituximab and bendamustine

3. A 46-year-old female with history of heart transplantation 5 years ago presents with inguinal lymphadenopathy. She undergoes an excisional lymph node biopsy, which reveals a monomorphic posttransplant lymphoproliferative disorder (PTLD). She denies any fevers, chills, or weight loss. Her labs reveal a white blood cell (WBC) count of 7.7/mcL, hemoglobin of 13 g/dL, and platelet count of 160/mcL. Her comprehensive metabolic panel is unremarkable. Her lactate dehydrogenase (LDH) is 165 U/L. She undergoes a PET scan, which shows low level uptake only in her right inguinal lymph nodes.
   What is the appropriate initial step in treatment of her PTLD?
   A. Reduce her immunosuppressives
   B. Observation and repeat her PET scan in 3 months
   C. Treat with rituximab alone
   D. Treat with R-CHOP
   E. Treat with radiation therapy only

4. A 25-year-old African male presents with a large palpable abdominal mass, which has been growing rapidly within the last 2 weeks. He has been experiencing night sweats, fevers, and weight loss. CT of the abdomen/pelvis demonstrates a large abdominal mass as well as diffuse mesenteric and retroperitoneal lymphadenopathy. His laboratory studies reveal a white blood cell (WBC) count of 20/mcL, hemoglobin of 9 g/dL, and platelet count of 90/mcL. A CT-guided core biopsy of the large mass reveals small monomorphic lymphocytes in a starry sky appearance. Ki67 staining is appreciated at 90%. By fluorescence in situ hybridization (FISH) he is found to have chromosomal translocation t(8;14).
   What is the main pathophysiology behind his lymphoma?
   A. A translocation causing overexpression of *MYC*
   B. A translocation causing overexpression of *BCL 6*
   C. A translocation causing overexpression of *BCL2*
   D. A translocation causing overexpression of Cyclin D1
   E. A translocation causing overexpression of *CIITA*

5. A 29-year-old male presents with night sweats and palpable lymphad-enopathy. He is referred to your clinic because he was recently diag-nosed with HIV last week and was found to have a CD4 count of 40. A PET scan reveals fluorodeoxyglucose (FDG) avid lymph nodes in his cervical, axillary, inguinal, and retroperitoneal lymph nodes. He under-goes an excisional lymph node biopsy, which reveals a CD20 positive diffuse large B-cell lymphoma.
   Which of the following has been shown to improve HIV lymphoma treatment outcomes?
   A. Use of antibiotic prophylaxis
   B. Incorporation of antiretroviral therapy prior to and during chemother-apy
   C. Delaying therapy until HIV viral load is undetectable
   D. Avoidance of rituximab during entire treatment course because of his low CD4 count
   E. Intrathecal prophylaxis to prevent central nervous system (CNS) involvement with his lymphoma

6. A 69-year-old male presents with night sweats and weight loss. He is found to have diffuse lymphadenopathy above and below the dia-phragm. He underdoes an excisional lymph node biopsy of an axillary node, which is consistent with diffuse large B-cell lymphoma.
   Which of the following tests are needed before considering initiating rituximab therapy?
   A. Cytomegalovirus (CMV) serologies
   B. Herpes simplex virus (HSV) serologies
   C. Hepatitis B surface antigen, hepatitis B surface antibody
   D. Respiratory virus panel
   E. Epstein–Barr virus (EBV) serologies

ANSWERS

1. **B. Overexpression of an antiapoptotic gene.** *BCL2* is an antiapoptotic gene that encodes one of the proteins involved in regulating cell death.

2. **C. Treatment with dose-adjusted EPOCH with rituximab.** Dose-adjusted EPOCH with rituximab has been shown to have a high cure rate and also obliviate the need for radiation therapy in patients with primary B-cell mediastinal lymphoma, and currently is a preferred regimen. The other treatment options are not appropriate or indicated in primary B-cell mediastinal lymphoma.

3. **A. Reduce her immunosuppressives.** Reduction of immunosuppressives is the most appropriate first step in the management of her posttransplant lymphoproliferative disorder. Observation is not appropriate in this situation. Other treatment modalities could be considered if she continues to have persistent disease after reducing her immunosuppressives first.

4. **A. A translocation causing overexpression of *MYC*.** Overexpression of cMYC is the major driver in the pathogenesis of Burkitt lymphoma/leukemia.

5. **B. Incorporation of antiretroviral therapy prior to and during chemotherapy.** Antiretroviral therapy has been shown to improve lymphoma therapy outcomes in patients with HIV-associated lymphomas. The other answer options have not demonstrated improved outcomes in HIV lymphoma therapy.

6. **C. Hepatitis B surface antigen, hepatitis B surface antibody.** Rituximab has a risk of reactivating hepatitis B and therefore hepatitis B infection needs to be checked prior to therapy.

Peripheral T-Cell Lymphomas

Sumana Devata and Ryan A. Wilcox

EPIDEMIOLOGY

1. **How common are the peripheral T-cell lymphomas (PTCLs) and what are their subtypes?**
   - PTCLs are a heterogeneous group of diseases that account for <15% of all non-Hodgkin lymphomas (NHLs) in Western countries, and 15% to 20% in Asia.
   - There are many PTCL subtypes, and the most common subtypes of nodal PTCL are:
     - Peripheral T-cell lymphoma, not otherwise specified (PTCL-NOS; 26%)
     - Angioimmunoblastic T-cell lymphoma (AITL; 19%)
     - Anaplastic large cell lymphoma, ALK+/− (ALCL; 12%)
       - ALK(+) (6.6%): median age of onset 34 years
       - ALK(−) (5.5%): median age of onset 58 years
   - Other subtypes include: extranodal NK/T-cell lymphoma (ENKL), nasal type; hepatosplenic T-cell lymphoma (HSTCL); subcutaneous panniculitis-like T-cell lymphoma (SPTCL); enteropathy-associated T-cell lymphoma (EATL); adult T-cell leukemia/lymphoma (ATLL).

RISK FACTORS

1. **What are the risk factors and associations for various subtypes of PTCL?**
   - Variable depending on the subtype:
     - HSTCL: chronic immunosuppression
     - ATLL: human T-cell leukemia virus type 1 (HTLV-1) infection, most common in Caribbean islands and southern Japan
     - EATL: celiac disease
     - ENKL: Epstein–Barr virus (EBV) infection, most common in Asia
     - ALK(−), ALCL: breast implants, lymphoma involving the fibrous capsule around the implant without invasion of underlying breast tissue

SIGNS AND SYMPTOMS

1. **What are the signs and symptoms of patients with PTCL?**
   - Lymphadenopathy (LAD), cytopenias, elevated lactate dehydrogenase (LDH), and advanced-stage disease at presentation are commonly seen. Unique features are as follows:

○ PTCL-NOS: 50% with concurrent extranodal disease (liver, bone marrow, skin, and gastrointestinal [GI] tract)

○ AITL: Acute onset LAD, B symptoms, organomegaly, also associated with eosinophilia, pruritic rash, autoimmune events (rheumatoid arthritis, thyroid disease, vasculitis), polyarthritis, effusions/ascites, polyclonal hypergammaglobulinemia, elevated erythrocyte sedimentation rate (ESR), hypoalbuminemia, positive Coombs test

STAGING

1. How is PTCL staged?

- Most subtypes of PTCL are staged according to the Ann Arbor lymphoma staging system (see Chapter 5).

- Cutaneous T-cell lymphoma (CTCL) employs a modified tumor, nodes, metastasis, and blood (TNMB) based staging approach.

PATHOLOGY

1. Are there any common genetic mutations seen in nodal PTCL?

- ALK(−) ALCL: DUSP22 (prevalence 30%, favorable prognosis) and TP63 (prevalence 8%, unfavorable prognosis) rearrangements have been described

- ALK(+) ALCL: t(2;5), ALK rearranged with NPM

2. What are the lymph node histopathological features of nodal PTCL?

- PTCL-NOS

  ○ Effacement of lymph nodes with cells of variable size; sheets of atypical lymphocytes in a paracortical or diffuse pattern; mixture of plasma calls and eosinophils; high mitotic rate

- ALCL

  ○ Sinusoidal growth pattern (and may mimic metastatic carcinoma)

  ○ Classical variant: large blastic cells with prominent nucleoli and abundant cytoplasm.

    ■ Hallmark cells: eccentric nuclei, eosinophilic paranuclear hof (Figure 8.1)

  ○ Immunophenotypic markers: CD30+

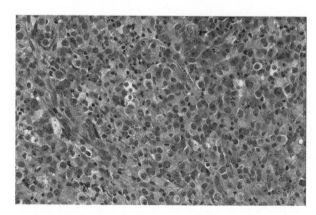

FIGURE 8.1 ■ Hallmark cells with eccentric nuclei and eosinophilic paranuclear hof as seen in anaplastic large cell lymphoma.
Courtesy of Nathaneal Bailey, University of Michigan Department of Pathology.

- AITL
  - Partial or complete effacement of lymph nodes; neovascularization or arborizing endothelial venules. AITL are derived from follicular helper T cells (explaining the B-cell and follicular dendritic cell expansion observed). Typified by a mixture of plasma cells, B-cell immunoblasts, small lymphocytes, eosinophils, follicular dendritic cells, and medium-sized malignant cells with abundant cytoplasm.

PROGNOSTIC FACTORS

1. How are patients with PTCL risk stratified?

- In general the International Prognostic Index (IPI) is applicable to PTCL.
- A similar Prognostic Index for T-cell lymphoma (PIT) can also be used.

IPI Prognostic Factors	PIT Prognostic Factors
Age >60	Age >60
LDH > ULN	LDH > ULN
ECOG PS ≥2	ECOG PS ≥2
Ann Arbor stage ≥3	Bone marrow involvement
Number of extranodal sites >2	

Number of IPI factors determines prognostic group: Low = 0–1; low–intermediate = 2; high–intermediate = 3; high = 4–5.

2. How does the prognosis of PTCL compare with aggressive B-cell NHL?

- Stage-for-stage outcomes are inferior for patients with PTCL compared to those with aggressive B-cell NHL.

3. What is an additional important prognostic factor for ALCL?

- The presence or absence of an ALK fusion protein significantly affects ALCL prognosis.
- ALK(+) ALCL has a 5-year overall survival (OS) rate of 70%, while ALK (–) ALCL has a 5-year OS rate of 49%.

INDICATIONS FOR TREATMENT

1. When should treatment be initiated for PTCL?

- Overall, the survival for patients with untreated PTCL is measured in months; treatment should be initiated once diagnosis is established.

TREATMENT

First-Line Therapy

1. What is standard first-line therapy for the common PTCL subtypes?

- ALK(+) ALCL
  - Multiagent, anthracycline-based therapy ± etoposide × 6 cycles, +/− radiation therapy (RT):

- Age >60 years, CHOP (cyclophosphamide, doxorubicin, vincristine, prednisone)
- Age <60 years, CHOEP (CHOP plus etoposide) or CHOP
  - Stage I–II disease: consider 3 to 4 cycles of chemotherapy followed by RT
- PTCL-NOS, ALK(−) ALCL, AITL
  - Consider clinical trial participation
  - Multiagent chemotherapy (CHOP or CHOEP) × six cycles. Abbreviated chemotherapy (three or four cycles) followed by RT (as in limited-stage diffuse large B-cell lymphoma [DLBCL]) may be considered in selected patients.

2. What is the role of consolidative autologous stem cell transplant (ASCT) after complete response with first-line therapy?

- Stage III/IV disease: In contrast to DLBCL, most transplant-eligible patients with stage III/IV PTCL-NOS, ALK(−) ALCL, and AITL achieving a complete remission with induction first-line therapy (CHOP or CHOEP) undergo consolidation with high-dose therapy and ASCT, as this approach appears to be associated with improved progression-free survival (PFS)/OS.
- Stage I/II disease: ASCT is considered for stage I–II (high–intermediate/high IPI) PTCL-NOS, ALK(−) ALCL, and AITL in first remission. Favorable outcomes have been reported in DUSP22 rearranged ALK(−) ALCL without ASCT in first remission.
- Patients with ALK(+) ALCL do not typically receive consolidative treatment in first remission due to favorable 5-year OS with chemotherapy.

Second-Line Therapy

1. What treatment options exist for relapsed or refractory PTCL?

- Consider clinical trial participation.
- Elderly AITL patients unable to tolerate chemotherapy: consider corticosteroids or immunosuppressive therapy with cyclosporine.
- No standard second-line treatment. Overall response rates in relapsed/refractory PTCL are ~20% to 50%; however, responses are not typically durable.
  - Single-agent regimens: brentuximab (ORR ~85% in ALCL), romidepsin, belinostat, pralatrexate (limited activity in AITL)
  - Multiagent chemotherapy is similar to aggressive B-cell lymphoma regimens without rituximab (eg, ICE, DHAP, GemOx)
- Stem cell transplantation
  - ASCT can be considered for patients who did not undergo transplant in first complete remission.
  - Allogeneic stem cell transplantation can lead to durable responses in up to 60% of relapsed/refractory cases, but is associated with up to a 30% rate of treatment-related mortality.

SPECIAL CONSIDERATIONS

1. What are notable aspects of other, less common subtypes of PTCL?

- ENKL, nasal type. EBV associated (EBER-positive):

- ○ Typically present with nasal obstruction or invasion of nose, palate, and sinuses
- ○ Multimodality treatment with concurrent chemotherapy and RT for patients with stage I/IIE disease. CHOP alone is ineffective:
  - RT with cisplatin followed by etoposide, ifosfamide, cisplatin, dexamethasone (VIPD) × three cycles or RT with dexamethasone, etoposide, ifosfamide, carboplatin (DeVIC) × three cycles or asparaginase-containing regimens prior to and following RT (in "sandwich" approach)
- ATLL, HTLV-1 associated:
  - ○ Clinically variable with acute, smoldering, lymphomatous and chronic types
  - ○ Peripheral blood lymphocytes have hyperlobated nuclei with condensed chromatin appearing as a clover leaf or flower
- CTCL:
  - ○ Most common subtype is mycosis fungoides (MF).
    - Typically pruritic patch/plaque skin lesions seen in non-sun-exposed areas.
    - Skin biopsy shows small–intermediate mononuclear cells with cerebriform nuclei in upper dermis and epidermal keratinocytes (also known as epidermotropism) or in intraepidermal aggregates (Pautrier microabscesses).
  - ○ A leukemic subtype is known as Sézary syndrome with classic circulating cerebriform cells seen on peripheral smear (Figure 8.2).
    - Clinically presents with erythroderma and pruritus
  - ○ Treatment includes a variety of agents (used as single agent or in combination) such as:
    - Skin directed: ultraviolet (UV) light, topical corticosteroids
    - Systemic: retinoids, histone deacetylase (HDAC) inhibitors, interferon alfa, pralatrexate, alemtuzumab, brentuximab (eg, in transformed MF)

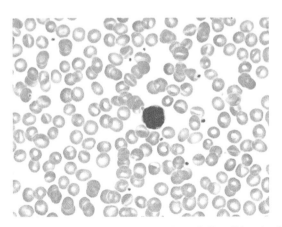

FIGURE 8.2 ■ Peripheral blood smear with cerebriform (Sézary) cell.
Courtesy of Nathaneal Bailey, University of Michigan Department of Pathology.

QUESTIONS

1. Which of the following peripheral T-cell lymphoma (PTCL) subtypes has the best prognosis?
   A. Angioimmunoblastic T-cell lymphoma (AITL)
   B. Anaplastic large cell lymphoma (ALCL), ALK(+)
   C. Extranodal NK/T-cell lymphoma
   D. ALCL, ALK(−)

2. A 47-year-old Jamaican man presents with an elevated lymphocyte count and peripheral blood shows some cells with hyperlobated nuclei appearing like clovers. Which pathogen is typically associated with this peripheral T-cell lymphoma (PTCL) subtype?
   A. *Helicobacter pylori*
   B. Epstein–Barr virus (EBV)
   C. Human T-cell leukemia virus type 1 (HTLV-1)
   D. Cytomegalovirus (CMV)

3. A 60-year-old man presents with years of pruritus with large scattered pink/erythematous patches on his chest, back, upper arms, and thighs. Past biopsies have showed eczema and folliculitis, and topical treatments have not resulted in improvement. Repeat biopsy shows mononuclear cells with cerebriform nuclei in upper dermis and epidermal keratinocytes with intraepidermal aggregates forming microabscess-like structures. What is the most likely diagnosis?
   A. Sézary syndrome
   B. Atopic dermatitis
   C. Psoriasis
   D. Mycosis fungoides
   E. Infection

4. A 68-year-old man develops joint pain and swelling, fatigue, shortness of breath, night sweats, lower extremity erythematous rash, and enlarged neck lymph nodes. Labs show a white blood cell count of 10 K/mcL with an absolute lymphocyte count of 0.5 K/mcL, hemoglobin of 6.5 g/dL, platelet count of 130 K/mcL, total bilirubin 4.5 mg/dL, and lactate dehydrogenase (LDH) >2 × the upper limit of normal. Chest x-ray shows bilateral pleural effusions. What is the most likely diagnosis?
   A. Angioimmunoblastic T-cell lymphoma (AITL)
   B. Mycosis fungoides
   C. Peripheral T-cell lymphoma, not otherwise specified (PTCL-NOS)
   D. Follicular lymphoma

5. A woman without a significant past medical history and only surgical history of bilateral breast implants presents with right-sided breast fullness. In addition to a primary breast carcinoma, which of the following is in the differential diagnosis?
   A. Angioimmunoblastic T-cell lymphoma (AITL)
   B. Peripheral T-cell lymphoma, not otherwise specified (PTCL-NOS)
   C. Metastatic disease
   D. Anaplastic large cell lymphoma (ALCL), ALK(−)

ANSWERS

1. **B. ALCL, ALK(+).** ALK(+) ALCL has the best overall prognosis of these PTCL subtypes with a 5-year overall survival rate of 70%. Note: The International Prognostic Index (IPI) risk group should also be taken into account and is still prognostic.

2. **C. HTLV-1.** This man most likely has adult T-cell leukemia/lymphoma (ATLL) given his heritage and peripheral blood features; this is associated with HTLV-1 infection.

3. **D. Mycosis fungoides.** The clinical history and pathology results with epidermotropism and Pautrier microabscess formation are consistent with mycosis fungoides.

4. **A. Angioimmunoblastic T-cell lymphoma (AITL).** AITL is the most likely diagnosis given the systemic symptoms of arthritis, effusions, B symptoms, and lymphadenopathy, as well as likely hemolytic anemia with an elevated bilirubin and LDH.

5. **D. ALCL, ALK(–).** ALK(–) ALCL has been associated with breast implants. Implant removal and capsulectomy followed by observation is associated with favorable long-term disease-free survival for patients without an associated mass.

9 Multiple Myeloma and Plasma Cell Dyscrasias

Maryann Shango and Erica Campagnaro

EPIDEMIOLOGY

1. **What are the plasma cell dyscrasias?**
   - Plasma cell myeloma (a.k.a. multiple myeloma [MM])
   - Monoclonal gammopathy of undetermined significance (MGUS)
   - Solitary plasmacytoma
   - Light and heavy chain deposition diseases
   - Primary (AL) amyloidosis
   - Polyneuropathy, organomegaly, endocrinopathy, M-spike, skin changes (POEMS)

2. **How common is MM?**
   - MM represents approximately 10% of hematologic malignancies, and 1% of all cancers.

3. **What is the significance of MM?**
   - MM is conventionally considered incurable, and accounts for 20% of hematological malignancy deaths and 2% of all cancer deaths.

ETIOLOGY AND RISK FACTORS

1. **What is the etiology of MM?**
   - MM is a cancer of plasma cells that arises from premalignant plasma cell dyscrasia, MGUS.

2. **What are the risk factors of MM?**
   - Advanced age, male gender, African American race, obesity, immunosuppression, and certain environmental exposures, including radiation and benzene, are associated with increased risk of myeloma.

SCREENING AND DIAGNOSTIC CRITERIA

1. **Who should be screened for MM?**
   - Myeloma should be considered when a patient has otherwise unexplained hypercalcemia, renal failure, anemia, bone pain, or lytic bone lesions on imaging.
   - Other potential reasons to consider the diagnosis of myeloma include high or low serum total protein, hyperviscosity, neuropathy, frequent infections, and generalized symptoms of advanced malignancy such as weight loss.

2. **What tests are important for assessing plasma cell dyscrasias, including MM?**
   - Complete blood count with differential and peripheral blood smear
   - Comprehensive metabolic panel to assess calcium and other electrolytes, renal and liver function
   - Serum beta-2 microglobulin (B2M) and lactate dehydrogenase (LDH)
   - Serum and 24-hour urine protein electrophoresis with immunofixation
   - Serum quantitative immunoglobulins, IgG, IgA, and IgM (IgD and IgE only if suspected)
   - Serum free light chain (FLC) quantification
   - Serum viscosity if: monoclonal immunoglobulin level is >5 g/dL or symptoms suggestive of hyperviscosity
   - Skeletal survey to screen for lytic bone lesions
     - Must include humeri and femoral bones
     - Bone lesions in POEMS are typically sclerotic
   - More sensitive imaging with CT, whole body MRI (total spine and pelvis if whole body unavailable), or PET/CT (correlates lytic lesions with metabolic activity) is recommended for patients with bone pain that is unexplained by plain radiographs. Other indications for more sensitive bone imaging include compression fractures, neurologic deficit, uncertainty of presence or burden of bone disease, or to rule out other sites of disease in suspected solitary plasmacytoma.
   - Bone marrow biopsy with flow cytometry, conventional cytogenetics, and fluorescence in situ hybridization (FISH) for commonly acquired genetic abnormalities
   - If AL amyloidosis is suspected, confirm diagnosis with Congo red staining and amyloid protein identification by immunohistochemistry or mass spectrometry on affected tissue (eg, bone marrow biopsy, fat pad aspirate, other affected organs).

3. **What are the diagnostic criteria for active MM (requiring treatment)?**
   - Soft tissue or bone plasmacytoma *or* ≥10% clonal bone marrow plasma cells *and* at least *one* of the following:
     - Clonal plasma cells ≥60% of bone marrow
     - Involved to uninvolved FLC ratio of 100 or more if the involved FLC is at least 100 mg/L
     - MRI with >1 focal lesion in the bone or bone marrow (≥5 mm)
     - Any plasma cell dyscrasia-related end-organ damage:
       - Anemia (hemoglobin <10 g/dL or >2 g/dL below lower normal limit)
       - Renal insufficiency (creatinine >2 mg/dL or creatinine clearance <40 mL/min)
       - Elevated serum calcium level (calcium >11 mg/dL)
       - Lytic bone lesions (one or more) on skeletal survey, CT, MRI, or PET/CT

4. **What are the diagnostic criteria and characteristics of other plasma cell dyscrasias?**
   - MGUS
     - Serum monoclonal (M) protein <3 g/dL
     - Clonal plasma cells <10% of bone marrow
     - Absence of end-organ damage attributed to plasma cell dyscrasia
   - Smoldering MM (SMM)
     - Serum M protein ≥3 g/dL
     - Clonal plasma cells 10% to 59% of bone marrow
     - No end-organ damage or other myeloma defining events
     - No amyloidosis
   - Solitary plasmacytoma
     - Clonal plasma cell mass without bone marrow involvement or evidence of end-organ damage attributable to monoclonal plasma cells
     - Patients with an apparently solitary plasmacytoma who have <10% clonal marrow plasma cells are considered to have "solitary plasmacytoma with minimal marrow involvement." They are treated as solitary plasmacytoma, but the risk of recurrence or progression to myeloma is somewhat higher.
   - POEMS
     - A syndrome that involves the following:
       - Polyneuropathy
       - Organomegaly
       - Endocrinopathy
       - Monoclonal gammopathy
       - Skin changes
     - Also known as osteosclerotic myeloma
     - Associated with increased circulation of vascular endothelial growth factor (VEGF)
   - Light and heavy chain deposition diseases (a.k.a. Randall disease)
     - Plasma cell neoplasia that secretes immunoglobulin that deposits in tissues and causes tissue damage but does not form an amyloid-type beta-pleated sheet
       - Nonfibrillary, amorphous eosinophilic material that is Congo red stain negative
       - Serum M protein (in 85%)
       - Monoclonal heavy and/or light chain deposition that causes organ dysfunction
       - Other, more common, diseases ruled out (eg, lymphoplasmacytic lymphoma with IgG deposition, chronic lymphocytic leukemia/small lymphocytic lymphoma [CLL/SLL] with IgM deposition, extranodal marginal zone lymphoma with IgA deposition)

- AL amyloidosis
  - ○ AL amyloidosis (a.k.a. "amyloid light chain" or primary amyloidosis) is characterized by systemic deposition of amyloid protein that is composed of immunoglobulin light chains.
  - ○ Amyloid protein deposition results in damage to the affected organ(s) (can be one or multiple), resulting in problems such as congestive heart failure, pulmonary infiltrates, malabsorption, nephrotic syndrome, neuropathy, and others.

PATHOLOGY

1. **What is the cell of origin for the malignant plasma cells of MM?**
   - MM cells are postgerminal center plasma cells identifiable by somatic mutations in the variable region of the immunoglobulin heavy chain gene.

SIGNS AND SYMPTOMS

1. **What are the most common symptoms of MM?**
   - Anemia (73%)
   - Bone pain due to lytic lesions (58%)
   - Increased creatinine (48%)
   - Fatigue (32%)
   - Hypercalcemia (28%)
   - Weight loss (24%)

2. **What are uncommon but important signs and symptoms?**
   - Plasmacytoma (7%)
   - Paresthesias (5%)
   - Spinal cord compression (5%—due to plasmacytoma or vertebral body fracture)

RISK STRATIFICATION

1. **Which features are associated with high-risk disease?**
   - FISH showing t(14;16), t(14;20), or del(17p13)
   - LDH >upper limit normal (ULN)
   - Evidence of primary plasma cell leukemia (≥20% plasma cells on manual differential or ≥2,000 plasma cells/mcL)
   - About 15% of MM are high risk with median survival 2 to 3 years despite standard therapy

2. **Which features are associated with intermediate-risk disease?**
   - FISH showing t(4;14), 1q+, deletion 13, or hypoploidy by conventional cytogenetics

3. **Which features are associated with standard-risk disease?**
   - Everyone who does not fit high- or intermediate-risk disease is considered to have standard-risk disease.
   - Median survival is 8 to 10 years.

4. **Do any genetic features predict response to specific therapies?**
   - Poor outcome previously associated with t(4;14) and monosomy 13/deletion 13 or hypoploidy is abrogated at least partially with early use of bortezomib-based therapy. This is why they are now classified as intermediate risk

5. **What are favorable prognostic factors?**
   - Hyperdiploidy, typically affecting the odd-numbered chromosomes, Eastern Cooperative Oncology Group Performance Status (ECOG PS) 0–2, age less than 70 years, and normal albumin

STAGING

1. **Which staging system is preferred for MM?**
   - The Revised International Staging System (R-ISS)

2. **How is MM staged according to the R-ISS?**
   - The R-ISS uses serum B2M, serum albumin, LDH, and genetics
   - Stage I: B2M <3.5 mg/L, albumin ≥3.5 g/dL, normal LDH, no del(17p), t(4;14), or t(14;16) (5-year progression-free survival [PFS] and overall survival [OS] 55% and 82%, respectively)
   - Stage II: neither stage I nor stage III (5-year PFS and OS 36% and 62%, respectively)
   - Stage III: B2M ≥5.5 mg/L, LDH greater than ULN, and/or del(17p), t(4;14), or t(14;16) by FISH (5-year PFS and OS 24% and 40%, respectively)

TREATMENT

General Treatment Principles

1. **Which plasma cell dyscrasias should be treated?**
   - There is no known benefit of treatment of MGUS or smoldering myeloma with standard chemotherapy; observation is the standard of care.
   - Patients with high-risk MGUS or smoldering myeloma are encouraged to participate in clinical trials to evaluate the possible utility of newer agents earlier in the disease course.
   - Patients with MM should be treated since, by definition, end-organ damage is present or imminent.

2. **What are the main factors in determining best frontline therapy for patients with newly diagnosed MM?**
   - Disease risk
   - Eligibility for high-dose chemotherapy followed by autologous hematopoietic cell transplantation (HCT)

3. **Which MM patients receive induction therapy?**
   - All

4. **Is there a standard induction therapy?**
   - No

5. How do you decide what induction therapy to use?

- Disease risk stratification, patient factors (performance status, comorbidities, psychosocial support), institutional resources (eg, infusion and clinical trial availability), eligibility for autologous HCT

6. What happens after induction therapy?

- Postinduction therapy is dependent on eligibility and timing of autologous HCT. Generally, if HCT is not pursued, patients are continued on therapy, which may be the same or a modified version of their induction regimen, until progression or therapy intolerance occurs.

7. What are some key agents used in first-line MM treatment and what are their common toxicities?

- Bortezomib
  - Mechanism: proteasome inhibition
  - Side effects: peripheral (sensory) neuropathy, thrombocytopenia, herpes zoster reactivation
  - Hepatic metabolism: liver dysfunction requires dose adjustment (useful in renal failure or chronic kidney disease [CKD] patients)
  - Viral prophylaxis with acyclovir or valacyclovir is required
- Thalidomide
  - Mechanism: immunomodulation
  - Side effects: peripheral neuropathy, constipation, fatigue, edema, somnolence, and venous thrombotic events (VTE)
  - If used in combination with high-dose dexamethasone, and/or patient is at high risk for thrombosis (ie, history of VTE, diabetes mellitus, coronary artery disease), VTE prophylaxis with warfarin to achieve international normalized ratio (INR) 2–3 or prophylactic or full dose low molecular weight heparin (LMWH) is recommended.
  - If used in combination with bortezomib or low-dose dexamethasone, and patient is without high baseline risk of VTE, prophylactic LMWH, fixed and low-dose warfarin, or low-dose aspirin, are all acceptable options for VTE prophylaxis.
- Lenalidomide
  - Mechanism: immunomodulation
  - Side effects: myelosuppression, venous thromboembolism, and fatigue
  - Renal metabolism: significant renal dysfunction requires dose adjustment
  - VTE prophylaxis same as that with thalidomide
  - This is a preferred agent in patients with preexisting peripheral neuropathy

8. What is the role of bisphosphonates in MM?

- Bisphosphonates decrease the risk of skeletal fractures and improve bone-related pain
- Recommended for patients with active myeloma, with or without known bone disease

- The two common intravenous formulations are pamidronate and zoledronate, which are dosed monthly
- Optimal duration is unknown, but current recommendations are monthly for 2 years after which the decision to continue can be reassessed, and treatment can be discontinued or continued on a less frequent schedule if myeloma is in remission
- Important side effects include hypocalcemia, renal insufficiency, and osteonecrosis of the jaw

Principles of Autologous HCT in MM

1. **What is the role of autologous HCT in MM therapy?**
   - Autologous HCT results in higher response rates and prolonged PFS compared to standard therapies; data from phase 3 studies describing its impact on OS are mixed.
   - Autologous HCT should be considered in all MM patients who are eligible.

2. **Who is eligible for an autologous HCT?**
   - The eligibility criteria for autologous HCT are not standardized; the decision for HCT is often individualized rather than based on standard eligibility criteria.
   - Age >75 years, ECOG PS ≥3, or other significant comorbidities (eg, heart failure, significant pulmonary disease) are generally considered too risky for autologous HCT.

3. **When are autologous hematopoietic stem cells collected after induction therapy for MM patients?**
   - Usually after 2 to 4 months of therapy and/or after cytoreduction of myeloma by 50% (partial remission [PR])

4. **When is the best time to complete an autologous HCT?**
   - Autologous HCT can be completed "early" (after first remission) or "late" (at the time of first relapse, after second remission).

5. **Can a patient undergo a second autologous HCT?**
   - Yes. Usually, enough hematopoietic stem cells are collected to perform two autologous HCTs. These can be used in the setting of "tandem" HCT for patients with a poor response (very good partial response [VGPR] not reached after first HCT), usually within 3 to 6 months of the first HCT, or at the time of relapse if it occurs at least 12 months after first HCT.

Principles of First-Line Therapy

1. **What are the initial treatment options for MM patients who are autologous HCT candidates?**
   - Key point: avoid prolonged treatment with alkylating agents (cyclophosphamide or melphalan), or lenalidomide, which can interfere with subsequent stem cell collection.

- *Standard-risk* MM:
  - ○ Induction therapy can be followed by autologous stem cell transplant (SCT) immediately ("early") or after relapse ("late").
  - ○ The most commonly used induction regimen for standard-risk myeloma is bortezomib, lenalidomide, and dexamethasone (VRD), though two-drug combinations, such as bortezomib or lenalidomide with dexamethasone (VD or RD), may be used in frail patients.
- *Intermediate or high-risk* MM:
  - ○ Use bortezomib-based regimens for frontline treatment if a clinical trial is not available or not preferred by the patient.
  - ○ The most commonly used induction regimen for high-risk myeloma is VRD.
  - ○ Induction therapy should be followed by HCT in most patients.
  - ○ Bortezomib should remain part of maintenance therapy after induction and HCT.

2. **What are the initial treatment options for MM patients who are not candidates for autologous HCT candidates?**
   - In general, the same induction regimens used for patients who are eligible for HCT are used for those ineligible for HCT. The main difference is that alkylating agents are acceptable as first-line therapy in patients who are not candidates for HCT.
   - For intermediate- or high-risk patients, a bortezomib-based regimen should be utilized regardless if an alkylating agent is used (eg, bortezomib, melphalan, and prednisone [VMP], or VRD).

Relapsed or Refractory Disease

1. **What is the definition of progressive disease after initial treatment?**
   - Twenty-five percent increase in any of the following:
     - ○ Serum or urine monoclonal immunoglobulin
     - ○ Bone marrow clonal plasma cell percentage
     - ○ Change in the kappa/lambda serum FLC ratio
     - ○ Progression should be confirmed over two separate lab draws
   - The appearance of new bony lesions or plasmacytomas
   - Increase in size of a preexisting bony lesion or plasmacytoma
   - New and otherwise unexplained serum calcium >11.5 mg/dL

2. **What treatment strategies are available for relapsed disease?**
   - If it has been ≥1 year since initial therapy, repeating the initial therapy is reasonable.
   - Combination therapy including agents of a different class should be considered, such as using a bortezomib-based regimen if a lenalidomide-based regimen was given first-line.

- Autologous HCT should be considered in suitable patients including previously transplanted patients relapsing more than 12 months after initial transplant.
- Myeloablative allogeneic stem cell transplantation is generally not recommended due to the high treatment-related morbidity and mortality, but can be considered in high-risk patients in the context of a clinical trial.
- Generally, the duration and quality of response to therapies subsequent to initial therapy tend to be shorter and poorer, respectively.

3. **How is relapsed disease risk-stratified?**
   - If relapse is <12 months since initial therapy, disease is now classified as high risk regardless of initial risk stratification.
   - For high-risk patients at diagnosis, if relapse is ≥2 years after initial therapy, disease is considered standard risk at time of relapse in the absence of any new high-risk cytogenetic findings.

4. **What additional drugs are available for relapsed/refractory disease?**
   - Immunomodulators:
     - Pomalidomide: approved for relapse within 60 days of third-line therapy after lenalidomide and bortezomib
   - Proteasome inhibitors:
     - Carfilzomib: approved for relapse within 60 days of first-line therapy if given alone after immunomodulatory therapy and bortezomib, or after 1 to 3 lines of therapy if given in combination with RD
       - Available as intravenous infusion only, less peripheral neuropathy than bortezomib
     - Ixazomib: approved in combination with RD after failure of first-line therapy
       - Oral drug, causes less peripheral neuropathy, but more gastrointestinal (GI) toxicity (eg, nausea and diarrhea) than bortezomib
   - Monoclonal antibodies:
     - Daratumumab: anti-CD38 antibody, which is an epitope that is highly expressed on malignant myeloma cells, and less so on normal cells. It is approved after third-line therapy in patients previously treated with a proteasome inhibitor and immunomodulatory drug.
       - Available as intravenous infusion only, infusion reactions common with first dose
     - Elotuzumab: anti-SLAMF7 antibody, which is a glycoprotein expressed on both natural killer (NK) and MM cells. It is approved after 1 to 3 lines of therapy in combination with RD.
       - Available as intravenous infusion only, infusion reactions common with first dose
   - Histone deacetylase inhibitors:
     - Panobinostat: approved with VD after two prior therapies that must have included bortezomib and an immunomodulatory drug
       - Oral drug, associated with GI toxicity (eg, nausea and diarrhea)

QUESTIONS

1. A 65-year-old man was referred to you after workup of anemia revealed an M protein of 5 g/dL with several lytic lesions on skeletal survey. Bone marrow biopsy showed 35% clonal plasma cells, with fluorescence in situ hybridization (FISH) showing t(4;14) and deletion 13. He is working full time as a construction manager, and runs about 5 miles per week. What is your treatment recommendation?
   A. Bortezomib, lenalidomide, and dexamethasone (VRD), with stem cell collection after four cycles and plan for early autologous hematopoietic cell transplantation (HCT)
   B. Carfilzomib, pomalidomide, and dexamethasone (KPD), with stem cell collection after four cycles and plan for early autologous HCT
   C. VRD without stem cell collection
   D. Lenalidomide and dexamethasone (RD) with stem cell collection after four cycles and plan for early autologous HCT

2. A 79-year-old woman was recently diagnosed with multiple myeloma and presents to you to initiate therapy with lenalidomide and low-dose dexamethasone. She lives independently, participating in a twice weekly swimming class. She has no history of peptic ulcer disease (PUD), gastritis or gastrointestinal (GI) bleed. She has no other comorbidities. What is the best way to reduce her risk of venous thrombotic events (VTE)?
   A. Dose-adjusted warfarin for international normalized ratio (INR) goal 2–3
   B. Fixed, low-dose warfarin, 1–2 mg daily
   C. Low-dose aspirin (81 or 100 mg daily)
   D. Enoxaparin 40 mg daily

3. Bisphosphonates in multiple myeloma patients do which of the following?
   A. Reduce skeletal-related events
   B. Improve bone pain
   C. Reduce risk of myeloma-related renal dysfunction
   D. A and B

4. A 55-year-old woman presents with left upper arm pain, and was found to have a 3 cm humeral mass on imaging. Humeral biopsy confirmed a monoclonal plasma cell population. Bone marrow biopsy showed 5% monoclonal plasma cells, and serum blood tests were negative for anemia, hypercalcemia, and renal dysfunction. No bone lesions were identified on skeletal survey or PET/CT. How would you treat this patient?
   A. Definitive radiation to the humeral plasmacytoma followed by observation
   B. Palliative radiation to the humeral plasmacytoma followed by bortezomib, lenalidomide, and dexamethasone (VRD) and autologous hematopoietic cell transplantation (HCT)

C. Surgical resection

D. VRD and autologous HCT followed by maintenance therapy as guided by her risk stratification

5. **Which of the following characterize high-risk multiple myeloma (MM)?**
   A. Relapse at 14 months after autologous hematopoietic cell transplantation (HCT)
   B. 1q+
   C. Trisomy 15
   D. t(14;20)

6. **A 65-year old woman was referred to you after her primary care physician (PCP) found an M protein of 3.3 g/dL during a workup for unexplained mild normocytic anemia, hemoglobin 11.2 g/dL. She has normal calcium levels, negative Bence Jones protein, normal renal function, and negative skeletal survey for lytic lesions. Bone marrow biopsy shows 35% monoclonal plasma cells. She owns her own bookstore and runs a dessert catering service on the side. What is your next step in management?**
   A. Obtain fluorescence in situ hybridization (FISH) studies from bone marrow aspirate to risk-stratify and determine therapy
   B. Start bortezomib, lenalidomide, and dexamethasone and refer to bone marrow transplant (BMT) in preparation for autologous stem cell transplant
   C. Continue observation, and recheck complete blood count (CBC), serum creatinine, serum calcium, urine protein electrophoresis (UPEP) with immunofixation, serum protein electrophoresis (SPEP), and free light chain ratio in 6 to 8 weeks
   D. Obtain an MRI of the spine and pelvis to rule out bone lesions missed by routine skeletal survey

ANSWERS

1. **A. Bortezomib, lenalidomide, and dexamethasone (VRD), with stem cell collection after four cycles and plan for early autologous hematopoietic cell transplantation (HCT).** This patient has intermediate-risk disease by FISH analysis (t(4;14) and deletion 13), which were classified as high risk until bortezomib-containing regimens brought their outcomes closer to that of standard-risk patients. The patient should therefore be treated with a bortezomib-containing regimen. This patient has a good performance status and should be considered for an autologous HCT, and therefore his stem cells should be collected after approximately the fourth cycle of induction therapy. KPD has not yet been approved in the frontline setting. Prolonged treatment with lenalidomide (generally, eight cycles or more) can interfere with the ability to mobilize and collect stem cells.

2. **C. Low-dose aspirin (81 or 100 mg daily).** This is a standard-risk patient for VTE on lenalidomide therapy as she is active without other VTE risk factors aside from lenalidomide being given with low-dose dexamethasone. For these patients, low-dose aspirin is sufficient for VTE prophylaxis.

3. **D. A and B.** Bisphosphonates have been shown in several studies to reduce risk of new skeletal events and reduce myeloma-related bone pain. Bisphosphonates may cause renal toxicity, so renal function must be monitored and doses adjusted as needed with treatment

4. **A. Definitive radiation to the humeral plasmacytoma followed by observation.** This patient has a solitary plasmacytoma of bone (SPB) with minimal (<10%) bone marrow involvement that does not meet the criteria for multiple myeloma (MM). Definitive radiation (total dose ≥40 Gy) is the standard of care for SPB, and after completing this, she would undergo surveillance for her underlying monoclonal gammopathy of undetermined significance (MGUS). PET/CT is important to rule out other possible bone lesions (ie, myeloma defining events) prior to a diagnosis of SPB with minimal marrow involvement.

5. **D. t(14;20).** Relapse within 1 year of HCT qualifies as high-risk MM. Trisomies and 1q+ qualify as low- and intermediate-risk disease, respectively. t(14;20), t(14;16), and del17p are cytogenetic markers of high-risk MM, along with lactate dehydrogenase (LDH) >upper limit normal (ULN) and evidence of plasma cell leukemia.

6. **D. Obtain an MRI of the spine and pelvis to rule out bone lesions missed by routine skeletal survey.** This patient has smoldering multiple myeloma based on her monoclonal serum protein of ≥3 g/dL and ≥10% clonal plasma cells in her bone marrow, but she has no evidence of end-organ damage. Prior to diagnosing her with smoldering myeloma and considering observation or clinical trial for smoldering myeloma, however,

she needs to be assessed for bone lesions that may have been missed by skeletal survey. This can be completed with whole body MRI, MRI total spine and pelvis (if whole body MRI is not available), or PET/CT. Up to 50% of patients without lytic lesions on skeletal survey demonstrate tumor-related lesions on more sensitive imaging.

AERODIGESTIVE MALIGNANCIES

II

10 | Non–Small Cell Lung Cancer

Manali Bhave and Gregory P. Kalemkerian

EPIDEMIOLOGY

- Poor prognostic factors include: male gender, older age, impaired performance status, and African American ethnicity.
- There is a decrease in large cell and small cell histologic subtypes and an increase in adenocarcinomas for both men and women.

ETIOLOGY AND RISK FACTORS

1. **What are the major risk factors for non–small cell lung cancer (NSCLC)?**
   - Smoking
   - Passive (second-hand) smoke
   - Radon and radioactive dust
   - Asbestos (synergistic with smoking)
   - Chronic obstructive pulmonary disease (COPD; emphysema), pulmonary fibrosis
   - Arsenic, chromium, nickel, cadmium
   - Polycyclic aromatic hydrocarbons
   - Prior history of lung cancer

2. **Do hereditary factors play a role in lung cancer development?**
   - Yes. Only 10% to 15% of smokers develop lung cancer, but the genetic mechanisms driving susceptibility to tobacco carcinogens are not known.
   - First-degree relatives of people with lung cancer have two- to threefold increased risk for lung cancer.
   - People with Li–Fraumeni syndrome who smoke have a threefold increased risk of lung cancer compared to smokers without an inherited mutation in p53.
   - Other rare genetic susceptibility syndromes have been identified, such as germline EGFR T790M mutation.

3. **What are the two most common mutations in NSCLC?**
   - p53 (inactivating mutations) in 50% to 60%
   - K-RAS (activating mutations) in 30% of adenocarcinomas

4. **What is the prevalence of sensitizing EGFR mutations (exon 19 deletion or L858R mutation)?**
   - About 10% in Western populations
   - 25% to 30% in the East Asian population

5. **Does NSCLC have simple chromosomal and molecular abnormalities?**
   - No. NSCLC is characterized by complex chromosomal and molecular abnormalities, with the complexity being directly related to the extent of tobacco smoke exposure.

6. **What is the major mechanism of smoking-induced carcinogenesis?**
   - Polycyclic aromatic hydrocarbons (benzopyrene), nitrosamines (NNK), and aromatic amines (4-aminobiphenyl) form DNA adducts by covalently binding to DNA, resulting in DNA misreplication and mutation.

SCREENING

1. **Who should undergo lung cancer screening with annual low-dose CT scan?**
   - High-risk subjects:
     - Current smokers or former smokers who quit within the last 15 years
     - 55 to 77 years of age
     - At least a 30-pack per year smoking history
   - CT screening in this population decreases lung-cancer-specific mortality by 20% and overall mortality by 7%.

PREVENTION

1. **Does beta-carotene prevent lung cancer in current smokers?**
   - No. In randomized trials, beta-carotene increased the incidence of lung cancer in smokers.

2. **Which medication/chemical compound has been shown to be effective in the prevention of lung cancer?**
   - None. Vitamin A does not provide a protective role. Smoking abstinence or cessation is the only intervention known to prevent lung cancer.

PATHOLOGY

1. **What are the major subtypes of NSCLC?**
   - Adenocarcinoma
     - Adenocarcinoma in situ (formerly bronchioloalveolar carcinoma)
   - Squamous cell carcinoma
   - Large cell undifferentiated carcinoma
   - Mixed tumors
     - Adenosquamous carcinoma

SIGNS AND SYMPTOMS

1. **What are the common paraneoplastic syndromes associated with NSCLC?**
   - Anorexia/cachexia
   - Humoral hypercalcemia (parathyroid hormone [PTH] related peptide)
   - Hypercoagulable state (Trousseau syndrome)

- Hypertrophic pulmonary osteoarthropathy (HPOA)
- Digital clubbing

DIAGNOSTIC WORKUP

1. **What is the first diagnostic step in the patient with incidentally found solitary pulmonary node (<3 cm in diameter)?**
   - Review of prior chest radiographs and/or CT scans

2. **What are the most critical decision-making points during diagnostic workup of NSCLC?**
   - Presence or absence of sites of disease that would preclude primary surgical resection or other potentially curative treatment options
     - Involvement of N2 or N3 lymph nodes; lymph nodes that are either enlarged by CT criteria or fluorodeoxyglucose (FDG)-PET-positive should be pathologically evaluated by endobronchial ultrasound or endoscopic ultrasound (EBUS/EUS) guided biopsy and/or mediastinoscopy/mediastinotomy. PET *does not* replace mediastinoscopy due to the incidence of false-positive and false-negative results. An exception can be made for a normal mediastinum on CT and PET imaging.
     - Presence of malignant pleural effusion or distant metastatic disease

3. **What immunohistochemical markers can be useful in the diagnosis or histologic subtyping of lung cancer?**
   - General
     - CK7+, CK20− (80% of primary lung cancers)
   - Adenocarcinoma
     - TTF-1+ (70% of primary lung adenocarcinoma)
     - Napsin A+ (>80% of primary lung adenocarcinoma)
     - Negative for mesothelioma markers (calretinin, WT1, CK 5/6, D2-40)
   - Squamous cell carcinoma
     - p63+, p40+
     - CK 5/6 (positive in squamous cell carcinoma and mesothelioma)

4. **What are the prognostic and predictive biomarkers for lung adenocarcinoma?**
   - Prognostic markers (define outcome regardless of specific therapy):
     - **EGFR** (mutation = better survival)
     - **K-RAS** (mutation = worse survival)
   - Predictive markers (predict outcome with a specific therapy):
     - **ERCC1** (high expression = resistance to platinum agents)
     - **RRM1** (high expression = resistance to gemcitabine)
     - **K-RAS** (mutation = resistance to EGFR-TKIs)
     - **EGFR** [del(19), L858R, L861Q, G719X] (sensitivity to EGFR tyrosine kinase inhibitors [TKIs])

- ○ **EGFR [T790M]** (resistance to first-generation EGFR-TKIs)
- ○ **EGFR [T790M]** (sensitivity to third-generation EGFR-TKIs)
- ○ **ALK** rearrangement (determined by fluorescence in situ hybridization [FISH]; sensitivity to crizotinib)
- ○ **ALK** [G2023R] (resistance to crizotinib)
- ○ **ROS1** rearrangement (determined by FISH; sensitivity to crizotinib)

5. **When should testing for EGFR mutation, ALK rearrangement, and ROS1 rearrangement be performed?**
   - Adenocarcinomas
   - Never smokers with any histologic subtype
   - Stage IV or incurable disease; there is no role for molecularly targeted therapy in stage I–III NSCLC, so routine testing will not be cost-effective.

STAGING

T/M		N	N0	N1	N2	N3
T1	**a** (<2 cm)		IA		IIA	
	b (2–3 cm)		IA			
T2	**a** (3–5 cm)		IB	IIA		
	b (5–7 cm)		IIA	IIB		
T3	• >7 cm • Invasion • Same lobe nodules		IIB	IIIA		IIIB
T4	• Extension • Ipsilateral lung					
M1a	• Pleural effusion • Contralateral lung		IV			
M1b	• Distant metastases					

Notes: Invasion = direct invasion of chest wall (including superior sulcus), diaphragm, phrenic nerve, mediastinal pleura, parietal pericardium; *or* tumor in main bronchus is <2 cm from carina (carina is *not* involved) or atelectasis/pneumonitis of entire lung. Extension = invades mediastinum, heart, great vessels, trachea, recurrent laryngeal nerve, esophagus, vertebral body, carina.

N1, lymph nodes within lobe up to and including hilum; N2, ipsilateral mediastinal/subcarinal lymph node(s); N3, contralateral mediastinal/hilar, ipsilateral or contralateral scalene, or supraclavicular lymph node(s); M1a, includes malignant pericardial effusion.

GENERAL TREATMENT PRINCIPLES

- For patients with stages IA, IB, IIA, IIB, IIIA, and IIIB disease, the intent of therapy is cure.
- A thoracic surgeon should evaluate every patient considered for curative surgical intervention.
- Completeness of resection: **R0**—complete; **R1**—*micro*scopic residual disease (positive margin); **R2**—*macro*scopic (gross) residual disease.
- Radiation therapy (RT) has a potential role in all stages of NSCLC: definitive in stages I–III; palliative in stage IV.
- Three-dimensional (3D)-conformal RT is a minimal standard for the delivery of thoracic RT.
- Chemotherapy can improve cure rates in early-stage NSCLC (stages IB–IIIB).
- Chemotherapy, molecularly targeted therapy, and immunotherapy can improve survival and improve quality of life in the palliative setting (stage IV).

1. **What are the general outcomes, as defined by 5-year survival rates, for patients with NSCLC?**
   - Stage IA = 70%
   - Stage IB = 60%
   - Stage IIA = 50%
   - Stage IIB = 40%
   - Stage IIIA = 20% to 30%
   - Stage IIIB = 15% to 25%
   - Stage IV <5%

TREATMENT BY STAGE

Clinical Stage IA, IB, IIA, and IIB

- Surgical resection is recommended (lobectomy or pneumonectomy plus mediastinal lymph node sampling or dissection).
- All patients being considered for lung resection should undergo preoperative pulmonary function testing with spirometry plus diffusing capacity (diffusing capacity of the lungs for carbon monoxide [DLCO]), as well as a general assessment of cardiac risk.
- Lobectomy or pneumonectomy yields better survival than sublobar resections (segmentectomy or wedge resection).
- Sublobar resection (segmentectomy or wedge resection) should be considered in patients who cannot tolerate lobectomy (medically inoperable due to poor pulmonary function or other comorbidities).
- For patients with IIB (T3-invasive N0) disease, en bloc resection is recommended.
- In patients who are medically inoperable or who decline surgery, 3D-conformal RT (stages I or II), stereotactic ablative radiotherapy (SABR; stage I), or radiofrequency ablation (RFA; stage I) should be considered with curative intent.
- What should be done if resection margins are positive?

○ R1: re-resect if possible (best option); RT (if re-resection is not possible or patient declines re-operation)
○ R2: concurrent chemotherapy plus RT

Pathologic Stage IA and IB After Complete Resection

- No proven benefit for adjuvant therapy for stage IA or IB (if <4 cm)
- Consider adjuvant chemotherapy in "high-risk" stage IB with tumor diameter >4 cm

Pathologic Stage IIA, IIB, IIIA, and IIIB After Complete Resection

- Adjuvant chemotherapy for patients with good performance status and uncomplicated surgical recovery within 6 to 12 weeks of resection.
- Cisplatin-based, two-drug regimens × 4 cycles can improve 5-year overall survival by 4% to 15% in patients with stage II and III NSCLC; cisplatin plus vinorelbine was the most commonly used regimen in trials of adjuvant chemotherapy that demonstrated a survival benefit. Cisplatin plus etoposide, gemcitabine or pemetrexed (nonsquamous only) can also be considered.
- Carboplatin-based, two-drug regimens × 4 cycles are acceptable in patients with contraindications to or intolerance of cisplatin.
- For patients with stage IIIA or IIIB, MRI or CT of the brain should be performed if not done as part of preoperative staging.
- For patients with stage IIIA (N2+), consider sequential RT after adjuvant chemotherapy is completed to decrease local recurrence and possibly improve overall survival.

Superior Sulcus (Pancoast) Tumors, Stage IIB, IIIA, or IIIB (T3–4 N0–1)

- Neoadjuvant concurrent chemotherapy plus RT followed by resection is recommended.
- If unresectable or medically inoperable, then recommend definitive chemotherapy plus RT.

Clinical Stage IIIA (Clinically Heterogeneous Group)

Stage IIIA (T3N1)
- Surgical resection with adjuvant chemotherapy.
- If unresectable or medically inoperable, recommend definitive chemotherapy plus RT (see stage IIIA-N2+ in the following).

Stage IIIA (T1-3N2)
- Confirm N2 lymph node involvement by biopsy of mediastinal lymph nodes by EBUS/EUS-guided biopsy, mediastinoscopy, or mediastinotomy.
- MRI or CT of brain is recommended as part of initial evaluation.
- Concurrent chemotherapy plus definitive RT yields better overall survival than sequential chemotherapy followed by RT.
- Sequential chemotherapy followed by definitive RT yields better overall survival than RT alone.
- Definitive RT dose with standard fractionation is 60 to 70 Gy in 2 Gy fractions.

- Reasonable regimens for use with concurrent RT are:
  - ○ Cisplatin plus etoposide × two cycles
  - ○ Carboplatin plus etoposide × two cycles
  - ○ Carboplatin plus paclitaxel (weekly) ± consolidation carboplatin plus paclitaxel × two cycles
  - ○ Cisplatin/carboplatin plus pemetrexed × three or four cycles (adenocarcinoma only)
- There is little evidence to support the use of induction or consolidation chemotherapy.
- There is little high-quality evidence supporting a role for surgery in stage IIIA NSCLC. Select patients with good performance status and nonbulky N2 disease who do not require pneumonectomy for complete resection may be candidates for neoadjuvant chemotherapy plus RT followed by lobectomy and mediastinal lymph node sampling/dissection.

Clinical Stage IIIB

- Confirm N2 or N3 lymph node involvement by biopsy of mediastinal lymph nodes by EBUS/EUS-guided biopsy, mediastinoscopy, or mediastinotomy.
- Concurrent chemotherapy plus definitive RT is recommended with curative intent per guidelines noted earlier for stage IIIA-N2+ disease.

1. **What is the role for prophylactic cranial irradiation (PCI) in patients with locally advanced (stage III) NSCLC?**
   - There is no role for PCI in locally advanced NSCLC as it does not improve overall survival.

Stage IV

- Stage IV NSCLC is incurable; all treatment is given with palliative intent with the primary goals of improving disease-related symptoms, maintaining quality of life, and prolonging survival.
- The addition of early palliative care consultation to standard oncologic care improves quality of life and overall survival.
- Cytologically confirmed malignant pleural or pericardial effusions indicate stage IV disease.
- Any solitary, FDG-PET-positive site that would preclude curative resection or define stage IV disease requires biopsy for pathological confirmation.
- All stage IV lung adenocarcinomas should be tested for *EGFR* mutation, *ALK* rearrangement, and *ROS1* rearrangement at the time of initial diagnosis.
- All stage IV NSCLCs should be tested for PD-L1 expression by immunohistochemistry.
- Unfit patients (Eastern Cooperative Oncology Group Performance Status [ECOG PS] 3–4) do *not* benefit from cytotoxic chemotherapy. Treatment with EGFR, ALK, or ROS1 inhibitors may be appropriate.

First-Line Therapy
DRIVER MUTATION POSITIVE

- For patients with tumors harboring an *EGFR* sensitizing mutation, treatment with an EGFR-TKI (erlotinib, gefitinib, afatinib) is the most appropriate first-line treatment option based on studies demonstrating improved response rates (60%–70%) and progression-free survival (9–12 months) when compared to chemotherapy.
- For patients with tumors harboring *ALK* or *ROS1* rearrangements, crizotinib is the most appropriate first-line treatment option based on studies demonstrating improved response rates (60%–70%) and progression-free survival (12–18 months).

DRIVER MUTATION NEGATIVE
Driver Mutation Negative, PD-L1 Positive

- For patients with tumors with high PD-L1 expression ($\geq$50% of tumor cells), pembrolizumab is superior to first-line chemotherapy with improved response rate and survival.

Driver Mutation Negative, PD-L1 Negative

- For first-line therapy, PD-L1 negative is defined as expression in less than 50% of tumor cells.
- Two-drug, platinum-based regimens are standard: carboplatin or cisplatin plus paclitaxel, docetaxel, pemetrexed (nonsquamous only), gemcitabine, vinorelbine, or etoposide.
- Cisplatin and carboplatin are equivalent in efficacy in stage IV NSCLC. Carboplatin is less toxic, so it is the more reasonable option in the palliative setting.
- There is no benefit to first-line combination chemotherapy beyond four to six cycles.
- Nonsquamous histology (adenocarcinoma, large cell carcinoma, non–small cell lung cancer, not otherwise specified [NSCLC-NOS]):
  - Cisplatin + pemetrexed are superior to cisplatin + gemcitabine.
  - Carboplatin, paclitaxel + bevacizumab (15 mg/kg every 3 weeks) followed by maintenance bevacizumab are superior to carboplatin + paclitaxel alone.
  - Carboplatin, pemetrexed + bevacizumab followed by maintenance pemetrexed + bevacizumab appear to be equivalent to carboplatin, paclitaxel + bevacizumab followed by bevacizumab.
  - Carboplatin + pemetrexed followed by maintenance pemetrexed are equivalent to carboplatin, paclitaxel + bevacizumab followed by maintenance bevacizumab.
- Squamous cell histology:
  - Pemetrexed is not indicated due to lack of efficacy in squamous cell carcinoma.
  - Bevacizumab should not be used due to excessive risk of massive hemoptysis.
  - Adding necitumumab (anti-EGFR monoclonal antibody) to cisplatin + gemcitabine led to a modest improvement in overall survival compared to cisplatin + gemcitabine alone.
  - Reasonable regimens include: carboplatin + gemcitabine; carboplatin + paclitaxel; carboplatin + *nab*-paclitaxel.

- Maintenance therapy:
  - ○ Consider maintenance therapy in patients with good performance status who have tolerated chemotherapy well.
  - ○ For patients with marginal performance status or significant toxicity from therapy, consider holding chemotherapy to allow recovery, with close surveillance and initiation of second-line therapy upon progression of disease.
  - ○ No clear role for maintenance therapy of any type in squamous cell carcinoma.
  - ○ Continuation maintenance:
    - ■ Bevacizumab after four to six cycles of chemotherapy plus bevacizumab
    - ■ Pemetrexed after four to six cycles of platinum plus pemetrexed may improve overall survival
  - ○ Switch maintenance:
    - ■ Pemetrexed after non-pemetrexed-containing chemotherapy for nonsquamous histology
    - ■ Erlotinib after platinum-based chemotherapy yields marginal clinical benefits
- Expected outcomes with platinum-based regimens:
  - ○ Objective response rate: 25% to 35%
  - ○ Median progression-free survival: 4 to 6 months
  - ○ Overall survival rate: 1 year = 30% to 40%; 2 years = 15% to 20%
- Carboplatin-based doublets should be considered for patients with advanced NSCLC with a performance status of 2.
- Fit elderly patients tolerate chemotherapy and treatment should be offered. They derive similar survival benefits as younger patients.

Subsequent Therapy at Relapse
DRIVER MUTATION POSITIVE

- For patients with EGFR mutation+ NSCLC, obtain repeat biopsy to evaluate for presence of T790M resistance mutation, which is present in 60% of tumors that progress on an EGFR-TKI. If T790M+, then osimertinib is the most appropriate second-line therapy with a response rate of 60%.
- For patients with ALK-rearranged NSCLC, second-generation ALK inhibitors, such as ceritinib or alectinib, are recommended upon progression on crizotinib.
- After progression on all available therapies targeting EGFR, ALK or ROS1, then patients should be treated with either first-line combination chemotherapy or immunotherapy as noted previously in the section on First-line Therapy, Driver Mutation Negative.

DRIVER MUTATION NEGATIVE

- Chemotherapy
  - ○ Docetaxel is superior to best supportive care or vinorelbine or ifosfamide.
  - ○ Docetaxel is equivalent to pemetrexed (all histologic subtypes included).
  - ○ Carboplatin plus pemetrexed is equivalent to pemetrexed alone (all histologic subtypes included).

- ○ Combination chemotherapy may improve response rate and progression-free survival, but also increases toxicity and does not improve overall survival.
- Molecularly targeted therapy
  - ○ Erlotinib is superior to best supportive care as second- or third-line therapy (*EGFR* mutational status not determined; all histologic subtypes included).
  - ○ Docetaxel plus ramucirumab (anti-VEGFR monoclonal antibody) provides a modest improvement in overall survival compared to docetaxel alone (all histologic subtypes included).
- Immunotherapy
  - ○ Nivolumab, an anti-PD1 monoclonal antibody, and atezolizumab, an anti-PD-L1 monoclonal antibody, induce response in 15% to 20% of patients and improve overall survival over docetaxel in patients who progress after first-line platinum-based chemotherapy without regard for level of PD-L1 expression. Therefore, PD-L1 testing is not required to use nivolumab or atezolizumab in the second-line setting.
  - ○ Pembrolizumab, an anti-PD1 monoclonal antibody, induces response in 40 to 45% of patients with metastatic NSCLC who do not have EGFR or ALK genetic tumor abnormalities and whose tumors have high PD-L1 expression (≥50%). Pembrolizumab can be used as first-line therapy in patients with metastatic non–small cell lung cancer whose tumors have high PD-L1 expression [tumor proportion score ≥50%].
  - ○ Pembrolizumab, an anti-PD1 monoclonal antibody, improves overall survival compared to docetaxel in patients who progress after first-line platinum-based chemotherapy and whose tumors express PD-L1 in ≥1% of tumor cells.

QUESTIONS

1. A 60-year-old man with a past medical history for hypertension and coronary artery disease with a 45 pack-year history of smoking presents to his primary care physician for his annual physical examination. He has no history of cancer, but continues to smoke. His father, a smoker, died of lung cancer at age 74 and his mother died of heart disease. He underwent his first screening colonoscopy approximately 10 years ago and was told the colonoscopy did not show any polyps.
In addition to referring the patient for his 10-year screening colonoscopy, what other age-appropriate cancer screening should be recommended for this patient?
   A. No other cancer screening is recommended at this time
   B. Ultrasound of the prostate
   C. Urinary cytology
   D. Low-dose helical CT scan

2. A 72-year-old woman with a past medical history of rheumatoid arthritis presents to the thoracic oncology clinic with a new diagnosis of lung cancer. CT scan shows a 4 cm right lower lobe mass, a 1 cm right lower lobe nodule, a 1.5 cm left upper lobe nodule, bilateral hilar and mediastinal lymphadenopathy, and three enhancing lesions in the liver

measuring up to 2.4 cm. Percutaneous core needle biopsy of one of the liver nodules revealed a poorly differentiated carcinoma that was immunohistochemically positive for CK7, TTF-1, and napsin A and negative for CK20, p63, and CK 5/6.

What molecular diagnostic studies would be useful in determining appropriate first-line therapy for this patient?

A. Immunohistochemistry for EGFR expression
B. Sequencing for PD-L1 mutation
C. Fluorescence in situ hybridization (FISH) analysis for *ALK* and *ROS1* rearrangement
D. Serum vascular endothelial growth factor (VEGF) concentration

3. A 63-year-old woman with a 60 pack-year smoking history presents to medical oncology to discuss treatment for newly diagnosed squamous cell carcinoma of the lung. CT of the chest shows a 7 cm right upper lobe mass with enlarged right hilar and bilateral mediastinal lymph nodes. PET/CT shows fluorodeoxyglucose (FDG) avidity in the right upper lobe mass and in the right hilar and bilateral mediastinal lymph nodes, but no evidence of distant metastases. MRI of the brain shows no metastases. Percutaneous biopsy of the right upper lobe nodule shows squamous cell carcinoma.

What is the next appropriate step in the management of this patient?

A. Endobronchial ultrasound guided biopsy of mediastinal lymph nodes
B. Definitive chemoradiotherapy
C. Palliative chemotherapy
D. Assessment of for *EGFR* mutation plus *ALK* and *ROS1* rearrangement

4. A 55-year-old man with a past medical history notable for tobacco abuse presents to the thoracic oncology clinic with a new diagnosis of lung cancer. He developed a productive cough a few weeks ago, which prompted a CT of the chest that showed a 3 cm right lower lobe spiculated mass with no lymphadenopathy. Pulmonary function testing revealed mild obstructive deficit with intact diffusing capacity. He underwent a right lower lobectomy with mediastinal lymph node sampling. Surgical pathology confirmed a 2.9 cm squamous cell carcinoma with negative margins and no involvement of hilar or mediastinal lymph nodes. He now presents to the thoracic oncology clinic to discuss further care.

What is the most appropriate next step in the treatment of this patient?

A. Adjuvant chemotherapy with cisplatin + gemcitabine × four cycles
B. Adjuvant chemotherapy with cisplatin + pemetrexed × four cycles
C. Adjuvant radiation to the right hilum and mediastinum
D. Active surveillance with thoracic CT scans

5. A 60-year-old man with a history of tobacco abuse presents to the emergency room with right upper quadrant abdominal pain. CT of the abdomen shows multiple masses within the liver suspicious for metastatic disease. CT of the chest is notable for a left lower lobe 5.5 cm

mass, multiple small bilateral pulmonary nodules, and enlarged ipsilateral hilar and mediastinal lymph nodes. MRI of the brain does not
show any evidence of intracranial metastases. Percutaneous biopsy
of one of the liver lesions reveals adenocarcinoma of lung primary.
Molecular studies for *EGFR* mutation and *ALK* and *ROS1* rearrangements are negative. PD-L1 expression is present in 20% of tumor cells.
His pain is controlled with hydrocodone–acetaminophen 10–325 mg
as needed and his Eastern Cooperative Oncology Group Performance
Status (ECOG PS) is 1.

What is the most appropriate next step in the management of this
patient's disease?

A. Palliative care plus chemotherapy with cisplatin, gemcitabine, and
   bevacizumab × four cycles
B. Palliative care plus chemotherapy with carboplatin + pemetrexed ×
   four cycles
C. PET/CT scan
D. Palliative immunotherapy with nivolumab every 2 weeks

6. A 62-year-old former smoker with a diagnosis of stage IV squamous
cell carcinoma of the lung completed four cycles of carboplatin +
gemcitabine 3 months ago with good partial response. He has recovered well from the side effects of treatment and he has an Eastern
Cooperative Oncology Group Performance Status (ECOG PS) of 1
with a stable cough and recent 8 lb weight loss. A repeat CT scan
shows growth of a right lower lobe mass from 3.0 to 4.5 cm, enlarging
mediastinal lymph nodes and left adrenal mass, and multiple new liver
lesions. His initial biopsy is inadequate for further immunohistochemical analysis and he declines repeat biopsy.

What is the most appropriate next step in treatment for this patient?

A. Cisplatin + paclitaxel
B. Pembrolizumab
C. Nivolumab
D. Prophylactic cranial irradiation to prevent intracranial metastases

ANSWERS

1. **D. Low-dose helical CT scan.** A low-dose helical CT scan should be recommended for lung cancer screening in current smokers or former smokers who quit within the last 15 years who are 55 to 77 years of age and have at least a 30 pack-year smoking history. Annual low-dose CT screening improves lung-cancer-specific and overall mortality. The screening process should include counseling on the risks and benefits of the procedure and assistance with smoking cessation.

2. **C. Fluorescence in situ hybridization (FISH) analysis for *ALK* and *ROS1* rearrangement.** Pathologic analysis of the patient's liver biopsy is consistent with metastatic lung adenocarcinoma. All metastatic lung adenocarcinomas should be tested for *EGFR* sensitizing mutations, *ALK* rearrangement, and *ROS1* rearrangement at the time of diagnosis to determine whether they are candidates for first-line targeted therapy. Expression of the EGFR protein is not useful for determining the utility of EGFR-TKI therapy. PD-L1 expression may correlate with response to anti-PD1 therapy, but PD-L1 mutations have no known predictive value for guiding treatment. There are no validated biomarkers to predict the clinical utility of antiangiogenic therapy, so evaluation of VEGF levels is not indicated.

3. **A. Endobronchial ultrasound guided biopsy of mediastinal lymph nodes.** Patients with clinical evidence of mediastinal lymph node involvement by CT or PET imaging should undergo pathologic confirmation of lymph node involvement prior to the initiation of therapy. The false-positive rate of PET in mediastinal lymph nodes is about 10%, so the decision to forego potentially curative surgical resection should not be based on imaging studies alone. If the patient is proven to have stage III non–small cell lung cancer (NSCLC) by biopsy of mediastinal lymph nodes then appropriate therapy would be definitive chemoradiotherapy. Molecular analysis does not have a role in the management of stage I, II, or III disease.

4. **D. Active surveillance with thoracic CT scans.** There is no role for adjuvant chemotherapy or radiotherapy for patients with stage IA (T1-2N0M0) non–small cell lung cancer (NSCLC). Adjuvant chemotherapy improves survival in patients with completely resected stage II and III NSCLC, and may also benefit those with "high-risk" stage IB disease with tumor diameter ≥4 cm. The benefits of postoperative radiotherapy are controversial, but it may benefit patients with completely resected stage III-N2 disease. Recommended follow-up for patients with pathologic stage IA NSCLC includes active surveillance with routine clinical evaluations and thoracic CT scans.

5. **B. Palliative care plus chemotherapy with carboplatin + pemetrexed × 4 cycles.** The patient has biopsy-proven metastatic lung adenocarcinoma. There is no need to obtain PET/CT in patients with confirmed metastatic disease. Early palliative care combined with standard oncologic care

improves quality of life and survival in patients with stage IV non–small cell lung cancer (NSCLC). Two-drug, platinum-based regimens are the standard treatment for stage IV disease with platinum + pemetrexed demonstrating superiority over platinum + gemcitabine in lung adenocarcinoma. The addition of bevacizumab does not improve the efficacy of cisplatin + gemcitabine. Pembrolizumab is approved for first-line therapy in metastatic NSCLC if additional immunohistochemical staining is performed on the biopsy and shows PD-L1 expression $\geq$50%.

6. **C. Nivolumab.** The patient has had progressive metastatic squamous cell carcinoma only 3 months after completion of first-line platinum-based therapy. Further combination therapy may induce response, but will not improve survival over single-agent therapy. Nivolumab, atezolizumab and pembrolizumab are approved for treatment of metastatic non–small cell lung cancer (NSCLC) that has progressed after platinum-based chemotherapy based on studies demonstrating improved overall survival when compared to docetaxel. However, pembrolizumab is only approved in patients with tumors that express PD-L1. PD-L1 testing would require additional immunohistochemical staining on a previously obtained or fresh biopsy. Since this patient does not have adequate tissue for such testing, he is not a candidate for pembrolizumab, but would be a candidate for nivolumab or atezolizumab. There is no role for prophylactic cranial irradiation in patients with any stage of NSCLC.

11 Small Cell Lung Cancer

Dana E. Angelini and Khaled A. Hassan

EPIDEMIOLOGY

1. **What is the incidence of small cell lung cancer (SCLC)?**
   - SCLC represents approximately 13% of new cases of lung cancers diagnosed annually.
   - The incidence of SCLC has decreased over the last few decades, and the proportion of males and females affected is roughly equal.

ETIOLOGY AND RISK FACTORS

1. **What is the main risk factor for SCLC?**
   - More than 90% of patients with SCLC are current or past smokers and the risk is related to magnitude of tobacco exposure.

2. **What are the most common molecular abnormalities of SCLC?**
   - The pathophysiology of SCLC follows a multistep carcinogenesis model, which is the accumulation of genetic abnormalities that ultimately result in malignant transformation. There are, however, several molecular abnormalities commonly seen in SCLC:
     - 3p deletion is almost ubiquitous in SCLC, which differentiates it from small cell cancer of extrapulmonary origin.
     - Mutation of tumor suppressor genes such as p53 (located on chromosome 17p13) and retinoblastoma (located on chromosome 13q14) is found in more than 80% of SCLC.
     - Upregulation of myc pathways and overexpression of c-kit are also common.

3. **What is the difference between non–small cell lung cancer (NSCLC) and SCLC?**
   - Compared to NSCLC, SCLC has rapid doubling time, higher growth fraction, and early widespread hematogenous metastases.
     - SCLC is typically centrally located and is highly sensitive to initial chemotherapy and radiation.
     - Despite high initial rates of response, most patients die from recurrent disease.
     - NSCLC can be associated with several genetic driver alterations, such as EGFR, ALK, and ROS1. SCLC does not have driver mutations amenable to currently available targeted drug therapies.

SCREENING

1. **Who should be screened with low-dose helical CT scan?**
   - Same population as those screened for NSCLC:
     - ○ High-risk patients: that is, current or former smokers 55 to 74 years old with ≥30 pack-year smoking history
     - ○ There is no clear impact on mortality for patients with SCLC (as opposed to 20% reduction in mortality for those with NSCLC)

PREVENTION

1. **Have there been any positive clinical trials to reduce the incidence of SCLC in smokers?**
   - No, the only known intervention for the prevention of NSCLC and SCLC is cessation of smoking.

SIGNS AND SYMPTOMS

1. **What are the common clinical presentations of SCLC?**
   - Symptoms of SCLC are similar to NSCLC; these are either local or systemic symptoms.
   - The primary tumor is more likely to be centrally located. Local symptoms related to intrathoracic bulk of disease include shortness of breath, persistent cough, hemoptysis, hoarseness, postobstructive pneumonia, as well as superior vena cava (SVC) syndrome (from local invasion in right paratracheal region).
   - Systemic symptoms related to hematogenous spread include fatigue, anorexia, weight loss, fever, and/or paraneoplastic syndromes.

2. **What are common sites of metastasis?**
   - Virtually any organ may be affected, yet favored sites are brain, liver, bone, and adrenal glands.
   - Central nervous system (CNS) metastasis are present in 15% of patients at presentation (can be silent or symptomatic).

3. **What are the common paraneoplastic syndromes related to SCLC?**
   - Up to 15% of SCLC patients will develop paraneoplastic syndromes due to ectopic production of polypeptides or antibodies irrespective of stage. SCLC is the most frequent cause of paraneoplastic syndromes.
   - The most common paraneoplastic syndromes are syndrome of inappropriate secretion of antidiuretic hormone (SIADH), ectopic adrenocorticotropic hormone (ACTH) production, and Lambert–Eaton syndrome.
   - Effective treatment of the underlying tumor usually controls peptide-related endocrine syndromes.
   - Hypercalcemia due to PTHrP is *rare* in SCLC; this paraneoplastic syndrome is more common in squamous histology.

Syndrome	Tumor Factor
Endocrine	
Cushing syndrome	ACTH
SIADH	Arginine vasopressin
Neurologic	
Central nervous system	
Subacute cerebellar degeneration	Anti-Hu Ab
Encephalomyelitis	Anti-Hu Ab
Myoclonus–opsoclonus	Unclear causative Ab
Cancer associated retinopathy	Antirecoverin Ab
Peripheral nervous system	
Subacute sensory neuropathy	Anti-Hu Ab
Subacute motor neuropathy	Anti-Hu antibody/anti-CV2 Ab
Autonomic neuropathy (Ogilvie syndrome)	Antibodies against myenteric plexuses
Neuromuscular junction	
Eaton–Lambert syndrome	Anti-P/Q calcium channel Ab

DIAGNOSIS

1. **What are the imaging modalities used for diagnosis and staging?**
   - CT of the chest extending through adrenal glands, and MRI of the brain are standards of care. PET/CT if limited stage is suspected as it will improve the accuracy of staging. If PET/CT cannot be performed, a nuclear medicine bone scan should be pursued.

2. **What are the pathologic features of SCLC?**
   - Macroscopically the tumor is typically soft, friable with extensive necrosis.
   - Histopathologic features include round small blue cells with high nuclear: cytoplasmic ratio.
   - SCLC generally stains positive for thyroid transcription factor-1, CK7, CD56 (NCAM), synaptophysin, chromogranin A, and neuron-specific enolase (NSE).

STAGING

1. **How is SCLC staged?**
   - The most widely used staging is the simplified two-stage system developed by the Veterans Administration Lung Cancer Study Group (VALCSG). The American Joint Committee on Cancer Tumor–Node–Metastasis (AJCC TNM) staging showed prognostic significance in SCLC.

Limited stage	Median survival	14–20 month
Disease confined to ipsilateral hemithorax within a single radiation port	2-year survival	40%
Extensive stage	Median survival	8–12 month
Disease beyond ipsilateral hemithorax or obvious metastatic disease	2-year survival	5%

PROGNOSTIC FACTORS

1. **What are prognostic factors for SCLC?**
   - Poor performance status (PS), extensive-stage disease, weight loss, presence of paraneoplastic syndrome, and increased lactate dehydrogenase (LDH) are adverse prognostic factors.
   - Most patients present with metastatic disease; only a third present with limited stage.

TREATMENT

1. **What is the role of chemotherapy in SCLC?**
   - Treatment of SCLC depends on stage; yet chemotherapy is an essential component of appropriate treatment and dramatically prolongs survival compared to best supportive care.
   - Main chemotherapeutic agents used: cisplatin/carboplatin; etoposide; topotecan/irinotecan.

2. **What is the goal of therapy in SCLC?**
   - In limited stage, the goal is to achieve cure with concurrent chemotherapy and thoracic radiation.
   - In extensive stage, the goal of therapy is palliation with chemotherapy.

3. **What is the treatment of limited-stage SCLC?**
   - Current standard of care for limited-stage SCLC is combination of cisplatin plus etoposide with concurrent thoracic radiation. Dual modality treatment in limited-stage disease has an overall response rate of >80%, complete response rate of 40% to 60%, and cure rate of 20%.
     - Addition of thoracic radiation to chemotherapy increases the absolute survival by approximately 5% at 3 years compared to chemotherapy alone.
   - Radiation administered concurrently with chemotherapy is more efficacious than sequential therapy. Early incorporation of radiation is recommended.
     - Twice daily radiation can be used for patients with good PS to a total of 45 Gy. However, daily radiation with total 60 to 70 Gy is an acceptable alternative.
     - A total of four to six chemotherapy cycles is standard practice, followed by prophylactic cranial irradiation (PCI) 4 to 6 weeks after completion of therapy.

4. What is the treatment of extensive-stage SCLC?

- For patients with extensive-stage disease, chemotherapy is the recommended treatment. Combination of a platinum (cisplatin or carboplatin) and etoposide is the most widely used frontline regimen. The response rates range from 60% to 70% (complete remission 10%), with median survival time of 9 to 11 months. However, overall survival remains poor with less than 5% of extensive-stage disease patients alive at 2 years.

- In patients with extensive stage and brain metastases, chemotherapy can be given either before or after whole-brain radiation therapy (WBRT) depending on the presence of neurologic symptoms, given increased toxicity with concurrent treatment.

5. When do we recommend PCI in SCLC?

- PCI decreases the incidence of brain metastasis and improves overall survival in limited-stage SCLC patients who achieve complete response after primary therapy, increasing 3-year survival by approximately 5%.

- PCI decreases the risk of symptomatic brain metastasis by about 25% in extensive-stage SCLC and also improves 1-year survival by 14%.
  - Dose of PCI: 25 to 36 Gy is optimal, delivered in 2 to 3 Gy daily
  - Need to balance side effects of PCI with benefit in elderly (ie, >70 years old) patients

6. What are the common complications of treatment?

- Concurrent chemoradiation has an increased risk of esophagitis, dysphagia, odynophagia, oropharyngeal/esophageal candidiasis, and pneumonitis.

7. Is there any role for maintenance chemotherapy in SCLC?

- No, maintenance therapy increases toxicity and has not shown significant survival benefit.

8. Can carboplatin be substituted for cisplatin in extensive-stage SCLC?

- Since chemotherapy in extensive-stage setting is palliative, carboplatin is often substituted for cisplatin to minimize toxicity with no significant difference in response rate or median survival time.

9. What is the treatment recommendation for progressive SCLC?

- Although SCLC is very sensitive to initial therapy, most patients relapse within a few months of completing initial therapy. Outcome of treatment of relapsed disease depends on duration of response to initial therapy.

Definitions of Disease Progression

Sensitive relapse	Tumor progression occurs 90 days or more after the last day of initial treatment
Resistant relapse	Tumor progression occurs within 90 days after the last day of initial treatment
Refractory	Tumor progresses during the initial therapy or did not respond to initial therapy

- Treatment of sensitive relapse: if relapse is >6 months from initial treatment, repeating the original regimen is preferred. If relapse occurs between 3 and 6 months, then topotecan is the Food and Drug Administration (FDA)-approved second line of treatment.
- There is no standard treatment for patients with resistant relapse or refractory disease; whenever possible, such patients should be enrolled in a clinical trial.
- Single-agent chemotherapy with activity for disease progression includes paclitaxel, docetaxel, oral etoposide, irinotecan, temozolomide, and gemcitabine.
- Relapsed SCLC has a median survival of approximately 6 months with therapy.

10. **How should we treat an elderly patient with good PS (Eastern Cooperative Oncology Group Performance Status [ECOG PS] 0 or 1)?**
    - Overall, elderly patients have a similar prognosis when compared to stage-matched younger patients. There is evidence that single agent etoposide is inferior to combination chemotherapy etoposide and cisplatin (EP) in elderly patients with good PS (0–2). Four cycles of carboplatin and etoposide appear to yield favorable results, as the area under the curve (AUC) dosing of carboplatin takes into account the declining renal function of the aging patient.

11. **What is the role of surgery in SCLC?**
    - In rare cases, SCLC is diagnosed at an early stage (ie, T1–2 N0). Surgical resection is recommended followed by adjuvant chemotherapy.

12. **What is the role of immunotherapy or molecular targets in SCLC?**
    - Trials evaluating targeted therapy in SCLC have not demonstrated benefit.
    - Immune checkpoint inhibitors have demonstrated encouraging results in early phase trials, showing a benefit in both platinum sensitive and platinum refractory SCLC. Several clinical trials are ongoing, the results of which are needed prior to making strong conclusions about the use of these agents.

13. **How do we follow SCLC following the completion of therapy?**
    - Follow-up physical examination and CT scan are recommended every 3 to 4 months during the first 2 years. The frequency of surveillance decreases with subsequent years in light of declining risk of recurrence.

QUESTIONS

1. A 65-year-old male with history of well-controlled hypertension, type 2 diabetes, chronic obstructive pulmonary disease (COPD), and 50 pack-year smoking history presents with cough and 15 lb weight loss over the past 2 months. CT of the chest, abdomen, and pelvis reveals a left upper lobe lung mass, mediastinal lymphadenopathy, and innumerable liver lesions. Biopsy of a liver lesion reveals small cell carcinoma consistent with lung primary. He denies headache, visual changes, and motor or sensory impairment. His performance status is 1 and he is motivated for therapy.
   Which of the following studies is needed to complete staging?
   A. MRI brain
   B. PET scan

C. Bone scan

D. None of these stagings is complete

2. A 57-year-old female with history of emphysema and 60 pack-year smoking history presents with fatigue, weight loss, and increased shortness of breath. CT of chest reveals a 13 cm right hilar mass, with mediastinal and right side hilar lymphadenopathy. Full staging imaging is pursued, which reveals multiple bone and liver lesions. Biopsy of a liver lesion returns as small cell carcinoma consistent with lung primary. Her performance status is 1.

Which of the following is the best treatment option for this patient?

A. Carboplatin/pemetrexed for four to six cycles followed by prophylactic cranial irradiation (PCI)

B. Concurrent chemoradiation to primary lesion followed by systemic therapy

C. Carboplatin/etoposide for four to six cycles followed by observation

D. Carboplatin/etoposide for four to six cycles followed by PCI

3. A 65-year-old female with a 45 pack-year smoking history underwent a CT of the chest following a motor vehicle accident. The CT incidentally noted a 1.5 cm suspicious lesion in her right upper lobe. After she recovered from her injuries, a biopsy of this lesion was pursued and returned as small cell lung cancer (SCLC). PET/CT imaging and brain MRI were performed to complete staging. The results of complete staging studies show a standardized uptake value (SUV) of 20 of the known neoplasm, but no evidence of distant metastatic disease. She undergoes right upper lobectomy and the final tumor size is 1.7 cm with no lymph node involvement. Which of the following is the most appropriate therapy following surgical resection?

A. Adjuvant chemotherapy with four cycles of platinum/etoposide

B. Radiation to mediastinum

C. Observation

D. Concurrent chemoradiotherapy

4. Which of the following molecular abnormalities is seen in the vast majority of small cell lung cancer (SCLC) cases?

A. EGFR mutation

B. 3p deletion

C. RAS mutation

D. ROS-1 rearrangement

5. A 53-year-old female presents to clinic for evaluation of cycle 1 carboplatin/etoposide for recently diagnosed extensive-stage small cell lung cancer (SCLC). Staging scans revealed primary lung mass in left upper lobe, mediastinal lymphadenopathy, and multiple liver lesions. Brain MRI from 2 weeks ago is negative for brain metastasis or other significant abnormalities. She describes irritability, confusion, headache, and right side paraparesis and states these symptoms have been present for the past 6 weeks.

Which of the following is likely the underlying pathophysiology of her neurologic complaints?

A. Development of new brain metastasis
B. Anti-Hu antibodies
C. Antirecoverin Ab
D. Antimyelin antibodies

6. A 64-year-old male with a 150 pack-year smoking history initially presented with cough and shortness of breath. Workup included CT of the chest, which showed a 3 cm left hilar lung mass and mediastinal lymphadenopathy. Subsequent mediastinoscopy showed a paratracheal node and biopsy of this node returned as small cell lung cancer. PET/CT showed several liver lesions and innumerable bone lesions throughout his skeleton. MRI of the brain was negative for brain metastasis. He completed four cycles of carboplatin/etoposide with an excellent partial response. Therapy was followed by prophylactic cranial irradiation (PCI). He returns for follow-up 8 months later with progressive fatigue and weight loss, and CT of chest, abdomen, and pelvis confirms recurrent disease.

What is the next best line of therapy for this patient?

A. Initiation of topotecan
B. Initiation of docetaxel
C. Reinitiation of carboplatin/etoposide
D. Initiation of vinorelbine

ANSWERS

1. **A. MRI brain.** Central nervous system (CNS) metastases are present in 15% of patients at diagnosis and can be asymptomatic. It is important to know the extent and burden of disease when designing the initial treatment plan. PET scan and bone scan will not give you more information, since it is already known he has extensive-stage disease.

2. **D. Carboplatin/etoposide for four to six cycles followed by PCI.** First-line treatment of extensive-stage small cell lung cancer (SCLC) consists of systemic chemotherapy with platinum and etoposide. PCI decreased the risk of symptomatic brain metastasis by about 25% in extensive-stage SCLC and improves 1-year survival by 14%.

3. **A. Adjuvant chemotherapy with four cycles of platinum/etoposide.** Surgery alone is inadequate therapy for limited-stage SCLC resulting in less than 5% long-term survival. Adjuvant chemotherapy after surgery results in prolonged survival and cure for a significant number of patients with surgically resected limited-stage SCLC.

4. **B. 3p deletion.** SCLC commonly has 3p deletion; however, the mechanism of this deletion is unknown.

5. **B. Anti-Hu antibodies.** The patient is describing symptoms of encephalomyelitis, a paraneoplastic syndrome associated with SCLC. Anti-Hu antibodies are associated with this disorder. New brain lesions are unlikely, given the timing of symptoms and the recent negative brain MRI.

6. **C. Reinitiation of carboplatin/etoposide.** The patient has sensitive relapse, defined as tumor progression ≥90 days after the last day of initial treatment. Since relapse has occurred beyond 6 months, repeating the original platinum/etoposide combination is recommended.

Malignant Pleural Mesothelioma

Jordan K. Schaefer and Gregory P. Kalemkerian

EPIDEMIOLOGY

1. **In what patient population does mesothelioma occur?**
   - Mesothelioma typically occurs in older men (median age at diagnosis is about 70 years) with a previous history of industrial asbestos exposure.

ETIOLOGY AND RISK FACTORS

1. **What are the most common risk factors for the development of mesothelioma?**
   - Occupational asbestos exposure is documented in 75% of patients with pleural mesothelioma
   - Prior thoracic therapeutic irradiation
   - Cigarette smoking is *not* associated with an increased risk of mesothelioma
   - Familial mesothelioma is rare and is caused by heritable germline mutations in BRCA1-associated protein (BAP1)

2. **What is the latency period between asbestos exposure and the development of mesothelioma?**
   - Three to four decades following exposure to asbestos

STAGING AND HISTOLOGICAL CLASSIFICATION

1. **Define the staging for malignant pleural mesothelioma.**
   - The International Mesothelioma Interest Group Staging System:

Stage	Criteria
I	Tumor involving ipsilateral parietal pleura with or without involvement of visceral pleura, without lymph node involvement or distant metastases
II	Tumor involving each of the ipsilateral pleural surfaces (parietal, mediastinal, diaphragmatic, visceral) with invasion of the pulmonary parenchyma and/or invasion of diaphragmatic muscle, without lymph node involvement or distant metastases

(continued)

(continued)

Stage	Criteria
III	Potentially resectable tumor involving all ipsilateral pleural surfaces (parietal, mediastinal, diaphragmatic, visceral) with at least one of the following: a solitary, resectable site of invasion of the chest wall; invasion of the endothoracic fascia; invasion of the mediastinal fat; or nontransmural involvement of the pericardium; and/or involvement of ipsilateral hilar, mediastinal or internal mammary lymph nodes without distant metastases
IV	Unresectable, locally advanced tumor involving one of the following: multifocal invasion of the chest wall, transdiaphragmatic extension to the peritoneum, contralateral pleura, mediastinal organs, spine, internal surface of pericardium, or pericardial effusion; or involvement of supraclavicular or contralateral mediastinal or internal mammary lymph nodes; or any distant metastatic disease

2. **What are the histological subtypes of pleural mesothelioma?**
   - Epithelioid (best prognosis)
   - Mixed (epithelioid plus sarcomatoid)
   - Sarcomatoid

SIGNS, SYMPTOMS, AND IMAGING FINDINGS

1. **What are the common signs and symptoms of malignant pleural mesothelioma?**
   - Chest pain
   - Cough
   - Dyspnea
   - Fatigue
   - Weight loss
   - Dullness to chest percussion or absent breath sounds
   - Chest x-ray demonstrating a unilateral pleural effusion

2. **What paraneoplastic syndromes are associated with mesothelioma?**
   - Thrombocytosis
   - Anorexia/cachexia
   - Hypercalcemia (secondary to production of parathyroid hormone-related peptide; PTHrp)
   - Hemolytic anemia
   - Disseminated intravascular coagulation
   - Neurologic syndromes

DIAGNOSIS

1. **Initial workup of a pleural effusion with suspicion for mesothelioma should include which diagnostic tests?**
   - Thoracentesis with cytological assessment
   - CT scan of chest with intravenous (IV) contrast
   - Thoracoscopic pleural biopsy (if cytology is negative or nonspecific)

2. **If mesothelioma is confirmed, what additional diagnostic testing is recommended?**
   - CT scan of abdomen with IV and oral contrast
   - PET/CT scan (if consideration for surgical resection)
   - Mediastinal lymph node biopsy (eg, mediastinoscopy, endobronchial/endoscopic ultrasound-guided biopsy—if consideration for surgical resection)

PROGNOSTIC FACTORS

1. **What histological features are associated with more favorable outcomes?**
   - The epithelioid histological subtype relative to either the mixed or sarcomatoid subtypes

2. **What are the other favorable prognostic factors?**
   - Early-stage, localized disease
   - Absence of lymph node or extensive chest wall involvement
   - Good performance status
   - Younger age
   - Female gender
   - Absence of a paraneoplastic syndrome

TREATMENT

1. **What are the initial treatment decisions for management?**
   - Determining if the mesothelioma is resectable
   - Determining the optimal intervention to control pleural effusion

2. **For patients with potentially resectable mesothelioma, what additional testing is recommended to determine whether the patient is a candidate for surgery?**
   - Histologic subtyping; patients with sarcomatoid and mixed tumors have poor outcomes with aggressive surgical procedures
   - PET/CT to evaluate extent of disease including mediastinal lymph node involvement and distant metastases
   - Pulmonary function testing
   - Quantitative ventilation/perfusion (V/Q) scan for patients with abnormal pulmonary function tests
   - Cardiac stress testing

Early-Stage and Locally Advanced (Stages I–II) Operable Disease

1. **What are the treatment options for operable stages I–II epithelioid mesothelioma?**
   - Induction chemotherapy (cisplatin/carboplatin plus pemetrexed) followed by surgery
   - Primary surgery

2. **What are the surgical options for operable malignant pleural mesothelioma?**
   - Pleurectomy/decortication (P/D) (removal of tumor and affected parietal and visceral pleura)
   - Extrapleural pneumonectomy (EPP) (en bloc removal of affected lung, parietal and visceral pleura, hemidiaphragm, and ipsilateral pericardium, with mediastinal lymph node sampling)

3. **What is the role of surgery in malignant pleural mesothelioma?**
   - The benefit of surgery remains controversial.
   - Retrospective data comparing EPP with P/D indicates a higher operative mortality with EPP compared to P/D (7% vs. 4%), with similar survival that favors P/D on multivariate analysis.
   - A randomized trial comparing EPP to nonoperative management in patients with early-stage, resectable disease showed increased mortality and decreased quality of life in patients randomized to EPP.
   - Trimodality approaches (surgery, chemotherapy, and radiation) should be considered for younger patients (good performance status) with an epithelioid variant, and negative mediastinal nodes.
   - Tumor debulking by thoracoscopic partial P/D does not improve survival, but is effective in controlling symptomatic pleural effusion.

4. **When is adjuvant therapy employed?**
   - Following EPP, consider radiation to the affected hemithorax and mediastinum; and sequential adjuvant chemotherapy (cisplatin/carboplatin plus pemetrexed), if not given preoperatively.
   - Following P/D, consider radiation to the mediastinum if lymph node involvement is found pathologically, and adjuvant chemotherapy (cisplatin/carboplatin plus pemetrexed), if not given preoperatively.

Inoperable (Stages I–III) and Advanced (Stage IV) Disease

1. **What are the treatment options for inoperable or advanced-stage mesothelioma?**
   - Observation with short interval imaging for progression
   - Systemic chemotherapy
   - Focal radiotherapy for control of localizable symptoms (eg, chest wall pain)
   - Supportive care alone (if marginal or poor performance status)

Chemotherapy

1. **What are the first-line chemotherapy regimens?**
   - Cisplatin/carboplatin plus pemetrexed (preferred); cisplatin/carboplatin plus pemetrexed plus bevacizumab
   - Cisplatin/carboplatin plus gemcitabine
   - Pemetrexed alone (for patients with marginal performance status)

2. **What are second-line chemotherapy options?**
   - Single-agent gemcitabine, vinorelbine, or doxorubicin/liposomal doxorubicin

Radiation Therapy

1. **When should radiation therapy be considered?**
   - After EPP
   - Palliatively for relief of localizable pain due to chest wall invasion
   - Prophylactically to prevent tracking through chest wall incisions, or chest tube or thoracentesis sites

SPECIAL CONSIDERATIONS

Pleural Effusions

1. **What is the management for pleural effusions associated with mesothelioma?**
   - P/D
   - Video-assisted thoracoscopic talc pleurodesis
   - Placement of a tunneled, indwelling pleural catheter

QUESTIONS

1. A 72-year-old retired pipefitter presents with progressive exertional dyspnea, chest wall pain, and cough. He has smoked one pack per day for 54 years. His medical history is notable for Hodgkin lymphoma in his 30s treated with chemotherapy and mantle field radiation with no evidence of recurrence. He has a family history of mesothelioma in a paternal uncle and ocular melanoma in his father. CT scan shows a left-pleural-based mass with a moderate left pleural effusion. Percutaneous pleural biopsy confirms malignant sarcomatoid mesothelioma. Which of the following is *not* a risk factor for the development of mesothelioma?
   A. Tobacco use
   B. Radiation exposure
   C. Family history of mesothelioma
   D. Occupational asbestos exposure

2. A 55-year-old, previously healthy man presents with progressive dyspnea, chest discomfort, fatigue, and peripheral edema. Clinical evaluation is notable for a blood pressure of 94/60, heart rate of 116,

and respiratory rate of 28. His neck veins are distended and heart sounds are distant with an audible rub. Echocardiogram shows a large pericardial effusion with early tamponade physiology. He undergoes pericardiocentesis with temporary catheter placement and cytologic evaluation of pericardial fluid reveals mesothelioma. CT shows diffuse left pleural thickening and a small pleural effusion with enlarged left hilar and mediastinal lymph nodes. After pericardial drainage, he is hemodynamically stable with a good performance status. What is the best next step in management?

A. Bronchoscopy with biopsy of mediastinal lymph nodes
B. PET/CT
C. Pleurectomy/decortication with mediastinal lymph node sampling
D. Cisplatin plus pemetrexed

3. A 58-year-old woman with hypertension and a 40 pack-year smoking history is evaluated for shortness of breath. Chest radiography and pulmonary function tests are normal. A CT of the chest is notable for nodular pleural thickening at the left lung base. There are no enlarged lymph nodes and no evidence of chest wall invasion. CT abdomen shows no evidence of metastatic disease. CT-guided pleural biopsy reveals malignant mesothelioma with sarcomatoid histology. She has a good performance status and is motivated for therapy. What is the best next step in management?

A. Chemotherapy
B. Radiation
C. Extrapleural pneumonectomy
D. Observation for progression

4. An 84-year-old man with a history of coronary artery disease, type 2 diabetes mellitus, hypertension, hyperlipidemia, chronic kidney disease, and moderate dementia is diagnosed with diffuse malignant pleural mesothelioma. His daily activities are significantly limited by shortness of breath from a recurrent right pleural effusion. He has modest improvement after a thoracentesis, but continues to have a performance status of 2. What is the most appropriate next recommendation for his care?

A. Palliative radiation to the affected lung
B. Palliative chemotherapy with cisplatin, pemetrexed, and bevacizumab
C. Placement of a pleural catheter
D. Surgical consultation for pleurectomy/decortication

5. A 57-year-old retired construction worker presented with 3 months of shortness of breath and is found to have a large right pleural effusion. Thoracentesis with cytologic evaluation reveals malignant epithelioid mesothelioma. CT scan after pleural drainage reveals patchy, nodular pleural thickening with a pleural-based mass in the cardiophrenic recess, but no evidence of intra-abdominal disease. He undergoes induction therapy with cisplatin plus pemetrexed for four cycles, which yields a

minor response. He undergoes an extrapleural pneumonectomy and surgical margins are positive, but hilar and mediastinal lymph nodes are negative for malignancy. What is the best next step in management?

A. Reoperation with resection of the positive margins

B. Postoperative hemithoracic radiotherapy

C. Adjuvant cisplatin plus gemcitabine for four cycles

D. Observation with serial CT scans

6. A 65-year-old man is found to have a pleural effusion on chest radiography during an insurance examination. He is eventually diagnosed with early-stage malignant pleural mesothelioma. He has hypertension, mild renal insufficiency, and chronic low back pain managed with ibuprofen 600 mg TID, but is otherwise healthy with a good performance status. He takes several alternative medications. He is started on cisplatin, pemetrexed, and bevacizumab, but will not take any of the chemotherapy premedications due to concerns for drug interactions. Prior to his third cycle of chemotherapy, he is found to be pancytopenic with a white blood cell (WBC) count of 1.3, absolute neutrophil count (ANC) of 0.4, hemoglobin of 10.4 g/dL, and platelet count of 92,000. What is the most likely explanation for these findings?

A. Interaction between chemotherapy and alternative medications

B. Involvement of bone marrow with mesothelioma

C. Chemotherapy-induced myelosuppression

D. Bevacizumab-induced myelosuppression

ANSWERS

1. **A. Tobacco use.** This elderly man was presumably exposed to asbestos while working as a pipefitter and occupational asbestos exposure is the primary cause of mesothelioma. Radiation exposure is also associated with an increased risk of mesothelioma. While extremely rare, germline mutations in *BRCA1*-associated protein (BAP1) have been associated with a familial risk of mesothelioma and melanocytic tumors. Smoking is not associated with the development of mesothelioma.

2. **D. Cisplatin plus pemetrexed.** This middle-aged man has stage IV mesothelioma with pericardial involvement and cardiac tamponade. Given his age and good performance status, treatment with palliative chemotherapy to preserve quality of life and prolong survival is the most appropriate option. Surgical staging or resection is not indicated. PET/CT would not be useful since he already has pathologically proven advanced disease. If he should develop symptoms from worsening pleural effusion, then pleurectomy/decortication or talc pleurodesis would be appropriate options to maintain pulmonary function.

3. **A. Chemotherapy.** This middle-aged woman has sarcomatoid histology, which generally predicts for a poor prognosis and poor outcome with aggressive surgical procedures. She is relatively young and in otherwise good health. Observation for progression can be considered, but in light of her symptoms and the aggressive histology of her tumor, chemotherapy would be the most appropriate treatment option. Palliative radiation could be an option if she develops localizable pain. Surgery is not indicated, given the sarcomatoid histology.

4. **C. Placement of a pleural catheter.** Insertion of a pleural catheter is the most reasonable supportive measure to maintain his functional status with minimal interventional morbidity. Given his advanced age, comorbidities, and debility, surgical interventions and cisplatin-based chemotherapy would be contraindicated as the risks would outweigh the benefits. The diffuse nature of his disease and lack of localizable symptoms argue against the benefits of palliative radiation.

5. **B. Postoperative hemithoracic radiotherapy.** The patient should be considered for radiation therapy in the setting of positive margins to improve local control. Further surgery will not be successful in obtaining negative resection margins. He has already had optimal chemotherapy with marginal response, so further chemotherapy is unlikely to provide significant benefit.

6. **C. Chemotherapy-induced myelosuppression.** Nonsteroidal anti-inflammatory drugs (NSAIDs) can decrease the renal clearance of pemetrexed thereby increasing toxicity, such as myelosuppression, fatigue, stomatitis, nausea, and diarrhea. Pemetrexed and cisplatin should also be used with caution in patients with renal insufficiency. In addition, his refusal of

vitamin B12 and folic acid supplementation would increase his risk for myelosuppression with pemetrexed. The use of bevacizumab along with chemotherapy can modestly increase the risk of cytopenia, but the prolonged and profound myelosuppression in this patient suggests another etiology. Involvement of bone marrow with mesothelioma would be exceedingly rare.

13 Thymoma and Thymic Carcinoma

Jordan K. Schaefer and Gregory P. Kalemkerian

EPIDEMIOLOGY

1. **What is the overall survival of thymoma?**
   - Survival is dependent on World Health Organization (WHO) classification, histologic subtype, stage, and completeness of resection (full resection provides an excellent prognosis).
   - Thymic carcinoma has a worse prognosis than thymoma, with an overall 5-year survival rate of 35%.

ETIOLOGY, RISK FACTORS, AND FEATURES

1. **What is the etiology of thymoma?**
   - Unknown. Most cases are detected incidentally during imaging of the chest for unrelated reasons.

2. **What are the common risk factors associated with the development of thymoma?**
   - African Americans, Asians, and Pacific Islanders have an increased risk
   - Older age
   - **Not associated** with thymoma risk: family history, radiation exposure, tobacco use, or immunosuppression

3. **What features are common to thymomas?**
   - Encapsulated
   - Well differentiated
   - Associated with paraneoplastic syndromes (myasthenia gravis)

STAGING AND HISTOLOGICAL CLASSIFICATION

1. **Define the staging for thymoma**
   - Masaoka Staging System

Masaoka Stage	Criteria
I	Completely encapsulated, both macroscopically and microscopically
II	Macroscopic invasion into adjacent fat or mediastinal pleura; or microscopic transcapsular invasion

(continued)

(*continued*)

Masaoka Stage	Criteria
III	Macroscopic invasion into adjacent structures (pericardium, great vessels, lung)
IV	Spread to pleura or pericardium; or lymph node involvement or distant metastatic disease

2. **Summarize the histological classification of thymoma**
   - WHO histologic classification is the most widely employed.

Histologic Type	Definition
A	Spindle- or oval-shaped cells without nuclear atypia and without nonneoplastic lymphocytes
AB	Mixed histology, with regions of type A and other regions of type B
B1	Epithelioid cells, enriched with nonneoplastic lymphocytes; features resemble normal thymus
B2	Increased numbers of plump epithelioid cells enriched with nonneoplastic lymphocytes
B3	Round or polygonal epithelial cells with mild atypia (well-differentiated thymic carcinoma)
C	Prominent cytologic atypia and nonthymic histologic features (thymic carcinoma)

3. **What are negative prognostic factors?**
   - Extent of resection by surgery (complete is best)
   - Tumor size >10 cm
   - Tracheal/vascular compromise
   - Young age (<30)
   - Hematologic paraneoplastic syndromes

4. **What are the common histologic subtypes of thymic carcinoma?**
   - Squamous cell carcinoma
   - Undifferentiated carcinoma
   - Lymphoepithelioma-like carcinoma
   - Sarcomatoid carcinoma
   - Neuroendocrine carcinoma: large cell and small cell

SIGNS AND SYMPTOMS

1. **What is the most common presentation of thymoma?**
   - Incidental anterior mediastinal mass (50%)

- Ninety percent of thymomas occur in the anterior mediastinum; conversely, the most common anterior mediastinal mass is thymoma

2. **What are the common signs and symptoms of thymoma?**
   - Fifty percent of patients with thymoma are asymptomatic.
   - Common symptoms are due to compression or direct invasion of neighboring structures, and include chest pain, cough, hoarseness, dyspnea, or superior vena cava syndrome.
   - Paraneoplastic syndromes commonly cause presenting symptoms in patients with thymoma, but are much less common with thymic carcinoma.

3. **What are the most common paraneoplastic syndromes associated with thymoma?**
   - Myasthenia gravis (30%–50%)
   - Hypogammaglobulinemia (Good syndrome) (2%–5%)
   - Pure red cell aplasia (<5%)

DIAGNOSIS

1. **Initial evaluation of a mediastinal mass, and assessment for presence of a thymoma, should include what initial diagnostic testing?**
   - CT scan of the chest with intravenous contrast
   - Serum beta-human chorionic gonadotropin (beta-HCG) and alpha-fetoprotein (AFP), if appropriate, to assess for germ cell tumors
   - Thyroid-stimulating hormone (TSH), T3, and T4
   - Complete blood count with platelets
   - Percutaneous biopsy is contraindicated in patients with an anterior mediastinal mass that is clinically and radiographically most consistent with primarily resectable thymoma. Biopsy may disrupt the capsule and foster tumor seeding.

PROGNOSTIC AND RISK FACTORS

1. **What clinical features of thymoma are associated with a more favorable outcome?**
   - Completeness of resection is a primary prognostic factor.
   - Patients who present with myasthenia gravis may fare better than patients without myasthenia gravis, as they are typically diagnosed at an earlier stage.

2. **What histological subtype has the worst prognosis?**
   - WHO histological type C, thymic carcinoma, has the worst overall prognosis, due to increased rates of local invasion and distant metastases.

3. **What is the most common site of metastatic disease for thymoma?**
   - The most common mode of spread is "drop metastases," via direct invasion into the pleural space.
   - Hematogenous metastases are uncommon, but may occur late in the course of the disease. Liver, lymph nodes, and bone are the most common extrathoracic sites of spread. Patients with thymic tumors can develop second primary tumors, so suspected metastatic disease should be pathologically confirmed.

TREATMENT

1. **What is the initial treatment decision for management of a mediastinal mass suspected to be a thymoma?**
   - The initial treatment decision is to determine if the tumor is resectable. If the tumor is resectable, then complete excision is carried out with total resection of the thymus.
   - If the tumor is not primarily resectable, tissue diagnosis is pursued with either a core needle biopsy or open biopsy, with care not to violate the pleural space.

2. **What further diagnostic evaluation is recommended prior to surgery for thymoma?**
   - Assessment for myasthenia gravis in order to prevent respiratory complications while under anesthesia. Testing includes a thorough neurologic examination and a serum assay for anti-acetylcholine receptor antibody levels. Control of myasthenia gravis is required prior to surgery.

Resectable Disease

1. **Following surgery for resectable disease, what are the primary considerations with regard to adjuvant therapy?**
   - Disease histology: thymoma (WHO types A, AB, and B) versus thymic carcinoma (WHO type C)
   - Presence of microscopic or macroscopic capsular invasion
   - Postsurgical residual disease classification: no residual disease (R0); microscopic residual disease (R1); macroscopic residual disease (R2)

2. **What is the postoperative management of resectable thymoma?**
   - R0 resection with no capsular invasion (stage I): no further therapy
   - R0 resection with capsular invasion (stage II/III): consider radiotherapy
   - R1 resection: radiotherapy
   - R2 resection: radiotherapy $\pm$ chemotherapy

3. **What is the appropriate surveillance after completion of therapy for resectable thymoma?**
   - Surveillance CT scan of the chest every 6 months for 2 years, then annually for 10 years

4. **What is the postoperative management of resectable thymic carcinoma?**
   - R0 resection with no capsular invasion (stage I): no further therapy
   - R0 resection with capsular invasion (stage II/III): consider radiotherapy
   - R1 or R2 resection: radiotherapy + chemotherapy

5. **What is the appropriate surveillance after completion of therapy for resectable thymic carcinoma?**
   - Surveillance CT scan of the chest every 6 months for 2 years, then annually for 5 years

Locally Advanced Unresectable, Metastatic, or Recurrent Disease

1. **What is the treatment of primarily unresectable or recurrent disease without distant metastases?**
   - Chemotherapy
   - If good response to chemotherapy, then reassess for resection
   - After resection, pursue radiotherapy to the tumor bed

2. **If unresectable thymoma remains unresectable following initial chemotherapy, what is the appropriate management?**
   - Radiotherapy ± chemotherapy

3. **What is the appropriate management of metastatic disease?**
   - For oligometastatic spread to the ipsilateral pleura: consider primary surgical resection, or chemotherapy with subsequent reassessment for resection
   - For more extensive pleural spread or extrathoracic metastases: palliative chemotherapy
   - For palliation of focal symptoms: radiotherapy

Chemotherapy

1. **What are appropriate first-line chemotherapy regimens that are used for thymoma?**
   - First-line regimens are platinum-based: cyclophosphamide, doxorubicin, and cisplatin (CAP); cisplatin, doxorubicin, vincristine, cyclophosphamide (ADOC); cisplatin, etoposide (PE); cisplatin, etoposide, ifosfamide (VIP).
   - Chemotherapy for thymic carcinoma should be tailored to histologic subtype (eg, small cell carcinoma should be treated with cisplatin/carboplatin plus etoposide).

2. **What is appropriate second-line chemotherapy for refractory or recurrent thymoma?**
   - Second-line therapy consists of single-agent chemotherapy or targeted therapy:
     - Chemotherapy: pemetrexed, paclitaxel, gemcitabine, 5FU/leucovorin or capecitabine
     - Targeted therapy: sunitinib (thymic carcinoma), everolimus, octreotide ± prednisone
   - Approximately 10% of thymic carcinomas harbor activating mutations of c-*KIT*. In such patients, imatinib has demonstrated clinical activity.

QUESTIONS

1. A 54-year-old, African American man presents with vague chest discomfort and progressive exertional dyspnea. Labs show hemoglobin of 4.6 g/dL, total leukocyte count of 8,400, and a platelet count of 169,000. Reticulocyte count is 0.1%. Chest radiography shows an anterior mediastinal mass. CT of the chest confirms a 5 cm, smoothly marginated, anterior mediastinal mass, which appears resectable.

Serum anti-acetylcholine receptor antibody testing is negative. After administering a blood transfusion, which of the following is the most appropriate next step in management?
A. Bone marrow biopsy with iron stains
B. Thymectomy
C. CT-guided biopsy of the anterior mediastinal mass
D. Palliative radiation

2. A 45-year-old woman is admitted to the intensive care unit with cough, fever, and hypotension due to *Streptococcus pneumoniae* and sepsis. Her hospital course is complicated by disseminated varicella zoster infection. Chest radiography identifies a large anterior medias-tinal mass. CT scan confirms the 8 cm anterior mediastinal mass and notes slightly enlarged mediastinal lymph nodes. Her infection is stabi-lized and she gradually improves. Additional evaluation is most likely to reveal which of the following?
A. Hyponatremia due to syndrome of inappropriate secretion of antidiuretic hormone (SIADH)
B. Hypercalcemia due to elevated parathyroid hormone related peptide (PTHrP)
C. Hypogammaglobulinemia
D. Monoclonal gammopathy

3. A 71-year-old man is incidentally found to have an anterior mediastinal mass during an evaluation for chest pain. After appropriate preop-erative evaluation, he undergoes attempted resection of the mass. Intraoperatively, the tumor is found to be encasing the great vessels and complete resection cannot be attained; he is left with macroscopic evidence of residual tumor (R2). Pathology shows undifferentiated thymic carcinoma. Which of the following is the next step in patient management?
A. Monitor with serial CT scans
B. Postoperative radiation therapy
C. Reoperation to obtain complete (R0) resection
D. Definitive radiation with chemotherapy

4. A 67-year-old man underwent resection of a stage II thymoma (World Health Organization [WHO] type B2) followed by postoperative radiotherapy 3 years ago. He now presents with progressive dyspnea on exertion and mild left chest discomfort. CT scan shows diffuse left pleural thickening and multiple pleural-based nodules measuring up to 3.6 cm. Percutaneous biopsy of a pleural nodule confirms recur-rent thymoma. He has a good performance status and is otherwise healthy. Which of the following would be an appropriate next choice for therapy?
A. 5-FU and leucovorin
B. Sunitinib
C. Pemetrexed
D. Cyclophosphamide, doxorubicin, and cisplatin (CAP)

5. A 55-year-old woman presents with double vision and ptosis. Her ophthalmologist suspects myasthenia gravis and serum anti-acetylcholine receptor antibodies are positive. CT scan of the chest shows a 3 cm, sharply marginated, anterior mediastinal mass concerning for thymoma. The mass appears to be resectable. Which of the following would be the most appropriate next step in management?
   A. Refer for surgical resection of the mass
   B. Refer to neurology for management of the myasthenia gravis
   C. Refer to interventional radiology for biopsy
   D. Initiate chemotherapy

6. A 64-year-old woman is diagnosed with locally advanced, unresectable thymoma (World Health Organization [WHO] type B1), confirmed by CT-guided biopsy. She completes four cycles of cisplatin, doxorubicin, and cyclophosphamide, and a restaging CT shows an excellent tumor response. There is no evidence of pleural or extrathoracic metastatic disease. Which of the following is the most appropriate next step in management?
   A. Consolidative radiation therapy to the primary tumor
   B. Maintenance chemotherapy with pemetrexed
   C. CT surveillance every 6 months for 2 years
   D. Surgical consultation to reconsider resection

ANSWERS

1. **B. Thymectomy.** This middle-aged man has a clinical presentation consistent with thymoma and secondary pure red cell aplasia. The low reticulocyte count suggests that the anemia is due to reduced red cell production. If the clinical and radiographic suspicion of resectable thymoma is high, then a biopsy should be avoided to prevent capsular disruption and tumor seeding. The patient should undergo primary surgical resection.

2. **C. Hypogammaglobulinemia.** This woman has Good syndrome associated with thymoma. Good syndrome is associated with secondary immunodeficiency due to hypogammaglobulinemia with anemia and leukopenia. Monoclonal gammopathy is uncommon. Patients with Good syndrome are at high risk for infection with encapsulated organisms.

3. **D. Definitive radiation with chemotherapy.** In the setting of an R2 resection (macroscopic residual disease), what distinguishes thymic cancer from thymoma is the recommendation for postoperative chemotherapy, in addition to radiation. Radiation is considered in all cases of microscopic or macroscopic residual disease. Chemotherapy is generally reserved for thymic carcinoma with residual disease based on the more aggressive and metastatic nature of this disease.

4. **D. Cyclophosphamide, doxorubicin, and cisplatin (CAP).** Platinum-based combination chemotherapy, such as CAP, or cisplatin and etoposide, would be an appropriate first-line chemotherapy option for stage IV thymoma in a patient with a good performance status. These regimens yield response rates of 40% to 50%. The other listed options could be considered for second-line therapy.

5. **B. Refer to neurology for management of the myasthenia gravis.** Patients with thymoma associated with myasthenia gravis should have a thorough neurologic evaluation, and the myasthenia gravis should be brought under good symptomatic control with medical management prior to undergoing surgical resection to avoid complications such as intraoperative respiratory failure.

6. **D. Surgical consultation to reconsider resection.** Patients with locally advanced, primarily unresectable thymic tumors who have had a good response to chemotherapy should be reassessed for surgery, since the completeness of resection is one of the strongest factors determining the prognosis of patients with thymic malignancies. If the tumor is still deemed unresectable, then radiation therapy should be considered.

Head and Neck Cancers and Salivary Gland Tumors

Paul L. Swiecicki and Francis P. Worden

ETIOLOGY AND RISK FACTORS

1. **What are the major risk factors for squamous cell cancer of the head and neck (SCCHN)?**
   - *Smoking* increases risk 5- to 25-fold.
   - Heavy *alcohol* consumption increases the risk 2- to 6-fold.
   - *Smoking combined with heavy alcohol* consumption increases the risk 15- to 40-fold.
   - *Human papillomavirus (HPV)* infection with high-risk serotypes 16 and 18 is an established cause of oropharyngeal cancer. p16 is an acceptable marker for HPV in oropharyngeal cancers only.
   - *Fanconi anemia*

2. **What is the incidence of secondary primary cancers, and where do these cancers occur?**
   - Three to seven percent, primarily in the lung, esophagus, head and neck

3. **What are the most common localizations of alcohol- and tobacco-related head and neck cancer?**
   - *Oral cavity* (floor of mouth, oral tongue, buccal mucosa, alveolar ridge, hard palate, retromolar trigone)
   - *Pharynx* (nasopharynx, oropharynx—soft palate, uvula, base of tongue, tonsil, posterior pharyngeal wall)
   - *Larynx* (supraglottic—false vocal cords, arytenoids, epiglottis; glottic—commissures; subglottic)
   - *Nasal cavity and paranasal sinuses* (nasal cavity maxillary sinuses, ethmoid sinuses, frontal sinuses, sphenoid sinuses)

4. **What are the most common localizations of HPV-related SCCHN?**
   - Lingual and palatine tonsils, and base of the tongue
   - Histologically identified by: **p16 staining**

5. **What is the role of epidermal growth factor receptor (EGFR) in SCCHN?**
   - *EGFR* gene copy number is increased in SCCHN and leads to the activation of growth pathways and resistance to apoptosis.

6. **Which virus is associated with nasopharyngeal nonkeratinizing and undifferentiated cancers and where does this cancer typically present?**
   - Epstein–Barr virus (EBV); histologically identified by **EBER staining**
   - Fossa of Rosenmuller

PREVENTION

- There is no effective chemoprevention for patients at risk for SCCHN.
- It has not been demonstrated yet that HPV vaccination can decrease the incidence of HPV-related SCCHN.

STAGING

1. **How is SCCHN staged?**
   - Staging of SCCHN is defined for the following specific regions:
     - Lip and oral cavity
     - Pharynx
       - Nasopharynx
       - Oropharynx
       - Hypopharynx
     - Larynx
     - Nasal cavity and paranasal sinuses
     - Major salivary glands
     - Mucosal melanoma of the head and neck

   Note: Mucosal melanoma of the head and neck is a very aggressive cancer and is not reviewed in this chapter.

   - Generic anatomic staging for SCCHN is:

Anatomic Stage/Prognostic Groups			
Stage 0	Tis	N0	M0
Stage I	T1	N0	M0
Stage II	*	*	M0
Stage III	*	*	M0
Stage IVA	*	*	M0
Stage IVB	*	*	M0
Stage IVC	Any T	Any N	M1

Relatively small primary tumor with no or minimal nodal involvement { Stage I, Stage II

Larger primary tumor and/or nodal involvement { Stage IVA, Stage IVB

*Specific for anatomic location.

2. **What is an initial goal of the therapy in a patient with "very advanced SCCHN" (T4b, any N, M0) in the absence of distant metastases?**
   - Cure, assuming that the patient is fit for chemoradiation or is a candidate for surgery

SIGNS AND SYMPTOMS

1. What are the most common signs and symptoms of head and neck cancer?

- Specific symptoms will depend on the cancer location with the most common symptoms as follows:
  - Nonhealing oral ulcers (painless and painful)—oral cavity
  - Difficulty with swallowing, odynophagia, change in speech—oropharynx
  - Hoarseness—larynx/pyriform sinus
  - Painless mass—adenoid cystic carcinoma
  - Unilateral otitis media or otalgia—nasopharynx, maxillary/paranasal sinus
  - Trismus—oral cavity
  - Persistent nasal congestion/fullness—nasopharynx, maxillary sinus

2. Who should be evaluated by a specialist for these symptoms?

- Any adult with any of the previously-mentioned symptoms lasting more than 2 to 4 weeks.

DIAGNOSTIC WORKUP

1. Why is the family history of cancers important?

- First-degree relatives have two- to fourfold increased risk of SCCHN.

2. What is the "field cancerization" concept?

- Diffuse epithelial injury within the aerodigestive tract (head, neck, lungs, and esophagus) due to chronic exposure to carcinogens

3. Why is the field cancerization concept clinically important?

- Patients with SCCHN may present with second metachronous and synchronous cancers of the aerodigestive tract.
- It dictates thorough examination of head and neck with laryngoscopy, nasopharyngoscopy, bronchoscopy, and esophagoscopy as indicated.
- It mandates chest imaging (chest x-ray [CXR], CT, or PET/CT) for all patients because of the risk of a concurrent lung malignancy.

PROGNOSIS

1. What is the most important prognostic factor for SCCHN cancer patients?

- Stage at the time of diagnosis

2. What is the 5-year survival rate for stage I patients?

- More than 80%

3. What is the 5-year survival rate for stages III and IV patients?

- Less than 40%

4. How does the presence of palpable lymph nodes in the neck affect survival rate compared to patients with the same T stage?

- It decreases the survival rate by 50%.

5. **What is the greatest survival risk for SCCHN cancer patients 3 years out of therapy?**
   - Development of recurrence or a second primary cancer

TREATMENT

General Approaches

1. **Can patients with an early stage of SCCHN cancer be clinically observed?**
   - No. There should be no delays in proper staging and therapy of head and neck cancer, as delays result in decreased survival.

2. **What percentage of patients present with early-stage cancer (stage I or II) and require single-modality therapy (surgery or radiation)?**
   - Thirty percent to 40% of patients present with early-stage cancer (stage I or II).
   - Survival is similar for both of these modalities.

3. **What percentage of patients present with locally advanced disease (stages III, IVA, and IVB) and require combined-modality therapy?**
   - About 60% of patients present with locally advanced disease (stages III, IVA, and IVB).
   - The exact sequence of treatment modality differs depending on cancer location and cancer center expertise (eg, surgery followed by radiation ± chemotherapy or chemoradiotherapy followed by surgery as needed [full extirpation/neck dissection]).

Surgical Therapy

1. **Which patients should receive surgery as a first-line therapy?**
   - Patients with limited disease (stage I or II); although lately, radiation is commonly used for these patients. Low bulk stage III—T1 to T2, N1 disease can also be surgically treated.
   - Patients with locoregionally advanced disease (higher volume stage III/IV without distant metastases) as an *alternative* to chemoradiotherapy.

2. **Who determines that an SCCHN tumor is surgically "unresectable?"**
   - A qualified head and neck surgeon

3. **Involvement of which structures makes the SCCHN tumor unresectable?**
   - Extension of tumor to the skull base
   - Direct extension to the superior nasopharynx or Eustachian tube
   - Encasement of the common or internal carotid artery
   - Direct extension to the mediastinum, prevertebral fascia, or cervical vertebra (there are exceptions)
   - Direct extension of neck disease to the external skin (there are exceptions)
   - Involvement of the pterygoid muscles (there are exceptions)

4. **What is a "classical radical neck dissection?"**
   - It includes resection of all lymph nodes from levels I to V, as well as resection of internal jugular vein, spinal accessory nerve, and sternocleidomastoid muscle.
   - It is rarely done nowadays due to severe morbidity.

5. **What are the current classifications of surgical neck dissection and what is their therapeutic intent?**
   - **Comprehensive** (removes all five lymph node levels that would be included in classical radical neck dissection, regardless of other structures resected or not)—curative intent
   - **Selective** (removes fewer than all five lymph node levels based on common pathways of spread of SCCHN)—performed electively to improve staging

6. **In which situations can selective neck dissection be used?**
   - Selective neck dissection is mostly used for N0 (no palpable lymph nodes) disease.
   - Selective neck dissection can be occasionally performed in certain patients with N1–N2 disease to prevent excessive morbidity.

7. **Is there a role for the surgery after radiation or chemoradiation therapy?**
   - Yes, if the patient has residual disease or suspected local progression; however, such surgery is complicated by poor wound healing, skin necrosis, or carotid exposure with risk for carotid blowout.

Radiation as a First-Line Therapy

1. **When may radiation be used as a first-line therapy?**
   - In early-stage (stage I or II) patients
   - When a patient's performance status is not suitable for upfront chemoradiotherapy or surgery

2. **What is the major advantage of radiation therapy in SCCHN?**
   - Organ preservation

3. **What is the major advantage of intensity-modulated radiation therapy (IMRT)?**
   - Decreased radiation-induced toxicity (especially xerostomia)
   - It has a similar overall survival compared to conventional radiation therapy.

4. **Is there any advantage to using accelerated fraction radiotherapy versus single fraction radiotherapy?**
   - Without chemotherapy: yes, accelerated fraction improves local control and survival.
   - With chemotherapy: no, local control and survival are the same.

5. **What is the traditional dose of radiation in SCCHN cancer?**
   - In general, 66 to 74 Gy in 1.8 to 2.0 Gy daily fractions to the bulk of the tumor and to the neck nodes (bilateral neck radiation is needed for stages III/IVA/B disease in oropharynx and nasopharynx cancers)

6. **What are common side effects of radiation?**
   - Dermatitis, xerostomia, mucositis, loss of taste, dysphagia, and loss of hair

7. **What is an important part of routine follow-up for patients who received radiation to the neck?**
   - Assessment of thyroid function (thyroid-stimulating hormone [TSH]) every 6 to 12 months (20%–25% of patients who received neck radiation have elevated TSH level)

8. **Should nonsurgically treated patients be examined by a head and neck surgical oncologist regularly?**
   - Yes, to evaluate for early detection of local or regional recurrences of cancer and early salvage surgery.

Concomitant Chemoradiation as a First-Line Therapy

1. **What is the role of concomitant chemoradiation as a first-line therapy?**
   - It may be used as a first-line therapy in locally advanced SCCHN (stage III/IVA/B) sparing some patients from surgical intervention.
   - It is a therapy of choice for "very advanced SCCHN" patients (T4b, any N, M0) who are usually not suitable candidates for surgery.
   - Salvage surgery is reserved for patients with residual or locally recurrent disease.

2. **Is sequential chemotherapy and radiation as effective as concomitant therapy?**
   - No. Concomitant chemoradiation is preferred for organ preservation; however, induction chemotherapy (cisplatin + 5-FU continuous infusion for three cycles) followed by radiotherapy (70 Gy) is an alternative for those with stage III/IVAB larynx cancer (laryngectomy-free survival rate is the same with chemoradiation and induction chemotherapy).

3. **What is the "standard" regimen for concomitant chemoradiation for SCCHN?**
   - 70 Gy at daily 2.0 Gy fractions for 7 weeks with cisplatin given every 3 weeks at 100 mg/m^2
   - Carboplatin can substitute for cisplatin in patients with contraindications to cisplatin, though prospective data comparing cisplatin and carboplatin with radiation are extremely limited.

4. **What is the role of cetuximab in SCCHN?**
   - Cetuximab can be used concomitantly with radiation for locally advanced SCCHN; there are currently no direct comparison data for cetuximab versus cisplatin concomitantly with radiation.
   - Cetuximab in addition to cisplatin and radiation is not superior to cisplatin and radiation; no improvements in local control or survival rate.
   - Metastatic disease: cetuximab in addition to platinum and 5-FU may be used as first-line treatment (improved survival rate over platinum and 5-FU).
   - Metastatic disease: cetuximab as a single agent may be used as second-line therapy after platinum failure.

Adjuvant Therapy

1. **What are the major and minor risk factors for local recurrence?**
   - **Major:**
     - ○ Positive margins
     - ○ Extracapsular nodal spread of tumor
   - **Minor:**
     - ○ Multiple positive nodes
     - ○ Vascular/lymphatic/perineural invasion
     - ○ pT3 or pT4 primary
     - ○ Oral cavity or oropharynx primary with level 4 or 5 nodal involvement

2. **Which patients should receive adjuvant radiation therapy alone?**
   - Patients with a single minor risk factor for local recurrence

3. **Which patients should receive adjuvant chemoradiation therapy?**
   - Patients with one major risk factor for recurrence
   - Patients with two or more minor risk factors for local recurrence can be considered for chemoradiotherapy

4. **Is there a role for adjuvant chemotherapy alone?**
   - No. Chemotherapy alone is not used in adjuvant settings for SCCHN.

5. **What is the standard chemoradiation regimen in the adjuvant setting?**
   - Cisplatin (100 mg/m^2) once every 21 days with concurrent radiation (66 Gy)

Chemotherapy

1. **When is chemotherapy used alone in SCCHN?**
   - For palliation in unresectable recurrent, metastatic SCCHN patients, or in patients with locally advanced SCCHN that are no longer amenable to surgery or radiotherapy

2. **Is combination therapy superior to monotherapy?**
   - Yes, platinum doublets are the standard of care. The responses are improved with cisplatin and 5-FU compared to carboplatin and 5-FU. Cisplatin and 5-FU are equivalent to cisplatin and paclitaxel.
   - The addition of cetuximab to cisplatin/5-FU or carboplatin/5-FU in nonnasopharyngeal cancers improves response rates and survival. Triplet therapy (platinum agent + 5-FU continuous infusion + cetuximab) can now be considered *first-line therapy.*

3. **What agents are used in patients who have failed platinum with radiation within 6 months of completing therapy or after platinum failures in the recurrent/metastatic setting?**
   - Nivolumab or pembrolizumab are now standard second-line therapy.
   - Single agent cetuximab, weekly docetaxel, and weekly methotrexate are acceptable in patients who are not candidates for immunotherapy.

4. When is radiation used in the palliative setting for SCCHN?

- Reirradiation and concurrent chemotherapy with radiation is not considered the standard of care. Reirradiation may improve local control but does not improve overall survival.

LOCATION-SPECIFIC CONSIDERATIONS

Cancer of the Lip and Oral Cancer

- Sun is an additional risk factor for cancer of the lip.
- Lower lip cancers are associated with low incidence of metastases.
- Cancer of the upper lip and commissural areas have higher incidence of metastases at the time of diagnosis.
- Surgery is the preferred therapeutic option for bulky and locally advanced resectable disease.

Cancer of the Nasopharynx

- World Health Organization (WHO) classification of nasopharyngeal carcinoma is as follows:
  - Type I (keratinizing squamous cell cancer [SCC])
  - Type II (nonkeratinizing SCC)
  - Type III (undifferentiated carcinoma)
- Neck mass is the most common presentation of nasopharyngeal carcinoma.
  - Nasopharyngeal carcinoma has a high metastatic potential (more in types II and III compared to type I).
- Type I has the worst prognosis, due to uncontrolled growth of primary tumor.
- Nasopharyngeal carcinoma is the only squamous cell carcinoma of the head and neck where surgery **is not** recommended as a first-line therapy.
- Standard therapy includes:
  - For stages I and IIA—radiation alone
  - For stages IIB, III, and IV—chemoradiation with cisplatin 100 mg/m^2 every 21 days or weekly cisplatin 40 mg/m^2 followed by three courses of adjuvant cisplatin with 5-FU
  - For stage IVC (metastatic disease)—cisplatin with gemcitabine or cisplatin with 5-FU or single agent docetaxel or paclitaxel

Cancer of the Oropharynx

- Management by stage:

Clinical Stage	T Stage	N Stage	M Stage	Treatment
Stage 0	Tis	N0	M0	Surgery
Stage I	T1	N0	M0	Surgery
				Or
Stage II	T2	N0	M0	Definitive radiation

(continued)

- Management by stage: (*continued*)

Clinical Stage	T Stage	N Stage	M Stage	Treatment
Stage III	T3	N0	M0	Surgery + radiation (±chemo)
	T1	N1	M0	
	T2	N1	M0	*Or*
	T3	N1	M0	Definitive
Stage IVA	T4a	N0	M0	chemoradiation
	T4a	N1	M0	*Or*
	T1	N2	M0	Induction
	T2	N2	M0	chemotherapy followed
	T3	N2	M0	by chemoradiation
	T4a	N2	M0	
Stage IVB	T4b	Any N	M0	Definitive chemoradiation
				Or
	Any T	N3	M0	Induction chemotherapy followed by chemoradiation
Stage IVC	Any T	Any N	M1	Chemotherapy

- When surgery is used as an initial modality in stages 0–IVA oropharyngeal cancer, a transoral resection (TORS) is typically employed.
- In locoregionally advanced oropharyngeal cancer (stage IVB) surgery is reserved for the management of residual regional lymph node metastases following chemo-radiotherapy and recurrent disease.

Cancer of the Hypopharynx

- May be treated with induction therapy (cisplatin + infusional 5-FU) × three cycles followed by radiotherapy or cisplatin (100 mg/m^2) every 21 days with radiation, if tumor is less than T4a (ie, no thyroid cartilage invasion)
- T4a tumors are treated with *total laryngectomy* followed by radiation ± chemo-therapy

Cancer of the Larynx

- Divided into supraglottic, glottic, and subglottic laryngeal cancers; glottis tumors have the best prognosis and supraglottic tumors have the worst prognosis.
- Management options in locally advanced resectable cancers (T3–4 or T2N+) include resection followed by radiation versus organ preservation.
- Organ preservation approaches include:
  ○ Induction chemotherapy (cisplatin + infusional 5-FU × three cycles) followed by definitive radiation

- ○ Combined chemoradiation: radiation with concurrent cisplatin (100 mg/m^2 every 21 days × three doses)

Note: Though organ preservation is highest with concomitant chemoradiation, laryngectomy-free survival is similar for both regimens.

- Patients with bulky (T4a) disease of larynx should have *total laryngectomy* followed by adjuvant radiation (+/− chemotherapy) as it is unlikely to spare the function of the larynx in these patients.

Cancer of the Nasal Cavity and Paranasal Sinuses

- Most of the tumors are symptomatic and present with advanced stage.
- Although surgical resection is generally preferred, it is difficult to perform due to advanced presentations, and patients are treated with chemoradiation (cisplatin and radiation).
- The most common histology is squamous cell carcinoma; other histologies are adenocarcinoma, esthesioneuroblastoma (a.k.a. olfactory neuroblastoma), sarcoma, and undifferentiated carcinoma.
- Esthesioneuroblastomas require surgery and radiation with long-term follow-up because recurrence can occur even after 15 years. Chemotherapy is generally not indicated.

Cancer of the Major Salivary Glands

- Tobacco and alcohol consumption are not risk factors.
- Ionizing radiation, rubber, and automotive industries are risk factors.
- Seventy-five percent of parotid gland neoplasms are benign.
- Seventy-five percent of submandibular, sublingual, and minor salivary glands are malignant.
- Most common histologies are:
  - ○ Mucoepidermoid (metastatic high-grade tumors can be treated with chemotherapy regimens used to treat SCCHN)
  - ○ Acinic
  - ○ Adenocarcinoma
  - ○ Adenoid cystic carcinoma (characterized by an indolent natural history, often followed with serial imaging)
  - ○ Malignant myoepithelial tumor
  - ○ Squamous carcinoma (rare)
- Squamous cell carcinomas of the surrounding skin frequently metastasize to the parotid glands (can be confused with primary parotid gland cancers).
- Complete surgical resection is a major therapeutic approach for all salivary gland tumors.
- The majority of cases require adjuvant radiation due to incomplete resection, close or positive margin, intermediate or high-grade histology, or neural/vascular/lymphatic invasion.
- Although chemoradiation could be considered, there is no role for adjuvant chemotherapy.

QUESTIONS

1. A healthy 67-year-old woman presents with the complaint of a slowly enlarging lump on her right face. A CT is performed demonstrating a 2.2 × 3.1 cm mass within the parotid gland without evidence of other masses, lymphadenopathy, or bone/muscle infiltration. An ultrasound-guided core needle biopsy is performed and demonstrates moderately differentiated adenoid cystic carcinoma.
   Which of the following is the most appropriate next step in this patient's management?
   A. Stereotactic beam radiation therapy to the mass
   B. Definitive chemoradiation utilizing cetuximab
   C. Docetaxel, cisplatin, and infusional 5-FU for three cycles followed by definitive radiation therapy to the mass
   D. Resection

2. A 55-year-old man with a history of type 2 diabetes and associated peripheral neuropathy presents to your clinic for consideration of adjuvant therapy in the setting of laryngeal cancer. He was found to have IVa (T4aN1M0) laryngeal cancer after 3 years of progressive hoarseness and underwent a laryngectomy 2 weeks ago. Pathology demonstrates a 5.1 × 4.5 poorly differentiated squamous cell carcinoma with negative margins. No perineural or vascular invasion was noted. Three of 23 lymph nodes were involved, one of which was noted to have extracapsular extension.
   Which of the following is the most appropriate recommendation for the management of this patient?
   A. Observation
   B. Radiation
   C. Concurrent chemoradiation therapy utilizing cisplatin 100 mg/m^2 once every 21 days
   D. Concurrent chemoradiation therapy utilizing weekly carboplatin
   E. Concurrent chemoradiation therapy utilizing weekly carboplatin and cetuximab

3. A 45-year-old man with a strong history of chewing tobacco use presents for a 6-month history of a progressively enlarging mass on the roof of the mouth. A CT was obtained demonstrating a 2.1 × 1.7 cm. Erosion of the hard palate is noted as well as right neck level I lymphadenopathy. A biopsy is obtained and demonstrates squamous cell carcinoma.
   Which of the following is the most appropriate next step in this patient's management?
   A. Surgical resection
   B. Irradiation of the oral cavity mass and bilateral necks
   C. Concurrent chemoradiation to the oral cavity mass and bilateral necks utilizing cisplatin 100 mg/m^2 once every 21 days
   D. Hospice referral

4. A 65-year-old man with a 100 pack-year history presents with a lump in his right neck noted while shaving. Eastern Cooperative Oncology

Group (ECOG) performance status is 0. CT of the neck is obtained and demonstrates large, matted, bilateral lymphadenopathy (largest lymph node conglomeration measuring 6.2 cm with cystic center) and a small 1.5 cm mass at the right tonsil. Fine needle aspiration of the lymph node conglomeration is performed and demonstrates poorly differentiated squamous cell carcinoma, p16 negative.

Which of the following is the most appropriate next step in this patient's management?

A. Transoral surgery resection of malignancy followed by selective neck dissection
B. Irradiation of primary tonsillar mass only with intensity-modulated radiation therapy
C. Irradiation of primary tonsillar mass only with intensity-modulated radiation therapy concurrent with cisplatin (100 mg/m²) every 21 days
D. Irradiation of mass and bilateral necks with intensity-modulated radiation therapy
E. Irradiation of the tonsillar mass and bilateral necks with intensity-modulated radiation therapy concurrent with cisplatin (100 mg/m²) every 21 days

5. A 62-year-old man with a history of stage IVA oropharyngeal squamous cell carcinoma presents 3 months after completion of chemoradiation for disease monitoring. He has noted fullness in the right neck and supraclavicular region but thought it was due to a muscle spasm. A PET/CT is obtained and demonstrates multiple lymph nodes with intense fluorodeoxyglucose (FDG) avidity in the right neck.

Which of the following is the most appropriate next step in this patient's management?

A. Close surveillance with repeat PET/CT in 3 months
B. Six cycles of chemotherapy with cisplatin + 5-FU + cetuximab
C. Reirradiation of the mass utilizing hyperfractionation and a nonplatinum radiosensitizing agent
D. Modified radical neck dissection

6. A 47-year-old woman with a history of stage IVB oropharyngeal cancer (p16 positive) presents 2 years after completion of chemoradiation for evaluation of axillary fullness. Axillary exam demonstrates gross lymphadenopathy. Restaging CT chest/abdomen/pelvis demonstrates multiple chest nodules bilaterally as well as right axillary lymphadenopathy. She is extremely active with an excellent performance status, working full time and taking care of her family.

Which of the following would be the most appropriate recommendation for first-line therapy for this patient's metastatic disease?

A. Weekly IV methotrexate
B. Cisplatin + 5-FU continuous infusion + cetuximab
C. Docetaxel + cisplatin + 5-FU continuous infusion
D. Cisplatin + 5-FU continuous Infusion
E. Carboplatin + paclitaxel

ANSWERS

1. **D. Resection.** Complete surgical resection is the first-line therapy for tumors of the major salivary glands. The remainder of the options listed here would not be appropriate therapeutic options.

2. **D. Concurrent chemoradiation therapy utilizing weekly carboplatin.** Concurrent chemoradiation utilizing weekly carboplatin is the preferred treatment modality in this patient with advanced laryngeal cancer. Given the advanced nature of the cancer, adjuvant radiation would be administered in this patient. With the pathological finding of extracapsular extension, concurrent chemotherapy would be added. Although cisplatin is the chemotherapeutic of choice given the patient's preexisting peripheral neuropathy this would not be an appropriate agent. Hence, weekly carboplatin would be utilized. There is no role for concurrent carboplatin and cetuximab with radiation therapy.

3. **A. Surgical resection.** Surgical resection would be the most appropriate management treatment modality in this patient with oral cavity cancer. Surgical management has superior outcomes when utilized in the first-line setting compared to chemoradiation. Hence it is the treatment of choice.

4. **E. Irradiation of the tonsillar mass and bilateral necks with intensity-modulated radiation therapy concurrent with cisplatin (100 mg/m^2) every 21 days.** First-line therapy of patients with oropharyngeal cancer, particularly those with advanced human papillomavirus tumors, consists of chemoradiation. In patients with advanced cancer, radiation is typically delivered to the bilateral necks.

5. **D. Modified radical neck dissection.** Persistent disease after completion of chemoradiation is typically managed by surgical resection, specifically a modified radical neck dissection. Given the short time since his last radiation therapy, reirradiation is unlikely to be effective and is associated with a high risk for severe toxicities. Chemotherapy alone is reserved for patients with inoperable recurrent or metastatic disease.

6. **B. Cisplatin + 5-FU continuous infusion + cetuximab.** In patients with good performance status, first-line treatment for unresectable recurrent or metastatic head and neck squamous cell carcinoma consists of a triplet containing a platinum agent, 5-FU continuous infusion, and cetuximab. This regimen has been shown to have the best response rate and overall survival to date.

III

ENDOCRINE MALIGNANCIES

15

Thyroid Cancer

Paul L. Swiecicki and Megan R. Haymart

EPIDEMIOLOGY

1. What are the histologic variants of thyroid cancer?

- There are three main variants: differentiated (approximately 94%), medullary (4%), and anaplastic (2%). Differentiated thyroid cancer is further subclassified into papillary (the most common thyroid cancer), follicular, and Hürthle cell.
- The distinction between differentiated and other types is crucial, as management is very different (see the section on Treatment).
- Approximately 50% of patients with anaplastic thyroid cancer have prior or concurrent differentiated thyroid cancer as well.

2. How common is thyroid cancer?

- Women are affected three times more often than men. Peak incidence for differentiated cancer (papillary, follicular, Hürthle cell) is around age 49.
- Undifferentiated thyroid cancer is seen mostly in older patients, with a mean age of 71 years.

ETIOLOGY AND RISK FACTORS

1. What are the common risk factors for thyroid cancer?

- Radiation exposure, especially in childhood, particularly under age 10
- Female sex (female:male ratio of 3:1)
- Familial syndromes: the risk of thyroid cancer is increased in MEN2A, MEN2B, Carney complex, Cowden syndrome, and familial adenomatous polyposis (FAP)

2. What fraction of medullary thyroid cancers are inherited?

- Eighty percent sporadic, 20% inherited (MEN2A, MEN2B)
- These are inherited in an autosomal dominant fashion
- Six percent of clinically sporadic cases of medullary thyroid cancer carry the germline *RET* gene mutation; therefore, genetic testing should be encouraged for all medullary thyroid cancer patients

3. What mutations are frequently seen in differentiated thyroid cancers?

- Up to 45% of patients with papillary thyroid cancer have V600E mutation in *BRAF* gene.
- De novo mutations in PI3-kinase pathway genes are often seen at the time of metastasis.

STAGING

1. Define the staging for thyroid cancer:

Stage	Definition
Follicular or papillary	**<45 years old:** stage I if no distant metastatic disease present, stage II if distant metastatic disease present
	≥45 years old:
	Stage I—if tumor ≤2 cm, limited to thyroid, no LN involvement
	Stage II—if tumor >2–4 cm, limited to thyroid, no LN involvement
	Stage III—tumor >4 cm with minimal extrathyroid extension (adjacent fat and muscle) or any tumor size with involvement of pretracheal, paratracheal, and prelaryngeal (level VI) LNs
	Stage IVa—tumor of any size that invades esophagus, recurrent laryngeal nerve, larynx, trachea, subcutaneous soft tissues, or any tumor size with involvement of levels I–V or level VII LNs
	Stage IVb—tumor of any size that encases carotid artery, mediastinal vessels, or involves prevertebral fascia, with or without LN involvement
	Stage IVc—distant metastatic disease present
Medullary carcinoma (all ages)	**Stage I**—if tumor ≤2 cm, limited to thyroid, no LN involvement
	Stage II—tumor >2 cm, but not more than 4 cm, that may involve minimal extrathyroid extension to adjacent fat and muscle, no LN involvement
	Stage III—tumor >4 cm or tumor of any size that may involve minimal extrathyroid extension to adjacent fat and muscle, with involvement of pretracheal, paratracheal, and prelaryngeal (level VI) LNs
	Stage IVa—tumor of any size that may involve esophagus, recurrent laryngeal nerve, larynx, trachea, subcutaneous soft tissues, or involvement of levels I–V or level VII LNs
	Stage IVb—tumor of any size that encases carotid artery, mediastinal vessels, or involves prevertebral fascia, with or without LN involvement
	Stage IVc—distant metastatic disease present
Anaplastic carcinoma (all ages)	**Stage IVa**—tumors that are intrathyroidal and surgically resectable, any LN involvement, no distant metastatic disease present
	Stage IVb—tumors that are extrathyroidal and surgically unresectable, any LN involvement, no distant metastatic disease present
	Stage IVc—distant metastatic disease present

LN, lymph node.

SIGNS AND SYMPTOMS

1. **What is the most common presentation of thyroid cancer?**
   - The nodules may be found on physical exam or are identified on radiologic studies performed for unrelated reasons.
   - Anaplastic thyroid cancer presents as widely metastatic disease in 15% to 50% of cases. In most cases it is also locally advanced at diagnosis, causing symptoms from compression of neck structures.

DIAGNOSTIC WORKUP

1. **How should a thyroid nodule be worked up?**
   - First, measure thyroid-stimulating hormone (TSH) and check ultrasound (US) of thyroid and central neck.
   - If the serum TSH is subnormal, a radionuclide scan should be performed to evaluate for hyperfunctioning nodules. If the nodule is found to be hyperfunctioning, no further workup is necessary.
   - If the TSH is normal, high, or thyroid nodule is not found to be hyperfunctioning, nodule characteristics and size on US determine need for fine needle aspiration (FNA).
   - Biopsy of smaller nodules should be considered in high-risk patients (family or personal history of thyroid cancer, history of radiation exposure as a child or adolescent, family history of genetic syndromes described earlier).

2. **How reliable is an FNA result?**
   - If FNA shows a follicular neoplasm, there is a 15% to 30% chance of cancer, and surgery is needed to make the diagnosis.
   - Between 2% and 20% of FNAs are nondiagnostic or unsatisfactory, and 3% to 6% show atypia of unknown significance. Molecular markers may be used to delineate risk of malignancy. Repeat FNA in 3 or more months if nondiagnostic or atypia of undetermined significance
   - If the FNA is interpreted as suspicious for malignancy: surgery is recommended and 60% to 75% end up malignant on final surgical pathology.
   - If FNA is read as malignant: surgery is recommended and 97% to 99% end up malignant on final surgical pathology.

3. **How should a newly diagnosed thyroid carcinoma be worked up?**
   - Neck US, including evaluation of the lateral neck
   - Consider neck MRI or CT if there are bulky, fixed lesions or substernal involvement is suspected
   - Routine preoperative serum thyroglobulin (Tg) measurement is *not* recommended
   - In a patient with medullary thyroid cancer, baseline serum calcitonin and carcinoembryonic antigen (CEA) should be measured
   - In a patient with medullary thyroid cancer, pheochromocytoma should always be ruled out by screening for metanephrines in plasma/urine, to avoid intraoperative hypertensive crisis

TREATMENT

1. **What initial surgical treatment modalities are used for differentiated thyroid cancer?**
   - Total thyroidectomy should be performed in patients with cancer >4 cm, gross extrathyroid extension, or clinically apparent metastatic disease to lymph nodes or distant sites.
   - Total thyroidectomy or lobectomy can be performed in patients with thyroid cancer >1 cm and <4 cm without extrathyroid extension and without clinical evidence of lymph node metastases.
   - Lobectomy should be performed as the surgery of choice in patients with thyroid cancer <1 cm without extrathyroidal extension and without clinical evidence of lymph node metastases in the absence of prior head and neck radiation and family history of thyroid cancer.
   - Total thyroidectomy should be pursued if postoperative radioactive iodine (RAI) imaging or ablation is planned because a large thyroid remnant can decrease the efficacy.
   - Total thyroidectomy with neck dissection should be performed in patients with clinically involved lymph nodes.

2. **What initial surgical treatment modalities are used for thyroid cancer other than differentiated (ie, medullary or anaplastic)?**
   - Total thyroidectomy with central neck dissection should be performed for *medullary thyroid cancer.*
   - Complete tumor excision is often impossible in *anaplastic thyroid cancer* because of locally advanced disease. Neoadjuvant external beam radiation therapy (EBRT) with radiosensitizing doses of doxorubicin, followed by resection in responders may allow more complete resection.
   - Clinical trial participation should be strongly encouraged, given dismal prognosis with anaplastic thyroid cancer.

3. **What is further management and follow-up after total thyroidectomy?**
   - Check TSH, Tg, and antithyroglobulin antibody (ATGAB) at 4 to 12 weeks after total thyroidectomy
   - RAI treatment in select differentiated thyroid cancer patients postoperatively
   - EBRT can be given if there is unresectable residual local disease

4. **What thyroid cancers are not RAI-avid?**
   - Medullary and anaplastic cancers are *not* RAI-avid.

5. **What are the indications for RAI ablation postthyroidectomy for differentiated thyroid cancers?**
   - RAI ablation should only be given for RAI-avid disease.
   - Ablation is only routinely recommended postthyroidectomy for patients with high-risk disease defined as:
     - Tumors (T4, any N, any M) of any size of which gross extrathyroid extension is noted
     - Patients with distant metastases

6. When can RAI treatment be omitted?

- In patients with non-RAI-avid disease (*medullary, anaplastic,* some cases of differentiated)
- In patients with low-risk disease defined as:
  - T1a tumors (size ≤1 cm) with no involved lymph nodes or distant metastases

7. How are patients prepared for RAI treatment?

- By withdrawal of thyroid supplementation until TSH >30 mU/L, or by administration of rhTSH (equivalent outcomes)
- Low iodine diet for 1 to 2 weeks before the treatment, no contrast CTs, no iodine-containing drugs (amiodarone)

8. What are some of the caveats of pretreatment RAI scans?

- May obviate RAI treatment if residual uptake is only in the thyroid bed
- Therapeutic RAI treatment with ^{131}I should always be followed by a posttreatment scan, as this accurately detects the extent of disease

9. What are the toxicities/risks of RAI therapy?

- Sialadenitis causing acute and/or chronic xerostomia
- Nasolacrimal duct stenosis
- Decrease of blood count is usually mild and transient with dose to bone marrow below 200 cGy
- Temporary amenorrhea is seen in up to 25% of women
- Women should avoid pregnancy for 6 to 12 months after RAI treatment to decrease the risk of miscarriage
- RAI should not be given to lactating mothers
- Transient decrease in fertility in men
- Gonadal exposure to RAI is decreased by vigorous hydration/frequent urination and frequent defecation/laxative use
- There is a dose-dependent, small increase in the risk of solid cancers and leukemic/myelodysplastic syndrome
- Renal dysfunction increases radiation exposure (and toxicities) by delaying excretion of RAI

10. What is the role of adjuvant EBRT in thyroid cancer?

- It may be given for macroscopic unresectable tumor or grossly positive margins in disease that does not concentrate RAI.

11. What is the initial follow-up after total thyroidectomy and RAI remnant ablation?

- RAI scan 1 week after the remnant ablation, which detects metastatic disease in up to 10% of the patients.
- Tg levels with suppressed TSH approximately 2 to 6 months after RAI; the same lab needs to be used over time to ensure comparability of results.

- In the absence of antithyroglobulin antibody (ATGAR), Tg <0.2 ng/mL during suppression or <1 ng/mL with stimulation implies a disease-free state.
- ATGABs are seen in 25% of the patients with thyroid cancer; it falsely lowers the Tg level.
- If present, ATGAB titer needs to be monitored over time. Persistence for over 1 year or rise after thyroidectomy and RAI ablation may indicate recurrence.
- Heterophile antibodies may cause falsely elevated Tg level.
- If Tg is >2, check the cervical neck US to look for recurrence.

12. **What is long-term follow-up in patients with differentiated thyroid cancer after total thyroidectomy and RAI remnant ablation?**
    - Tg every 6 to 12 months for the first 5 years
    - ATGAB titer every 6 to 12 months for the first 5 years
    - RAI scan at 6 to 12 months after ablation in intermediate- or high-risk patients
    - Cervical neck US at 6 to 12 months postsurgery, then depending on risk of recurrence and Tg level
    - PET/CT may be used in Tg-positive, RAI-scan-negative relapse of differentiated thyroid cancer, or for follow-up in Hürthle cell carcinoma

13. **What is the follow-up in patients with differentiated thyroid cancer who did not undergo postoperative RAI ablation, or if less than total thyroidectomy?**
    - Periodic neck US every 6 to 12 months
    - Serial thyroglobulins

14. **What is the surveillance for patients with resected medullary thyroid cancer?**
    - Serum calcitonin and CEA should be checked 2 to 3 months postoperatively, and then every 6 to 12 months. Patients with detectable calcitonin or elevated CEA levels should undergo imaging to identify residual disease/recurrence; frequency can be adjusted based on calcitonin doubling time.
    - Patients with MEN2A should undergo annual screening for pheochromocytoma and hyperparathyroidism; patients with MEN2B, annual screening for pheochromocytoma.

15. **What is the role of TSH suppression in differentiated thyroid cancer?**
    - Decreases mortality in patients with stages II to IV disease up to 15%.
    - Initial TSH suppression to >0.1 mU/L is recommended for patients with high-risk differentiated thyroid cancer, and 0.1 to 0.5 mU/L in intermediate-risk patients.
    - For low-risk patients who have undergone lobectomy, TSH may be maintained in the mid to lower reference range (0.5–2 mU/L).
    - Subsequently, TSH should be maintained:
      ○ Below 0.1 mU/L indefinitely in patients with a structural incomplete response to therapy by neck US or pathology

○ Between 0.1 and 0.5 mU/L indefinitely in patients with an incomplete bio-chemical response to therapy evidenced by persistently elevated Tg

○ Between 0.1 and 0.5 mU/L for up to 5 years in patients with high-risk disease and considered free of disease

○ Within the lower end of the reference range (between 0.5 and 2 mU/L) for patients with low risk of relapse and are considered free of disease

- Patients managed with TSH suppression should receive calcium (1,200 mg/day) and vitamin D (1,000 IU/day) supplementation to minimize the risk of bone loss.

16. What are the risks of TSH suppression therapy?

- Increased risk of atrial fibrillation
- Increase risk of osteoporosis in postmenopausal women and older men
- Symptomatic exacerbation of coronary artery disease

17. What thyroid cancers should not be managed with TSH suppression?

- Medullary and anaplastic cancers should not be managed with TSH suppression, just with thyroid supplementation to maintain euthyroid state after thyroidectomy.

18. What should be done if Tg rises but RAI scan is negative?

- Newly elevated stimulated serum Tg above 2 ng/mL in an ablated patient is concerning for relapse. Up to 25% to 50% of cases of metastatic spread in initially RAI-avid disease may be RAI-refractory.
- Consider checking for heterophile antibodies, as these, albeit rare, can cause falsely elevated Tg level.
- Bedside US. If this is not revealing, consider CT neck, chest.
- Consider PET scan.
- If cross-sectional imaging detects metastatic disease, consider observation with ongoing thyroid suppression, surgery, EBRT, radiofrequency ablation (RFA), clinical trial, or initiation of tyrosine kinase inhibitor if progressive disease.
- If cross-sectional imaging does not detect metastatic disease, and Tg is >10 ng/mL in a patient with prior history of RAI-avid disease, consider empiric therapeutic RAI treatment, with a diagnostic scan 5 to 8 days afterward (more sensitive than a low-dose, diagnostic scan), although this is controversial. If Tg is stable and bedside US is negative, consider continuation of thyroid suppression therapy with ongoing Tg and US/cross-sectional surveillance.

19. What are the most common sites of local recurrence in patients with thyroid cancer?

- Cervical lymph nodes

20. What are the most common sites of distant metastases in patients with thyroid cancers?

- Differentiated thyroid cancers: lungs and bones; rarely brain
- Medullary thyroid cancers: lungs, liver, and bones

21. **How is metastatic differentiated thyroid cancer managed?**
    - Locoregional metastases, in the absence of distant disease, should be managed surgically whenever technically feasible; RAI may be used adjuvantly after the surgery.
    - Even though this would not affect distant disease, surgical treatment of locoregional disease should be considered in patients with metastases with symptomatic cervical disease or at risk from symptomatic disease, including physician concern for airway compromise.
    - RAI-avid pulmonary metastases should be treated with RAI, possibly with repeated treatments every 6 to 12 months as long as disease remains RAI-avid; prognosis is much better for RAI-avid pulmonary micrometastases. RAI dose may be limited by risk of radiation pneumonitis; consider dosimetry.
    - RAI treatment may cause acute swelling in metastatic areas, thus causing compression of nearby structures; steroids may alleviate this.
    - RAI is of no benefit in non-RAI-avid metastatic disease.
    - TSH suppression to <0.1 mU/L should be maintained in patients with metastatic (distant or local unresectable) differentiated thyroid cancer.
    - EBRT may be used palliatively for metastatic lesions.
    - For RAI-avid brain lesions, pretreatment with glucocorticoids and EBRT, followed by RAI treatment, may yield best response and minimize acute swelling.
    - Clinical trial participation is encouraged.
    - Pharmacotherapy with tyrosine kinase inhibitors may be considered (sorafenib or lenvatinib). Of note, thyroid supplementation must be monitored regularly with these drugs.
    - Chemotherapy is usually ineffective.
    - Combination chemotherapy is not better than single-agent, and response rates to chemotherapeutic agents are generally low.

22. **How do you define RAI-refractory disease?**
    - At least one target lesion without iodine uptake on thyroid scan (RAI pretreatment imaging)
    - Progression following treatment dosage of RAI (lack of iodine uptake on thyroid scan; ie, RAI imaging)
    - Cumulative RAI treatment of >600 mCi

23. **How is recurrent/metastatic medullary thyroid cancer managed?**
    - Resectable locoregional recurrences should be managed surgically, ± adjuvant EBRT
    - Palliative EBRT to symptomatic distant lesions
    - Clinical trial participation should be encouraged
    - Pharmacotherapy with tyrosine kinase inhibitors may be considered (vandetanib or cabozantinib)

24. What are the Food and Drug Administration (FDA) approved pharma-cotherapeutics of recurrent/metastatic thyroid cancer?
    - Differentiated thyroid cancer: Sorafenib and lenvatinib have both been approved; the appropriate sequencing has yet to be determined.
    - Medullary thyroid cancer: Vandetanib and cabozantinib have both been approved; the appropriate sequencing has yet to be determined.
    - Anaplastic thyroid cancer: There are no FDA-approved therapeutics for the treatment of anaplastic thyroid cancer.

25. What are the most serious side effects for the following tyrosine kinase inhibitors?
    - Lenvatinib: hypertension and bleeding
    - Vandetanib: prolonged QT interval (black box warning)
    - Cabozantinib: tracheoesophageal fistulas and gastrointestinal perforations (black box warning)
    - Sorafenib: hypertension and hand/foot syndrome

QUESTIONS

1. A 69-year-old man presents with the complaint of a dysphagia and wheezing. A CT is performed demonstrating a heterogeneously enhancing 10.4 × 8.7 cm mass arising from the thyroid gland encasing and causing compression of the larynx and esophagus. An ultrasound-guided fine needle aspiration (FNA) is performed and demonstrates poorly differentiated anaplastic thyroid carcinoma.
   Which of the following is the most appropriate next step in this patient's management?
   A. External beam radiation therapy to the mass with radiosensitizing doxorubicin
   B. Total thyroidectomy
   C. Vandetanib
   D. Sorafenib

2. A 67-year-old woman with recently diagnosed thyroid cancer presents to you for evaluation. She was undergoing an evaluation for fatigue during which an ultrasound of her thyroid gland was performed and demonstrated a 2 × 3 cm nodule. Fine needle aspiration (FNA) was performed and demonstrated medullary thyroid cancer.
   Which of the following is the most appropriate recommendation for the management of this patient?
   A. Lobectomy
   B. Radiation
   C. Total thyroidectomy
   D. Total thyroidectomy with central neck dissection
   E. Neoadjuvant chemoradiation followed by total thyroidectomy and central neck dissection

3. A 49-year-woman presents in follow-up for medullary thyroid cancer. She has successfully undergone a thyroidectomy and is currently being observed. She requests evaluation for possible inheritable causes of her malignancies as she has six children.
   Which of the familial syndromes is associated with an increased risk of medullary thyroid cancer?
   A. Cowden syndrome
   B. Familial adenomatous polyposis
   C. MEN2B
   D. Birt–Hogg–Dube syndrome

4. A 37-year-old man with recently diagnosed thyroid cancer presents to establish care. A large thyroid mass was noted by his primary care physician during a yearly physical exam. Fine needle aspiration (FNA) established the diagnosis of papillary thyroid cancer and ^{131}I scan demonstrated no evidence of distant metastases. He underwent a total thyroidectomy, of which pathology demonstrated a 4.3 × 3.7 cm well-differentiated thyroid carcinoma focally muscle invasive.
   Which of the following is the most appropriate next step in this patient's management?
   A. Observation with an ultrasound in 12 months for monitoring of disease recurrence
   B. Adjuvant external beam radiation therapy
   C. Sorafenib for adjuvant therapy
   D. PET/CT scan
   E. Radionuclide scan followed by radioactive iodine (RAI) ablation

5. A 52-year-old woman with a history of thyroid cancer reports to your clinic for evaluation. She underwent a thyroidectomy 10 years ago for neck discomfort, and pathology demonstrated medullary thyroid cancer. Two years ago she had an episode of pneumonia and was found to have an obstructive lesion. Carcinoembryonic antigen (CEA) was 20 ng/mL and she was treated with external beam radiation. CEA 3 months after therapy was <2 ng/mL. She now presents with severe diarrhea and 30 lb weight loss with a CEA = 700 ng/mL. CT demonstrates innumerable pulmonary metastases and a 3 × 4 cm thyroid bed mass.
   Which of the following is the most appropriate next step in this patient's management?
   A. Supportive care and hospice referral
   B. Doxorubicin
   C. Radionuclide scan followed by radioactive iodine (RAI) therapy
   D. Cabozatinib

6. A 64-year-old man presents to your medical oncology practice to transfer his care for metastatic thyroid cancer. Seven years ago he underwent a total thyroidectomy for a 6 cm mass, pathologically shown to be papillary thyroid cancer. He was treated with radioactive iodine (RAI) therapy (200 millicuries) and levothyroxine suppression.

Over the ensuing years he was found to have slowly progressive metastases involving the neck, thoracic inlet, and innumerable pulmonary metastases. Seven months ago, radionuclide scan was repeated demonstrating innumerable metastases and he was treated with repeat RAI therapy (353 millicuries). In the past two months, the patient complains of progressive chest fullness. Prior to your consultation, a radionuclide scan was repeated and demonstrates no evidence of disease. You order a CT, which demonstrates a large thyroid bed mass with progressive narrowing of the thoracic inlet and interval enlargement of the pulmonary metastases.

Which of the following would be the most appropriate recommendation for treatment of this patient's disease?

A. Repeat RAI therapy (200 millicuries)
B. Doxorubicin
C. Lenvatinib
D. Cabozatinib
E. Observation

ANSWERS

1. **A. External beam radiation therapy to the mass with radiosensitizing doxorubicin.** External beam radiation therapy to the mass with radiosensitizing doxorubicin is the treatment of choice for anaplastic thyroid cancer. Excision is often impossible due to invasion of local structures; however, this may be considered after neoadjuvant chemoradiation.

2. **D. Total thyroidectomy with central neck dissection.** Total thyroidectomy with central neck dissection is the treatment of choice for medullary thyroid cancer.

3. **C. MEN2B.** MEN2A and 2B are associated with an increased risk of medullary thyroid cancer. Other syndromes associated with increased risk of thyroid cancer include Cowden syndrome and familial adenomatous polyposis, which are associated with differentiated thyroid cancers.

4. **E. Radionuclide scan followed by radioactive iodine (RAI) ablation.** Radionuclide scan followed by RAI therapy is utilized for remnant ablation in this setting. The absolute indications for RAI ablation postthyroidectomy are tumors that have gross extrathyroidal extension as well as those with distant metastases.

5. **D. Cabozatinib.** Cabozatinib is the treatment of choice for metastatic medullary thyroid cancer. Doxorubicin is a Food and Drug Administration (FDA) approved cytotoxic agent approved for the treatment of metastatic differentiated thyroid cancer and does not have a role in the management of medullary thyroid cancer. RAI therapy does not have a role in the management of medullary thyroid cancer.

6. **C. Lenvatinib.** Lenvatinib would be the appropriate treatment for this patient with iodine refractory metastatic papillary thyroid cancer. Food and Drug Administration (FDA) approved therapeutics in this setting include lenvatinib and sorafenib. Cabozatinib is an approved therapeutic for metastatic medullary thyroid cancer and does not have a role in the management of differentiated thyroid cancer.

16

Adrenocortical Carcinoma

Frank C. Cackowski and Tobias Else

EPIDEMIOLOGY, PATHOGENESIS, AND RISK FACTORS

1. **What is the most common adrenocortical tumor?**
   - Unilateral, benign, adrenocortical adenoma, usually less than 4 cm in size

2. **What is the peak age of incidence for adrenocortical carcinoma?**
   - Two peaks: early childhood and the fifth decade of life

3. **What hereditary cancer syndromes are associated with increased risk of adrenocortical carcinoma (ACC)?**
   - Li–Fraumeni syndrome
   - Lynch syndrome
   - Multiple endocrine neoplasia type 1
   - Beckwith–Wiedemann syndrome (children)
   - Offer genetic counseling and TP53 germline testing to all patients with ACC (Chompret criteria) and consider screening of tumor tissue for absence of DNA mismatch repair proteins

4. **Which signaling pathways are commonly altered in hereditary or spontaneous ACC?**
   - IGF2, TP53, and Wnt/beta-catenin

STAGING

1. **Define the staging for adrenal gland tumors European Network for the Study of Adrenal Tumors (ENSAT).**

Stage	Definition
I	Primary tumor ≤5 cm in greatest dimension, limited to the adrenal, and no LN involvement
II	Primary tumor >5 cm in greatest dimension, limited to the adrenal, and no LN involvement
III	Tumor of any size with invasion of periadrenal fat or adjacent organs or involvement of regional LN
IV	Any local tumor extent when distal metastases are present

LN, lymph node.

SIGNS AND SYMPTOMS

1. **What are common manifestations of ACC?**
   - Sixty percent of patients with ACC present with symptoms of excess steroid hormone production.
     - Cushing syndrome presents as weight gain, proximal muscle weakness, supraclavicular fat pad enlargement, hyperglycemia, truncal obesity, hypertension, hypokalemia, purple striae, "buffalo hump," and diabetes.
     - Hirsutism and virilization due to androgen excess in women are common.
     - Mineralocorticoid excess manifests as hypertension, hypokalemia (rare in ACC).
     - Estrogen-secreting tumors may cause gynecomastia, testicular atrophy in men.
   - Nonsecreting adrenal cancer may present with pain or abdominal discomfort due to compression of nearby structures.

DIAGNOSIS

1. **How should an adrenal mass be worked up?**
   - Biochemical evaluation should always precede imaging.
   - Endocrine evaluation for secretory versus nonsecretory tumor:
     - One milligram dexamethasone suppression test; 24-hour urine cortisol is less sensitive.
     - Serum dehydroepiandrosterone sulfate (DHEAS) and total testosterone
     - Plasma aldosterone and renin activity
     - Other hormone measurements, such as 11-deoxycortisol, 17-OH-progesterone, or estradiol can help in some settings
     - To exclude adrenomedullary tumors (pheochromocytoma): fractionated plasma free metanephrines (levels above twofold upper limit of normal are concerning for pheochromocytoma), 24-hour urine fractionated metanephrines, drugs that may affect testing for metanephrines and should be avoided include caffeine, appetite suppressants, acetaminophen, clonidine, dexamethasone, diuretics, MAOIs, nicotine, tricyclic antidepressants, serotonin reuptake inhibitors, adrenergic agonists, alcohol, tetracycline, and amphetamines
     - Serum electrolytes
   - Adrenal protocol CT abdomen or MRI abdomen allows evaluation for signs of malignancy of an adrenal tumor.
   - If malignant tumor is suspected, CT chest, abdomen, and pelvis should be performed to evaluate extent of disease.

2. **Which radiographic features help distinguish adrenal adenoma versus ACC?**
   - Attenuation of <10 Hounsfield units (HU) on noncontrast CT is reassuring for a lipid-rich benign adenoma; not valid if the tumor is heterogeneous.

- On a contrast CT, a contrast washout >60% at 15 minutes is reassuring for a benign adenoma.
- Irregular borders, internally heterogeneous tumor, local invasion on cross-sectional imaging are features concerning for ACC.
- Activity on ^{18}FDG-PET/CT is useful in ambiguous cases. However, ~10% of adenomas are FDG-avid.

TREATMENT OF LOCALIZED DISEASE

1. **What surgery is recommended for ACC?**
   - Complete removal of the ACC in its entirety, following surgical oncology principles, preferably by open adrenalectomy at a large volume medical center. Avoidance of capsule rupture is essential.

2. **What are key perioperative management points at time of adrenalectomy for ACC?**
   - If Cushing syndrome (even subclinical Cushing syndrome) is caused by the tumor, glucocorticoid replacement should be started promptly postoperatively to avoid acute adrenal insufficiency.

3. **What adjuvant treatments can be given for localized ACC?**
   - Adjuvant radiation therapy improves local control, but the effects on progression-free survival and overall survival are unclear.
   - Adjuvant mitotane is the traditional adjuvant therapy, although benefits are controversial. Current prospective studies are trying to answer this question.

4. **What is the role of partial resection in advanced ACC?**
   - In patients with advanced, secretory ACC, resection should be considered if a significant bulk of the primary tumor and the metastatic mass can be removed to improve symptomatic/hormonal control and the speed of tumor growth justifies this intervention.

SURVEILLANCE

1. **What surveillance measures should be taken for resected adrenal cancer?**
   - History and physical exam every 3 to 6 months with special attention to signs of hormone insufficiency
   - Imaging with CT scans (chest, abdomen, and pelvis) every 3 to 6 months
   - Repeat tumor markers (if secretory tumor) every 3 to 6 months.

TREATMENT OF METASTATIC DISEASE

1. **What are the systemic treatment options for locally advanced or metastatic ACC?**
   - **Mitotane** monotherapy:
     - Partial response in 10% to 30%
     - Mitotane should be given with replacement dose hydrocortisone (may be required lifelong).

- **Cisplatin (or carboplatin) + etoposide + doxorubicin ± mitotane** produced a 49% response rate in a large, single-arm phase 2 trial and demonstrated significant improvements in response and progression-free survival (but not overall survival) when compared to **streptozocin ± mitotane**.
- **Streptozocin ± mitotane** is generally considered after failures with platinum, etoposide, and cisplatin ± mitotane.
- Consider clinical trials. Many targeted agents are in development.
- Observation is appropriate for indolent disease.
- Control of hormone excess symptoms:
  - Patients with hormone-producing tumors need antihormonal therapy to treat often debilitating symptoms (particularly with glucocorticoid production)
    - Receptor antagonists (eg, spironolactone or mifepristone)
    - Synthesis inhibitors (eg, ketoconazole, metyrapone)
    - Adrenolytic agents (eg, mitotane)

QUESTIONS

1. A 28-year-old woman presents with nausea and abdominal pain. Blood is present on her urinalysis, so a stone protocol CT is ordered, which shows the presence of a left kidney stone. The scan also demonstrates the presence of a 2 cm well-circumscribed, homogeneous right adrenal lesion with an attenuation of 8 Hounsfield units.
   What follow-up is most appropriate for her right adrenal lesion?
   A. Adrenal protocol CT abdomen now
   B. MRI abdomen
   C. Repeat CT abdomen in 3 months
   D. No follow-up is necessary

2. A 56-year-old woman presents with mild hyperglycemia, and facial swelling, and is found to have a 7 cm right adrenal tumor. She proceeds to radical adrenalectomy, which is performed without complications.
   How should her glucocorticoids be managed after surgery?
   A. Start hydrocortisone replacement following surgery (eg, 50 mg IV tid) and transition to 20 mg in the a.m. and 10 mg in the early afternoon
   B. Give 200 mg IV hydrocortisone once
   C. Measure 8 a.m. cortisol the next morning
   D. Order an adrenocorticotropic hormone (ACTH) stimulation test for the next day

3. A 39-year-old otherwise healthy man presents with left flank pain and hyperglycemia. He is found to have a 12 cm left adrenal mass with a 4 cm right upper lobe lung nodule. A 1 mg dexamethasone suppression test is abnormal (8 a.m. cortisol following 1 mg dexamethasone is 14 mcg/dL).
   What is the most appropriate initial management?
   A. Left open radical adrenalectomy
   B. Left open radical adrenalectomy and right upper lobe lung wedge resection

C. Medical therapy with mitotane
D. Medical therapy with sunitinib

4. A 32-year-old woman presents with right flank pain and is found to have a right 13 cm non-hormone-secreting adrenocortical carcinoma (ACC) and multiple, bilateral lung metastases. She has a right radical adrenalectomy without complications. She is thought to have too many metastases to benefit from cytoreductive surgery. She has a 2-year-old daughter that she would really like to see enter kindergarten and wants to be as aggressive as possible with her treatment. What is the most appropriate medical therapy?
   A. Sunitinib
   B. Mitotane
   C. Mitotane and streptozocin
   D. Cisplatin, etoposide, doxorubicin, and mitotane

5. A 43-year-old man presents with left abdominal pain and hyperglycemia. He is found to have a 15 cm left adrenal mass. A dexamethasone suppression test confirms the presence of elevated cortisol. Imaging does not reveal distant metastases. He proceeds to a radical adrenalectomy. A lymph node dissection is also performed and reveals three positive nodes.
   What if any additional therapy would you recommend?
   A. Observation
   B. Adjuvant radiation therapy and/or adjuvant mitotane
   C. Wide surgical reexcision
   D. Adjuvant cyclophosphamide, etoposide, doxorubicin, and mitotane

6. A 26-year-old woman is found to have a 7 cm localized adrenocortical carcinoma (ACC). She has no family history of ACC or other cancers. If germline testing were performed, a mutation is most likely to be found in which gene?
   A. *TP53*
   B. *RET*
   C. *VHL*
   D. *IDH*

ANSWERS

1. **D. No follow-up is necessary.** The adrenal lesion is most likely benign because of the size and Hounsfield units <10.

2. **A. Start hydrocortisone replacement following surgery (eg, 50 mg IV tid) and transition to 20 mg in the a.m. and 10 mg in the early afternoon.** Patients with adrenal tumors with Cushing syndrome will have adrenal insufficiency after surgery (suppression of adrenal axis due to long-standing cortisol excess) and should be given replacement dose glucocorticoids. Later replacement therapy can be tapered as recovery of adrenal function is assessed.

3. **B. Left open radical adrenalectomy and right upper lobe lung wedge resection.** If feasible, cytoreductive surgery is preferred in adrenocortical carcinoma (ACC), particularly if the tumor is hormone secreting. The decision for the therapeutic approach is largely dependent on the speed of disease. Another consideration would be to initiate neoadjuvant chemotherapy (EDP+M) and follow patient to assess for speed of disease and to control hormone excess prior to surgery.

4. **D. Cisplatin, etoposide, doxorubicin, and mitotane.** According to the FIRM-ACT trial the regimen of cisplatin, etoposide, doxorubicin, and mitotane is probably the most active and is in keeping with her goal of intensive therapy.

5. **B. Adjuvant radiation therapy and/or adjuvant mitotane.** Adjuvant radiation does prevent local recurrence, although the effect on progression-free or overall survival is unclear. Adjuvant mitotane should also be considered.

6. **A. TP53.** Mutations in TP53 are very common in ACC and therefore all newly diagnosed patients should be offered genetic counseling and TP53 testing. A recent series showed a frequency of TP53 mutations of approximately 2% to 5% in patients with no family history to suggest a genetic syndrome. More than 50% of children with ACC have a germline TP53 mutation. It is also worthwhile to conduct germline testing or tumor analysis for Lynch syndrome, which is present in 3% to 4% of all ACC patients.

17 Pheochromocytomas and Paragangliomas

Frank C. Cackowski and Tobias Else

EPIDEMIOLOGY

1. **What is the peak age of incidence of pheochromocytoma?**
   - Between the third and fifth decades of life, usually earlier in genetic syndromes

ETIOLOGY AND RISK FACTORS

1. **What is the cell of origin of a pheochromocytoma?**
   - Pheochromocytoma: chromaffin cell of the adrenal medulla.
   - Paraganglioma: extra-adrenal paraganglial cell (cells associated with paraganglia of the autonomous nervous system). Common locations are head, neck, and abdomen.

2. **What genetic syndromes are associated with pheochromocytoma?**
   - All pheochromocytoma/paraganglioma patients should be sent for genetic counseling since more than 25% are caused by genetic syndromes
   - MEN2A and 2B (RET)
   - Neurofibromatosis type 1 (NF1)
   - Von Hippel–Lindau (VHL)
   - Succinate dehydrogenase subunit A, B, C, and D gene mutations (*SDHA, SDHB, SDHC, SDHD,* and *SDHAF2*)
   - Transmembrane protein 127 (TMEM127), myc-associated protein X (MAX)

3. **What clinical/biochemical features distinguish pheochromocytomas of various genetic causes?**

Genetic Condition	Catecholamines Secreted by Pheo	Proportion of Malignant Pheo (%)	Location of Pheo
MEN2	Epi	<5	Adrenal
Neurofibromatosis-1	Epi, NE	<5	Adrenal
Von Hippel–Lindau	NE	<5	Adrenal
SDH subunit mutation	NE, dopamine	>20 (SDHB)	Adrenal, extra-adrenal
Sporadic	NE, Epi	10	Adrenal

epi, epinephrine; NE, norepinephrine; Pheo, pheochromocytoma.

   - Some pheochromocytomas (especially paragangliomas) are nonfunctional.

4. **Which two classes do pheochromocytoma driver mutations fall into?**
   - Hypoxia/pseudohypoxia: including HIF2A, VHL, SDHx, and succinate dehydrogenase
   - Kinase pathways: including RET, NF1, and TMEM127

SIGNS AND SYMPTOMS

1. **What are common manifestations of pheochromocytomas and paragangliomas?**
   - Autonomic symptoms: episodic hypertension, perspiration, headache, pallor, orthostatic hypotension, arrhythmias, and hyperglycemia. (*classic triad = headache, diaphoresis, and tachycardia*)
   - Compressive symptoms from primary tumor or metastases

2. **What are common locations of metastases?**
   - Lymph nodes, liver, lung, and bone

DIAGNOSIS

1. **How is pheochromocytoma diagnosed?**
   - Biochemical evaluation should always precede imaging.
   - Endocrine evaluation for secretory versus nonsecretory tumor:
     - Fractionated plasma free metanephrines (levels above twofold upper limit of normal are concerning for pheochromocytoma)
     - Twenty-four hour urine fractionated metanephrines
   - Drugs that may affect testing for metanephrines and should be avoided include monoamine oxidase inhibitors (MAOIs), tricyclic antidepressants (TCAs) (and atypical TCAs, eg, cyclobenzaprine), serotonin and norepinephrine reuptake inhibitors (selective serotonin reuptake inhibitors [SSRIs] and serotonin and norepinephrine reuptake inhibitors [SNRIs]), adrenergic agonists, and amphetamines.
     - For adrenal tumors (to exclude adrenocortical tumors): plasma aldosterone and renin activity, 1 mg of dexamethasone suppression test; 24-hour urine cortisol is less sensitive, serum dehydroepiandrosterone sulfate (DHEAS) and total testosterone
     - Adrenal protocol CT abdomen or MRI abdomen allows characterization of the adrenal tumor
   - If malignant tumor is suspected, CT chest, abdomen, and pelvis should be performed to evaluate extent of disease.
   - Cross-sectional imaging (CT or MRI) should be used before functional imaging.

2. **Which functional imaging modalities are used for pheochromocytoma/ paraganglioma?**
   - Metaiodobenzylguanidine (MIBG) scan (MIBG is a ^{131}I- or ^{123}I-labeled molecule similar to norepinephrine) is most commonly used. MIBG scans confirm the diagnosis of a pheochromocytoma or paraganglioma, which usually is obvious on cross-sectional imaging.

- Other useful functional imaging modalities are ^{18}F-FDG-PET/CT (eg, SDHB-related tumors) or 18F-DOPA PET/CT for tumors with mutations in kinase pathways. Most pheochromocytomas and paragangliomas, particularly head and neck paragangliomas, will be positive in Ga68 DOTATATE scans.

PROGNOSTIC FACTORS

1. **What are adverse prognostic features of pheochromocytoma?**
   - Metastatic disease
   - Symptoms due to elevated catecholamines

TREATMENT OF LOCALIZED DISEASE

1. **What surgery is recommended for pheochromocytoma?**
   - Laparoscopic surgery is preferred.
   - Cytoreduction of distant metastases with chemotherapy, if feasible, should be considered.

2. **What are key perioperative management points at time of adrenalectomy for pheochromocytoma?**
   - Preoperative alpha-1 blockade with phenoxybenzamine or doxazosin must be started at least 7 days before surgery, and perioperative additional alpha- and beta-blockers should be considered (the latter only after alpha-blockade has been achieved). Patients are sufficiently alpha-blocked once they develop orthostatic hypotension and nasal congestion.
   - Salt and volume supplementation should be encouraged to ameliorate orthostatic symptoms and to prevent hypotension postoperatively.

3. **What surveillance measures should be taken for completely resected pheochromocytoma?**
   - Physical exam, tumor markers at 3 to 6 months after the surgery, then every 6 months for 3 years, then annually
   - Biannually metanephrine/normetanephrine plasma—even slightly elevated above normal range should provoke concern (do not wait for a twofold increase)
   - Imaging as clinically indicated (always in genetic cases)
   - Carriers of genetic mutations need lifelong surveillance with at least yearly plasma metanephrine levels and adequate imaging (yearly abdomen MRI for VHL, whole body MRI every 2 years for patients with SDHx mutations)

TREATMENT OF METASTATIC DISEASE

1. **What are treatment options in metastatic, unresectable pheochromocytoma?**
   - Symptom control with alpha- and beta-blockers
   - Clinical trial participation
   - Chemotherapy with cyclophosphamide + vincristine + dacarbazine yielded an overall response rate of 57% (biochemical overall response rate 79%), with median duration of response 21 to 22 months in a single-arm, phase 2 study
   - Alternatively, temozolomide and capecitabine are promising agents

- Radioactive ^{131}I-MIBG at specialized centers
- Other radiopharmaceuticals such as somatostatin analogs can be used if their uptake is demonstrated on functional imaging

QUESTIONS

1. A 25-year-old man is found to have concurrent medullary thyroid cancer and pheochromocytoma. He does not know the family history on his father's side but otherwise has no family history of cancer. Genetic testing is most likely to find a mutation in which gene?
   A. *VHL*
   B. *RET*
   C. *SDHB*
   D. *NF1*

2. A 37-year-old otherwise healthy woman develops hypertension that is not controlled with hydrochlorothiazide and lisinopril. Laboratory testing reveals elevated plasma metanephrines.
   Which antihypertensive should be added to her regimen?
   A. Doxazosin
   B. Amlodipine
   C. Metoprolol
   D. Losartan

3. A 52-year-old man presents with diaphoresis and episodic hypertension and is found to have elevated levels of metanephrines in a 24-hour urine. An adrenal protocol CT abdomen demonstrates a 7 cm left adrenal mass. His CT chest and CT pelvis are normal.
   What additional imaging is most appropriate?
   A. No additional
   B. MRI abdomen
   C. ^{18}F-FDG-PET/CT
   D. ^{131}I-MIBG scan

4. A 33-year-old otherwise healthy woman presents with hypertension and palpitations and is found to have elevated plasma metanephrines and a 6 cm left adrenal mass on CT of her abdomen. A ^{131}I-MIBG scan demonstrates the left adrenal mass and an additional 3 cm area of uptake in the left lobe of her liver.
   In addition to an alpha-blocker, what is the most appropriate management?
   A. Laparoscopic left adrenalectomy and liver wedge resection
   B. Laparoscopic left adrenalectomy only
   C. Cyclophosphamide, vincristine, and dacarbazine
   D. Medical therapy with ^{131}I-MIBG

5. A 42-year-old man with a history of an adrenal incidentaloma is admitted to the hospital with diaphoresis and atrial fibrillation with rapid ventricular response. The morning after admission his rate is controlled with diltiazem. He is also taking aspirin, ibuprofen, and cyclobenzaprine.

Which of the following medications should be held during the upcoming evaluation?

A. Diltiazem

B. Aspirin

C. Ibuprofen

D. Cyclobenzaprine

6. **A 37-year-old woman presents with pain from a 16 cm left pheochromocytoma and at least five liver metastases that are not causing symptoms, but showed growth over the last 3 months. What is the most appropriate plan of treatment?**

A. Adrenalectomy and liver tumor debulking

B. Adrenalectomy followed by chemotherapy with cyclophosphamide, vincristine, and dacarbazine

C. Adrenalectomy alone

D. ^{131}I-MIBG therapy alone

ANSWERS

1. **B. RET.** Pheochromocytoma and medullary thyroid cancer are characteristic of multiple endocrine neoplasia type 2, which is characterized by mutations in the RET oncogene.

2. **A. Doxazosin.** This patient's presentation is suspicious for a pheochromocytoma as the cause of her hypertension. Metanephrine levels are usually elevated more than twofold at initial presentation. The catecholamines released by a pheochromocytoma are best inhibited with an alpha-blocker such as doxazosin. In addition, the patient should be worked up with cross-sectional imaging to find the tumor.

3. **D. ^{131}I-MIBG scan.** ^{131}I-MIBG scan can be considered to prove the adrenal mass as the source of elevated catecholamines. In the setting of vastly elevated metanephrine levels (eg, >4–5-fold), one could argue to not conduct confirmatory functional imaging and make the diagnosis by biochemistry and cross-sectional imaging only. Due to the size of his pheochromocytoma, this patient is at increased risk of metastases. Thus, a functional imaging modality can help to detect occult metastasis, for example, bone metastasis. The ^{131}I-MIBG scan is often more sensitive than an ^{18}F-FDG-PET/CT.

4. **A. Laparoscopic left adrenalectomy and liver wedge resection.** Adrenalectomy and metastasectomy. Patients presenting with metastatic pheochromocytoma should have resection of their primary tumor and cytoreduction of metastases if feasible to provide palliation of symptoms and ease of medical management.

5. **D. Cyclobenzaprine.** This patient may have a pheochromocytoma and requires laboratory testing for metanephrines. Many drugs can interfere with this evaluation including selective serotonin reuptake inhibitors (SSRIs), serotonin and norepinephrine reuptake inhibitors (SNRIs), tricyclic antidepressants (TCAs), and atypical tricyclics such as cyclobenzaprine.

6. **B. Adrenalectomy followed by chemotherapy with cyclophosphamide, vincristine, and dacarbazine.** She should have an adrenalectomy for symptom control. Her metastases are unlikely to be amenable to cytoreductive surgery. Therefore the regimen of cyclophosphamide, vincristine, and dacarbazine is the most reasonable choice (alternatively temozolomide and capecitabine or ^{131}I-MIBG). Alternatively, adrenalectomy and surveillance of liver metastasis are another option for slow growing neoplasms. Some pheochromocytomas grow very slowly and chemotherapeutic intervention can be delayed until growth or biochemical progression is obvious. MIBG therapy is a consideration, but only after surgery.

IV

BREAST CANCER

Breast Cancer

18

Kunal C. Kadakia, Erin F. Cobain, and Monika Burness

EPIDEMIOLOGY

1. **What is the most frequently diagnosed cancer among females?**
   - In the United States, as well as worldwide, breast cancer is the most frequently diagnosed cancer among females. Annual incidence is approximately 230,000 cases per year.

2. **Where does breast cancer rank as a cause of cancer death?**
   - In the United States, breast cancer is the second most frequent cause of cancer-related death among women overall behind lung cancer; among women in their fifth and sixth decades of life, it is the most frequent cause of cancer-related deaths. Worldwide, breast cancer is the leading cause of cancer deaths among women.

3. **Among women in the United States, what is the lifetime risk of developing breast cancer?**
   - There is a 12% (approximately one in eight) lifetime risk of developing breast cancer.

ETIOLOGY AND RISK FACTORS

1. **What risk factors are associated with the development of breast cancer?**
   - Female gender
   - Older age: the median age of female breast cancer diagnosis is 61 years
   - Predisposing genetic mutations such as *BRCA1* and *BRCA2*
   - Personal history of breast cancer (in situ or invasive)
   - Family history of breast cancer in a first-degree relative (especially if diagnosed under age 50 or in a male)
   - History of chest irradiation
   - Race: the highest rates of breast cancer occur among White females
   - Younger age at menarche ($\leq$ age 12)
   - Older age at menopause ($\geq$ age 55)
   - Nulliparity or pauciparity
   - Older age at first birth ($\geq$ age 30)
   - History of certain benign breast lesions
   - High mammographic breast density

- Alcohol use
- Postmenopausal hormonal replacement therapy: specifically combination estrogen and progestin therapy for >5 years

2. **What is the Gail model and what factors are incorporated into this model?**
   - The Gail model, also known as the Breast Cancer Risk Assessment Tool, is used to estimate a woman's risk of developing invasive breast cancer.
   - The Gail model incorporates current age, age at menarche, age at first birth, race, number of first-degree relatives diagnosed with breast cancer, total number of previous breast biopsies, and presence or absence of atypical hyperplasia on a previous breast biopsy to report estimated 5-year risk and lifetime risk of developing breast cancer.

STAGING AND HISTOLOGY

1. **American Joint Committee on Cancer (AJCC) Staging for breast cancer:**

Stage	Criteria
0	Carcinoma in situ
I	Tumor ≤20 mm in greatest dimension with negative or micrometastatic lymph node disease (ie, lymph node metastasis >0.2 mm and/or >200 metastatic cells, but ≤2.0 mm)
	No distant metastatic disease
II	Tumor >20 mm in greatest dimension without surface skin involvement and without nodal disease
	or
	Tumor ≤50 mm in greatest dimension with 1–3 three positive lymph node metastases
	No distant metastatic disease
III	Any size tumor with ≥4 axillary lymph node metastases or any clinically diagnosed internal mammary lymph node metastases
	or
	Tumor >50 mm in greatest dimension with ≥1 axillary nodal metastases
	or
	Any size tumor with direct extension to the chest wall or skin regardless of nodal status
	or
	Any inflammatory breast cancer regardless of nodal status
	No distant metastatic disease
IV	Any breast cancer with distant metastatic disease

2. Nottingham combined histologic grading of breast cancer:

Nottingham Combined Grade	Definition	Prognosis
G1	Well differentiated	Most favorable
G2	Moderately differentiated	Intermediate
G3	Poorly differentiated	Least favorable

3. **Define the histologic subtypes of in situ breast cancers.**
   - The in situ breast cancers can have ductal or lobular phenotype.

4. **Define the histologic subtypes of invasive breast cancer. Which is the most common?**
   - The invasive breast cancers include ductal, lobular, mixed, mucinous, tubular, medullary, metaplastic, papillary, and cribriform.
   - Infiltrating ductal carcinoma is the most frequent, accounting for >75% of cases of invasive breast cancers. Infiltrating lobular carcinomas are second most common (5%–10%), primarily found in the elderly, and are more often multicentric. The vast majority of lobular carcinomas are estrogen receptor (ER) positive and display loss of E-cadherin; some are associated with hereditary diffuse gastric cancer (E-cadherin [CDH1] germline mutation).

5. **Among the histologic subtypes of invasive breast cancer, which are the more favorable?**
   - Tubular and mucinous represent favorable histologies due to decreased propensity to metastasize.

SIGNS AND SYMPTOMS

1. **What are the common signs and symptoms of breast cancer?**
   - Breast lump
   - Nipple discharge
   - Inversion of the nipple
   - Distortion of shape or size of breast
   - Associated skin changes including dimpling, scaling, flaking, erythema, and pitting

DIAGNOSIS

Screening

1. **How are most breast cancers diagnosed?**
   - Most breast cancers are diagnosed as a result of an abnormal finding on screening mammography.

2. **At what ages should women undergo screening mammography for breast cancer?**
   - Screening guidelines are based on an individual's breast cancer risk. Guidelines differ slightly by organization. For women at average risk, routine screening

for breast cancer is well accepted for women 50 to 69 years age. The benefit of screening in women between ages 40 and 49 is less than that for older women; some guidelines favor screening this population and some recommend against screening. The benefit of screening above age 70 is less well established; screening is generally recommended for women above age 70 who could benefit from treatment of a discovered cancer based on life expectancy and comorbidities.

3. **How often should screening mammography be performed?**
   - Every 1 to 2 years

4. **What is the role of clinical breast exam in breast cancer screening?**
   - Some organizations recommend clinical breast self-exam yearly after age 40. Breast self-exam is not recommended for screening.

Diagnostic Workup of the Abnormal Mammography or Clinical Exam

1. **What is the initial approach to an abnormal finding on mammography or clinical examination?**
   - Detection of a breast mass by the patient or on clinical exam should prompt additional workup by mammography and/or ultrasound. Abnormal screening mammographic findings can lead directly to biopsy or may require additional assessment with diagnostic mammography, ultrasound, or MRI.

2. **What features on a mammogram are suspicious for malignancy?**
   - Dense mass, which is often spiculated
   - Microcalcifications

3. **Ultrasound assessment is particularly useful for assessment of what features?**
   - Ultrasound is useful in distinguishing between cystic and solid masses detected on mammography or clinical examination.
   - Ultrasound may also provide additional information on whether a solid mass is more or less likely to be malignant.

4. **When should the breast abnormality on imaging or clinical exam be biopsied?**
   - Any palpable mass should be biopsied.
   - Any mass that is suspicious on imaging studies should be biopsied.

Diagnostic Workup for Pathologically Confirmed Breast Cancer

1. **Once a diagnosis of invasive breast cancer has been made on biopsy, what are the next appropriate steps in the diagnostic workup of the patient?**
   - Complete physical exam including clinical staging of the cancer
   - Bilateral mammography to assess for any additional breast lesions
   - Surgical staging of the ipsilateral axillary lymph nodes if the results will affect therapeutic decisions for the patient
   - Consideration of testing for a genetic predisposition to breast cancer in patients that meet criteria

2. **What additional imaging studies are required for staging once a diagnosis of breast cancer has been made?**
   - All clinically suspicious symptoms such as bone pain that might suggest metastatic disease should be assessed with appropriate imaging.
   - Early-stage disease (stages I and II) generally does not require further imaging assessment.
   - Stage III disease should prompt additional imaging studies to assess for metastatic disease; this is usually accomplished with CT scan in combination with bone scan, or whole body PET scan.

3. **For whom should assessment of cardiac function be performed?**
   - For patients who are at risk of developing cardiac dysfunction, including those who will be receiving chemotherapy that includes anthracyclines and/or anti-human epidermal growth factor receptor 2 (anti-HER2) therapy (eg, trastuzumab and/or pertuzumab)

4. **What molecular assessments should be performed on pathologically positive breast cancer specimens?**
   - Testing should be performed to determine expression of ER, progesterone receptor (PR), and HER2, to direct subsequent systemic therapy decisions.

5. **What constitutes a positive, equivocal, and negative HER2 result?**
   - HER2 status can be assessed by immunohistochemistry (IHC) and in situ hybridization (ISH). A positive result is defined as IHC 3+ or dual-probe ISH HER2/CEP17 ratio of more than ≥2.0 or a HER2/CEP17 ratio <2.0 with an average HER2 copy number 6.0 signals/cell. An equivocal result is defined as IHC 2+ or single-probe ISH average HER2 copy number ≥4.0 and <6.0 signals/cell or dual-probe HER2/CEP17 ratio <2.0 with an average HER2 copy number ≥4.0 and <6.0 signals/cell. A negative result is defined as IHC 1+ or 0 or single-probe average HER2 copy number <4.0 signals/cell or a dual-probe HER2/CEP17 ratio <2.0 with an average HER2 copy number <4.0 signals/cell.

6. **When is MRI assessment useful for diagnostic assessment of breast cancer?**
   - To detect multifocal, multicentric disease in the ipsilateral breast
   - To assess the contralateral breast when primary cancer has been detected
   - To assess response to neoadjuvant therapy
   - In cases of axillary lymph node adenocarcinoma or Paget disease of the nipple, to identify a primary breast cancer when other imaging modalities or clinical exam fail to identify the primary lesion

Diagnostic Assessment of Recurrent Breast Cancer

1. **In addition to history, physical exam, and laboratory assessment, what additional diagnostic testing is appropriate for patients with distant recurrence of breast cancer?**
   - Biopsy of first recurrence of disease
   - Determination of ER, PR, and HER2 receptor status of the recurrent cancer

- Imaging (CT chest/abdomen/pelvis and bone scan or PET) to assess the extent of disease

PROGNOSTIC AND PREDICTIVE FACTORS

1. **What are the anatomic and histologic factors in breast cancer that confer a poorer prognosis?**
   - Increasing number of positive lymph nodes
   - Increasing size of tumor
   - Increasing histologic grade
   - Aggressive histologic tumor type

2. **What is the effect of ER and PR status on breast cancer prognosis?**
   - In general, ER/PR-negative tumors have a worse prognosis compared with ER/PR-positive tumors.

3. **What is the effect of increased proliferative rate on breast cancer prognosis?**
   - Increased proliferative rate, usually assessed by mitotic index and staining for Ki67, is associated with a worse prognosis. However, current methods for measuring proliferative status are not standardized.

4. **What are the molecular prognostic tools that are commonly utilized for breast cancer and how are they applied?**
   - Oncotype DX® is a 21-gene assay that provides a numerical score to quantify the 10-year risk of disease recurrence for ER-positive breast cancer. Oncotype DX is currently a standard test incorporated into the treatment algorithm for ER/PR-positive, HER2-negative, lymph node negative breast cancer and is prognostic and predictive of adjuvant chemotherapy benefit. As per American Society of Clinical Oncology (ASCO) guidelines, the EndoPredict 12-gene recurrence score and the PAM50 risk of recurrence score may be used as well.

5. **How is receptor expression employed as a predictive factor (ie, variable that predicts clinical response to proposed therapy)?**
   - ER and PR expression predicts which patients will benefit from endocrine therapy.
   - HER2 overexpression predicts response to HER2 targeted therapies.

TREATMENT: LOCOREGIONAL MANAGEMENT OF BREAST CANCER

Management of Noninvasive Breast Cancer

Lobular Carcinoma In Situ

1. **If the original diagnosis of lobular carcinoma in situ (LCIS) is made with a core needle biopsy, what further intervention is recommended?**
   - Surgical excision

2. **Following pathological confirmation of LCIS, what further management is recommended?**
   - Interval surveillance, implementation of risk reduction strategies including consideration of the use of tamoxifen, raloxifene, aromatase inhibitors, or bilateral prophylactic mastectomy

3. **What is the risk of future invasive breast cancer in a patient with LCIS?**
   - One percent per year

Ductal Carcinoma In Situ

1. **When a diagnosis of ductal carcinoma in situ (DCIS) is made, what are the appropriate treatment options?**
   - Surgical management: mastectomy or lumpectomy with radiation therapy
   - Sentinel lymph node biopsy (SLNB) can be considered and should be performed if a patient is undergoing mastectomy, as SLNB will not be possible at a later time if invasive disease is found
   - Consideration of tamoxifen to decrease risk of recurrence and as chemoprevention in ER-positive DCIS, although no survival benefit has been demonstrated. Tamoxifen not indicated in patients who have undergone bilateral mastectomy

Management of Invasive Breast Cancer

Locoregional Stage I, II or T3, N1, M0 Breast Cancer

1. **What are the initial treatment options for operable, early-stage breast cancer?**
   - Lumpectomy with surgical staging of the axillary lymph nodes

     or
   - Total mastectomy with surgical staging of the lymph nodes

     or
   - Neoadjuvant chemotherapy for tumor size reduction to permit breast-conserving therapy

2. **Is there a survival benefit of mastectomy versus lumpectomy?**
   - No

3. **In the case of lumpectomy, what radiation therapy is recommended following appropriate chemotherapy?**
   - Radiation therapy is recommended to the whole breast, ± radiation boost to tumor bed.
   - In the case of one to three positive lymph nodes, consideration should be given to radiation therapy to the infraclavicular and supraclavicular regions and the internal mammary nodes.
   - In the case of four or greater positive lymph nodes, radiation therapy is recommended to the infraclavicular and supraclavicular regions and consideration is given to radiation to the internal mammary nodes.

4. **In the case of a total mastectomy, what radiation therapy is indicated following appropriate chemotherapy?**
   - For negative axillary lymph nodes:
     - When the tumor is <5 cm and the margins ≥1 mm, no radiation therapy is recommended.
     - When the tumor is <5 cm and the margins are <1 mm, radiation to the chest wall is indicated.
     - When the tumor is >5 cm and the margins are positive, radiation should be considered to the chest wall, and the infraclavicular, supraclavicular, and internal mammary nodes.
   - In the case of one to three positive axillary lymph nodes:
     - Consideration should be given to radiation therapy to the chest wall and the infraclavicular, supraclavicular, and internal mammary lymph nodes.
   - In the case of four or greater positive lymph nodes:
     - Radiation therapy is indicated to the chest wall and infraclavicular and supraclavicular lymph nodes.

PREOPERATIVE CHEMOTHERAPY

1. **For which patients is preoperative chemotherapy considered an option?**
   - Patients with early-stage, resectable disease who wish to consider breast conservation surgery, that is, stages IIA (T2N0M0), IIB (T2N1M0, T3N0M0), and IIIA (T3N1M0) and who would otherwise qualify for breast-conserving surgery except for tumor size
   - Patients with locally advanced breast cancer whose disease is not resectable at the time of diagnosis but might be rendered resectable with preoperative chemotherapy, that is, stage III (except T3N1M0) disease

Preoperative Therapy for Early-Stage, Operable Breast Cancer, Stages IIA (T2N0M0), IIB (T2N1M0, T3N0M0), and IIIA (T3N1M0)

1. **What chemotherapy regimens are appropriate for preoperative therapy?**
   - The same regimens that are used for adjuvant chemotherapy are acceptable for preoperative therapy.
   - An acceptable option is endocrine therapy alone in postmenopausal ER- and/or PR-positive patients.
   - If endocrine therapy is employed, an aromatase inhibitor is recommended in postmenopausal patients.
   - For patients with HER2-positive tumors, preoperative chemotherapy is recommended to include a minimum of 9 weeks of trastuzumab (with or without pertuzumab) therapy.

2. **For patients who will be receiving preoperative chemotherapy, what portion of the chemotherapy regimen should be completed prior to surgery?**
   - It is recommended to administer all chemotherapy prior to surgery.

Treatment of Locoregional Recurrence

1. **What are the indicated treatments for patients who experience local recurrence of their breast cancer?**
   - For patients initially treated with lumpectomy and radiation, they are recommended to undergo a total mastectomy plus axillary lymph node staging with consideration of systemic therapy.
   - For patients initially treated with mastectomy, axillary lymph node dissection, and radiation, they are recommended to undergo surgical resection with consideration of systemic therapy.
   - For patients initially treated with mastectomy and axillary lymph node dissection without radiation, they are recommended to undergo surgical resection, radiation to the chest wall, supraclavicular lymph nodes, and infraclavicular lymph nodes with consideration of systemic therapy.

2. **What are the indicated treatments for patients with regional recurrence of their breast cancer?**
   - For patients with an axillary recurrence, they are recommended to undergo axillary lymph node dissection and radiation therapy to the chest wall, the axilla, and supraclavicular and infraclavicular lymph nodes with consideration of systemic therapy.
   - For patients with a supraclavicular recurrence, they are recommended to undergo radiation therapy to the chest wall, the axilla, and supraclavicular and infraclavicular lymph nodes with consideration of systemic therapy.
   - For patients with an internal mammary node recurrence, they are recommended to undergo radiation therapy to the chest wall, supraclavicular, infraclavicular, and internal mammary lymph nodes with consideration of systemic therapy.

TREATMENT: SYSTEMIC THERAPY

Adjuvant Endocrine Therapy

1. **What are aromatase inhibitors?**
   - Aromatase inhibitors are a class of drugs that inhibit the enzyme aromatase, which converts circulating androgens to estrogen. Anastrozole and letrozole are nonsteroidal reversible aromatase inhibitors, and exemestane is a steroidal irreversible aromatase inactivator.

2. **What is tamoxifen?**
   - Tamoxifen is a selective ER modulator.

3. **For premenopausal breast cancer patients who will be receiving adjuvant endocrine therapy, what is the recommended regimen (multiple options exist)?**
   - Tamoxifen for at least 5 years or if sufficiently high risk (ie, received adjuvant chemotherapy), current ASCO guidelines (based largely on the SOFT/TEXT trials) suggest consideration of ovarian suppression with tamoxifen or an aromatase inhibitor.

- After 5 years, if treated with tamoxifen alone, women should receive additional therapy based on menopausal status. If they remain pre- or perimenopausal, they should be offered continued tamoxifen for a total duration of 10 years. If postmenopausal, they should be offered the choice of continuing tamoxifen for a total duration of 10 years or switching to an aromatase inhibitor, for a total duration of up to 10 years of adjuvant endocrine therapy.

4. **For postmenopausal breast cancer patients who will be receiving adjuvant endocrine therapy, what is the recommended regimen?**
   - Aromatase inhibitors have greater benefit in postmenopausal women compared to tamoxifen. They can be administered up front for a total of 10 years. Tamoxifen should be used in postmenopausal women with contraindications to or intolerance of aromatase inhibitors.

Neoadjuvant/Adjuvant Chemotherapies

1. **For favorable histology (tubular and colloid) invasive breast cancers, what are the recommendations for adjuvant therapy?**
   - For ER- and/or PR-positive tumors:
     - For tumors <1 cm, no adjuvant therapy is indicated.
     - For tumors 1 cm to less than or equal to 3 cm, consideration can be given to adjuvant endocrine therapy.
     - For tumors 3 cm or greater, adjuvant endocrine therapy is recommended.
   - For node-positive disease, adjuvant endocrine therapy is recommended with or without chemotherapy.
   - For ER- and PR-negative tumors, receptor status should be verified and if still negative, these tumors should be treated as breast cancers with less favorable histology (ductal, lobular, mixed, and metaplastic).

2. **For the less favorable histologies (ductal, lobular, mixed, and metaplastic), what are the recommendations for adjuvant therapy?**
   - Choice of therapy is based on tumor receptor status and stage.
   - ER- and/or PR-positive and HER2-positive tumors:
     - For node-negative disease with a tumor ≤0.5 cm, consideration of endocrine therapy is recommended.
     - For all other diseases, adjuvant endocrine therapy is recommended.
     - Adjuvant chemotherapy with trastuzumab can be considered for tumors 0.6 to 1 cm with negative nodes, and is recommended for tumors >1.0 cm or with nodal disease.
   - ER- and/or PR-positive and HER2-negative tumors:
     - For node-negative disease with a tumor ≤0.5 cm, consideration of endocrine therapy is recommended.
     - For all other diseases, adjuvant endocrine therapy is recommended.
     - For node-negative disease with a tumor >0.5 cm, consideration should be given to performing one of several biomarker assays to guide decision regarding addition of chemotherapy.

○ Adjuvant chemotherapy is recommended for all patients with node-positive disease, pending results of ongoing clinical trials.

- For ER/PR-negative and HER2-positive tumors:
  ○ For node-negative disease with a tumor ≤0.5 cm, no adjuvant therapy is recommended.
  ○ Adjuvant chemotherapy with trastuzumab can be considered for tumors 0.6 to 1 cm with negative nodes, and is recommended for tumors >1.0 cm or with node-positive disease.

- For ER-, PR-, and HER2-negative tumors:
  ○ For node-negative disease with a tumor ≤0.5 cm, no adjuvant therapy is recommended.
  ○ Adjuvant chemotherapy should be considered for tumors 0.6 to 1 cm with negative nodes, and is recommended for tumors >1.0 cm or with node-positive disease.

3. **What are some of the more common non-trastuzumab-based regimens employed for the neoadjuvant and adjuvant treatment of breast cancer?**
   - TAC (combination docetaxel, doxorubicin, and cyclophosphamide); 21-day cycles × six cycles
   - Dose-dense AC (doxorubicin/cyclophosphamide) every 2 weeks × four cycles followed by dose-dense paclitaxel (every 2 weeks × four cycles) or paclitaxel every week × 12 cycles
   - TC (docetaxel/cyclophosphamide) every 3 weeks × four cycles

4. **What are some of the more common trastuzumab-based regimens employed for neoadjuvant and adjuvant treatment of breast cancer?**
   - Dose-dense AC followed by TH (paclitaxel/trastuzumab with or without pertuzumab) weekly × 12 weeks, with trastuzumab continued every 3 weeks for the duration of 1 year
   - TCH (docetaxel/carboplatin/trastuzumab with or without pertuzumab) every 3 weeks × six cycles (or weekly trastuzumab) with trastuzumab continued every 3 weeks for the duration of 1 year
   - If <3 cm and lymph node negative, TH (paclitaxel/trastuzumab) weekly × 12 cycles alone, with trastuzumab continued every 3 weeks for the duration of 1 year is reasonable

Treatment of Metastatic Disease

1. **What is the indicated treatment for ER- and/or PR-positive metastatic breast cancer?**
   - If visceral crisis, consider initial chemotherapy followed by endocrine therapy.
   - Patients without visceral crisis should be started on endocrine therapy.

2. **What is the indicated treatment for patients with ER, PR, HER2 (triple) negative or endocrine refractory, HER2-negative systemic breast cancer?**

- These patients should receive chemotherapy; early incorporation of palliative care should be considered during therapy. If performance status does not permit additional chemotherapy, referral for hospice care is indicated.

3. **What are some of the common chemotherapy regimens for recurrent or metastatic breast cancers?**
   - The goal of therapy for metastatic breast cancer is palliation. Thus, single-agent chemotherapy is commonly used to achieve tumor response while minimizing side effects. Anthracyclines, taxanes, or antimetabolites are frequently used.

4. **What is the indicated treatment for patients with ER/PR-negative or endocrine refractory, and HER2-positive disease?**
   - Therapy in HER2-positive disease should include a HER2 targeted agent. Initial therapy should consist of trastuzumab, pertuzumab, and a taxane, given until maximum tumor response, followed by administration of trastuzumab/pertuzumab alone until disease progression. Second-line therapy should include ado-trastuzumab emtansine, and later regimens can include lapatinib or trastuzumab.

5. **What orally administered inhibitor of cyclin-dependent kinases 4 and 6 has been approved for ER/PR+ metastatic breast cancer in postmenopausal women?**
   - Palbociclib. If endocrine naïve or >12 months since adjuvant therapy, give palbociclib with letrozole. If progressive disease on endocrine therapy, give palbociclib with fulvestrant.

6. **What is the indicated treatment for stage IV breast cancer that has spread to the bone?**
   - If spread to the bone has occurred, in addition to systemic therapy, the patient is recommended to receive osteoclast inhibition with a bisphosphonate or denosumab for prevention of skeletal-related events.

Targeted Agents Employed in Breast Cancer

1. **What is trastuzumab?**
   - Trastuzumab is a humanized monoclonal antibody directed against HER2. Trastuzumab is used in the adjuvant and metastatic settings in patients with HER2-positive tumors. A second monoclonal antibody targeting the extracellular domain of HER2, pertuzumab, has now been approved for use in combination with trastuzumab and chemotherapy in the neoadjuvant setting as well as for metastatic disease.

2. **What is lapatinib?**
   - Lapatinib is a dual tyrosine kinase inhibitor that targets signaling via the EGFR and HER2 pathways.

3. **When is lapatinib used in the treatment of breast cancer?**
   - Lapatinib is used to treat metastatic HER2-positive breast cancer that is resistant to trastuzumab.

4. **What is ado-trastuzumab emtansine and when is it indicated?**
   - Ado-trastuzumab emtansine (TDM-1) is an antibody–drug conjugate composed of the microtubule inhibitor DM1 linked to trastuzumab. It is given as monotherapy and most often used in the second- or third-line setting in metastatic HER2 patients.

Follow-Up/Surveillance

1. **After treatment of breast cancer, how should surveillance be performed?**
   - Clinical assessment every 4 to 6 months for first 5 years and then annually thereafter
   - Annual mammography
   - Annual gynecologic assessment for patients receiving tamoxifen
   - Baseline and periodic evaluation of bone mineral density for patients receiving an aromatase inhibitor or experiencing premature ovarian failure

SPECIAL CONSIDERATIONS

Management of Breast Cancer During Pregnancy

1. **When may chemotherapy be safely instituted in the pregnant breast cancer patient?**
   - Chemotherapy may safely be instituted after the first trimester of pregnancy, and before 35 weeks of pregnancy or 3 weeks of anticipated delivery date (so as to avoid a peripartum bleeding diathesis).

2. **What chemotherapies may be used during pregnancy?**
   - Cyclophosphamide and doxorubicin are considered safe during pregnancy. Fewer safety data are available for taxanes. Trastuzumab is contraindicated during pregnancy.

3. **When may radiation therapy be used during pregnancy?**
   - Radiation therapy is contraindicated during pregnancy.

4. **At what point in the pregnancy may endocrine therapy be employed?**
   - Endocrine therapy is contraindicated during pregnancy and with breastfeeding. It is recommended that endocrine therapy be instituted in the postpartum period once breastfeeding, if used, is complete.

5. **What is the recommended treatment for breast cancer discovered in the first trimester of pregnancy?**
   - With a continued pregnancy, mastectomy with axillary staging is recommended with institution of adjuvant chemotherapy in the second trimester and radiation and endocrine therapy in the postpartum period.

6. **After the first trimester of pregnancy what is the recommended treatment for breast cancer?**
   - A mastectomy or breast-conserving surgery with staging of the axillary lymph nodes followed by adjuvant chemotherapy and institution of adjuvant radiation

and endocrine therapy in the postpartum period, or initiation of neoadjuvant chemotherapy, with surgery and radiation after delivery

- In the later third trimester, after 35 weeks, neoadjuvant therapy should not be given and mastectomy or breast-conserving surgery with staging of the axillary lymph nodes followed by adjuvant chemotherapy and institution of adjuvant radiation and endocrine therapy in the postpartum period is recommended

Fertility Preservation

1. Who should be informed of the impact of chemotherapy on fertility?

- All premenopausal women who will receive chemotherapy should be counseled regarding the potential decline in fertility related to this therapy. These women should be offered referral for fertility preservation prior to initiating therapy.

2. Do most premenopausal women regain menses after chemotherapy?

- The likelihood of resuming menses is related to age. Most women <35 years old will regain menses; however, it is suspected that fertility can be decreased due to early ovarian failure even in women who resume menses.

Management of Inflammatory Breast Cancer

1. What is inflammatory breast cancer?

- Inflammatory breast cancer is a locally advanced form of invasive breast cancer defined by a clinical presentation of peau d'orange skin changes characterized by a well-circumscribed region of edema and erythema, in which the dermal lymphatics are frequently involved. It is associated with high risk of recurrence and a generally poor prognosis.

2. What is the appropriate management of inflammatory breast cancer?

- Neoadjuvant chemotherapy including an anthracycline and taxane, with trastuzumab if the tumor is HER2-positive, is recommended.

- If the patient responds to neoadjuvant therapy, a total mastectomy with level I and II axillary lymph node dissection and radiation therapy to the chest wall and supraclavicular and internal mammary lymph nodes is recommended. Postsurgery, chemotherapy should be completed with inclusion of endocrine therapy as indicated. Trastuzumab should be administered for one full year if the tumor is HER2-positive.

- If there is no response to neoadjuvant chemotherapy, consideration should be given to alternative chemotherapy and the use of radiation.

Management of Paget Disease of the Breast

1. What is Paget disease of the breast?

- Paget disease of the breast is an infrequent malignancy characterized by proliferation of malignant Paget cells in the epidermis leading to areolar eczema with associated scaling, flaking, ulceration, bleeding, and itching. It is important to diagnose Paget disease as it is associated with underlying carcinoma of the breast.

2. **When Paget disease is suspected what is the appropriate diagnostic approach?**
   - Assessment for the presence of an underlying breast lesion with clinical exam and imaging

3. **If no underlying breast lesion is detected what are the next diagnostic and therapeutic steps?**
   - A full thickness biopsy of the affected nipple–areola complex to assess for Paget disease is recommended. If this biopsy is negative for Paget disease, interval follow-up is recommended with consideration of rebiopsy if breast skin alterations do not resolve. If this biopsy is positive for Paget disease, consideration can be given to further imaging and breast tissue assessment. Ultimately a mastectomy with axillary lymph node staging or resection of the nipple–areola complex with whole breast radiation therapy is recommended; this is followed by adjuvant treatment as needed.

4. **If an underlying breast lesion is detected, what are the next diagnostic and therapeutic steps?**
   - A core biopsy of the breast lesion should be performed together with biopsy of the affected skin of the nipple–areola complex.
   - If both the breast and skin biopsies are without evidence of malignancy, interval follow-up is recommended with consideration of rebiopsy if breast skin alterations do not resolve.
   - If DCIS is detected in the breast and Paget disease in the skin, the treatment is the same as for invasive breast cancer with Paget disease except that axillary lymph node staging is not mandatory.

Management of Phyllodes Tumor

1. **What is a phyllodes tumor?**
   - Phyllodes tumor is a quickly growing, typically large tumor consisting of epithelial and stromal components arising from the periductal cells of the breast. The phyllodes tumor may be pathologically classified as benign, borderline, or malignant.

2. **What characteristics of a mass are suspicious for a phyllodes tumor?**
   - Features suspicious for a phyllodes tumor are large size exceeding 2 cm, swift growth, and ultrasound imaging with features similar to a fibroadenoma.

3. **If a diagnosis of a phyllodes tumor is made on excisional or core biopsy what is the next therapeutic step?**
   - Wide excision of the mass; further staging is not required.

4. **If a diagnosis of a fibroadenoma is made on a core biopsy what is the next appropriate diagnostic step?**
   - Wide excision with pathologic assessment is recommended to rule out phyllodes tumor.

QUESTIONS

1. A 63-year-old White woman is diagnosed with a left breast unilateral ER/PR-positive, HER2-negative 3.5 cm invasive ductal carcinoma. Axillary lymph node dissection confirms 2 of 16 lymph nodes involved with invasive carcinoma. She is recovering well and is otherwise asymptomatic with normal labs. What staging studies are indicated at this time?
   A. PET/CT
   B. Bone scan
   C. CT scan of chest, abdomen, and pelvis
   D. No further imaging

2. A 68-year-old woman with stage III ER-positive breast cancer develops metastatic disease involving the bones while on adjuvant exemestane therapy. Her performance status is 0. She is asymptomatic. Which of the choices is optimal as next line therapy?
   A. Tamoxifen
   B. Ovarian suppression
   C. Palbociclib with fulvestrant
   D. Palbociclib with letrozole
   E. Combination cytotoxic chemotherapy

3. A 56-year-old woman is diagnosed with a right breast triple negative 4 cm invasive ductal carcinoma invading through the skin with palpable axillary lymphadenopathy. Staging for metastatic disease is negative. What is the optimal treatment course?
   A. Neoadjuvant chemotherapy followed by mastectomy with axillary lymph node dissection and postmastectomy radiation
   B. Neoadjuvant chemotherapy followed by mastectomy with axillary lymph node dissection
   C. Mastectomy with axillary lymph node dissection followed by radiation
   D. Palliative chemotherapy

4. A 42-year-old female is found to have a right-sided 4 cm breast mass without associated palpable lymphadenopathy. Core biopsy reveals carcinoma and sentinel lymph node biopsy is negative. Her 38-year-old brother is currently undergoing palliative chemotherapy for unresectable gastric cancer. What is the most likely histological subtype of the patient's breast cancer and associated germline genetic abnormality?
   A. Medullary carcinoma and BRCA1 mutation
   B. Lobular carcinoma and cadherin (CDH1) mutation
   C. Metaplastic carcinoma and STK11
   D. Invasive ductal and BRCA2 mutation

5. A 44-year-old woman is evaluated for a left-sided breast mass that has doubled in size over the last 30 days. Exam reveals a large 8 cm smooth, multinodular mass without associated palpable axillary lymphadenopathy. Core biopsy reveals characteristic leaf-like architecture containing papillary projections of epithelial-lined stroma with low

mitotic rate and lack of stromal overgrowth. She undergoes wide local excision with negative margins. What is the next step in management?

A. Complete staging with sentinel lymph node biopsy
B. Adjuvant radiation therapy
C. Adjuvant endocrine therapy
D. Surveillance

6. A 68-year-old female is diagnosed with metastatic ER/PR-negative, HER2+ breast cancer involving the lungs. Her disease is well controlled on docetaxel, trastuzumab, and pertuzumab for 1.5 years until she has multifocal progression in her liver. She is treated with ado-trastuzumab for 1 year when she presents with altered mental status and is found to have multiple (>5) brain metastases. Restaging reveals progression in her liver. She undergoes whole-brain radiotherapy. Performance status is 1 and she has preserved organ function. Which of the following options is most reasonable?

A. Combination chemotherapy that includes an anthracycline
B. Retrial trastuzumab and pertuzumab
C. Capecitabine with lapatinib
D. Lapatinib alone
E. Hospice care

ANSWERS

1. **D. No further imaging.** Patient has T2N1 breast cancer (stage IIB). In the absence of symptoms or abnormal labs concerning for metastatic disease, evaluating for distant disease is not indicated for stages I–II breast cancers.

2. **C. Palbociclib with fulvestrant.** Palbociclib, an oral CDK4/6 inhibitor, is well tolerated and improves progression-free survival when combined with fulvestrant compared to fulvestrant alone in postmenopausal patients who have progressed on endocrine therapy, including an aromatase inhibitor.

3. **A. Neoadjuvant chemotherapy followed by mastectomy with axillary lymph node dissection and postmastectomy radiation.** The patient has what appears to be a locally advanced T4 breast cancer with clinical adenopathy (stage IIIB disease). For stage IIIB disease, neoadjuvant multiagent chemotherapy followed by mastectomy with axillary lymph node dissection and postmastectomy radiation is associated with the highest chance of cure.

4. **B. Lobular carcinoma and cadherin (CDH1) mutation.** This patient's family history is strongly suspicious for hereditary diffuse gastric cancer, which is associated with a germline mutation in the *CDH1* gene. Lobular breast cancers are found in 25% to 50% of families with hereditary diffuse gastric cancer. In women with known CDH1 germline mutations, guidelines suggest annual breast MRI starting at age 30. If this patient is found to harbor a germline CHD1 mutation, she should be considered for prophylactic gastrectomy.

5. **D. Surveillance.** The pathologic description is characteristic of a benign phyllodes tumor. In the absence of high mitotic rate, marked stomal cellularity and atypia, the tumors are treated like fibroadenomas with wide local excision to negative margins (at least 1 cm) without adjuvant therapy. Adjuvant radiation can be considered for borderline or malignant phyllodes and adjuvant chemotherapy is reserved for select high-risk, recurrent, or large tumors.

6. **C. Capecitabine with lapatinib.** Central nervous system (CNS) progression is not uncommon (8%–12%) in HER2+ metastatic breast cancer likely due to the inability of trastuzumab to cross the blood–brain barrier along with the increased survival of these patients. Although this patient has progressed on three anti-HER2 therapies (trastuzumab, pertuzumab, and ado-trastuzumab), additional anti-HER2 therapy should be considered and includes lapatinib, a small molecule inhibitor of EGFR and HER2. The combination of lapatinib and capecitabine is particularly active in CNS disease with reported partial responses of greater than 60% (LANDSCAPE trial).

GENITOURINARY MALIGNANCIES

19 Bladder Cancer

Sarah Yentz, Alon Weizer, and Ajjai Alva

EPIDEMIOLOGY

- Average age at diagnosis is 73 years
- Fourth most common cancer in men
- Approximately 75% of urothelial carcinomas are non-muscle-invasive
- Primary upper urinary tract urothelial cancer carries a 20% to 50% risk of synchronous or metachronous bladder cancer
- Primary bladder cancer carries a 1% to 4% risk of synchronous or metachronous upper urinary tract tumors

ETIOLOGY AND RISK FACTORS

1. **What are the major environmental risk factors for bladder cancer?**
   - Smoking (3× higher risk compared to never smokers)
   - Occupational exposure
     - Metal workers, painters, rubber industry workers, leather workers, textile and electrical workers, miners, cement workers
   - Schistosoma haematobium (squamous)
   - Chronic cystitis (squamous)
   - Cyclophosphamide

2. **Do hereditary factors play a role in urothelial malignancy?**
   - The hereditary nonpolyposis colorectal cancer (HNPCC) gene *MSH2* is associated with an increased risk of upper urologic tract malignancies.

3. **What are the most common mutations in urothelial bladder cancer?**
   - Different genomic alterations are seen in different stages of bladder cancer
     - Low-grade, noninvasive
       - HRAS mutation 30% to 40%
       - FGFR3 alterations 70%
     - Invasive
       - Rb loss
       - P53 loss

PATHOLOGY

1. **What are the histologic types of bladder cancer?**
   - Urothelial (90%–95%)

- Squamous (5%)
- Adenocarcinoma (1%–2%)
- Small cell (<1%)

SIGNS AND SYMPTOMS

1. **What is the most common presenting symptom of bladder cancer?**
   - Gross painless hematuria (85%)

2. **What are other common symptoms of bladder cancer?**
   - Hematuria (microscopic), dysuria, nocturia, urinary frequency, and urgency
   - Incomplete bladder emptying
   - Suprapubic, hypogastric, flank pain, or heaviness
   - Pain (locally advanced disease)

DIAGNOSTIC TESTS

1. **How is bladder cancer diagnosed?**
   - CT urogram
   - Urine cytology is often used prior to cystoscopy, but is not sufficient
   - Cystoscopy with bladder biopsy or transurethral resection of bladder tumor (TURBT)

2. **What tests are used for staging of muscle-invasive bladder cancer?**
   - History, physical exam (with bimanual exam under anesthesia)
   - CT abdomen/pelvis with contrast or MRI with gadolinium:
     - Imaging is preferably done prior to TURBT since the procedure can cause bladder wall thickening or perivesical stranding that can be interpreted as extravesical disease in the absence of a procedure.
   - Chest x-ray (CXR) or CT chest
   - Bone scan (if bone pain or high alkaline phosphatase/calcium)

3. **When is restaging TURBT needed after initial diagnosis of non-muscle-invasive bladder cancer (NMIBC)? Why?**
   - When?
     - All stages except Tis, low-grade Ta and low-volume, high-grade Ta with muscle in specimen
   - Why?
     - Risk of understaging with a single TURBT can be up to 30%.
     - Complete endoscopic resection improves disease outcomes for noninvasive disease treated with intravesical therapy and invasive disease with neoadjuvant chemotherapy or chemo-radiation.

STAGING

1. **Define Tx through T4 and N0 to N3 in bladder cancer.**
   - Tx: primary tumor cannot be assessed

- T0: no evidence of primary tumor
- Ta: noninvasive papillary lesion
- Tis: carcinoma in situ (CIS)
- T1: invasion into the subepithelial connective tissue (lamina propria, muscularis mucosa, submucosa)
- T2a: invasion into the muscle (superficial)
- T2b: invasion into the muscle (deep)
- T3a: invasion into perivesical tissue (microscopic)
- T3b: invasion into perivesical tissue (macroscopic)
- T4a: invasion to prostate stroma, uterus, and vagina
- T4b: invasion to pelvic/abdominal wall
- N0: no lymph nodes
- N1: single lymph node in the true pelvis (hypogastric, obturator, external iliac, or presacral node)
- N2: multiple lymph nodes in the true pelvis
- N3: common iliac lymph node

2. **How is bladder cancer staged?**
   - Stage 0a = TaN0M0
   - Stage 0is = TisN0M0
   - Stage I = T1N0M0
   - Stage II = T2N0M0
   - Stage IIIA = T3 or T4a/N0/M0 OR T1-T4a/N1/M0
   - Stage IIIB = T1-T4a/N2-or-N3/M0
   - Stage IVA = T4b/any N/M0 OR Any T/Any N/M1a (Distant metastasis limited to lymph nodes beyond the common iliacs)
   - Stage IVB = Any T/Any N/M1b (Non-lymph-node distant metastases)

3. **How common is NMIBC?**
   - Seventy-five percent of all bladder tumors; Ta (60%), Tis (10%), T1 (30%)

4. **What is the 5-year risk of recurrence and risk of muscle invasion for NMIBC?**

Tumor (All <3 cm)	Recurrence	Progression
Low-grade Ta	31%	0.8%
High-grade Ta	46%	6%
High-grade T1	46%	17%
CIS	46%	Variable depending on T stage, up to 45% with T1, high-grade tumor
Overall	70%	15%

PROGNOSTIC FACTORS

1. **What are the main prognostic factors in localized bladder cancer?**
   - Stage and grade

2. **What are the main prognostic factors for poor outcomes in metastatic bladder cancer?**
   - Performance status <80%
   - Visceral (lung, liver, or bone) metastases

3. **What other factors may affect the outcome in bladder cancer?**
   - Associated CIS
   - Incomplete response to bacillus Calmette–Guérin (BCG) for high-grade NMIBC
   - Tumor multifocality for NMIBC
   - Early/frequent recurrence for NMIBC
   - Tumor size >3 cm for NMIBC

TREATMENT

1. **How is NMIBC treated?**
   Low Risk Tumors (Ta, low grade): TURBT plus a single dose of intravesical mitomycin within 24 hours after TURBT

   High Risk Tumors (T1, High Grade, CIS): TURBT + intravesical BCG (6 weekly doses) followed by maintenance BCG. Cystectomy is an alternative in patients with high grade T1 disease and associated CIS in some patients

   Recurrent Low Grade: Intravesical mitomycin or gemcitabine

   Recurrent High Grade: Intravesical chemotherapy, clinical trial or cystectomy

2. **What is the surveillance after treatment of NMIBC?**
   - Low-grade Ta
     - Cystoscopy at 3 months, then annually
   - High grade
     - Cystoscopy and urine cytology every 3 months for 1 year; every 6 months for next 1 year; then yearly for life
     - Upper urinary tract imaging every 1 to 2 years

3. **How is stage II/III (T2-4aN0M0) muscle-invasive bladder cancer treated?**
   - Neoadjuvant platinum-based chemotherapy followed by:
     - Radical cystectomy + bilateral pelvic lymph node dissection
     - Or chemoradiation

4. **What are the urinary diversion options?**
   - Ileal conduit that drains to an ostomy bag on the anterior abdominal wall

- Continent cutaneous reservoir constructed from detubularized bowel
- Orthotopic neobladder

5. **Why is it preferred to give chemotherapy neoadjuvantly in bladder cancer?**
   - Early treatment of micrometastases and possible tumor downstaging leading to a less complicated surgery
   - When given postoperatively, patients frequently need delays or treatment breaks due to complications from postop recovery

6. **How much does neoadjuvant chemo improve outcomes?**
   - Phase III trial showed that neoadjuvant MVAC (methotrexate, vinblastine, Adriamycin, cisplatin) prior to cystectomy leads to a 77-month median survival as compared to 46 months with cystectomy alone ($P = .06$).
   - A 3,000 patient meta-analysis showed that the absolute survival benefit at 5 years was 5% with overall survival (OS) increasing from 45% to 50%.

7. **In patients who did not receive neoadjuvant chemotherapy, can chemotherapy be given adjuvantly?**
   - Yes. However, many adjuvant trials were underpowered and terminated early, hence no level 1 evidence.
   - Some data show a prolonged progression-free survival (PFS) but no improvement in OS in immediate versus deferred adjuvant chemotherapy.

8. **When can a bladder-sparing approach be considered? What modalities of treatment does this involve?**
   - Considered if the treatment can completely eradicate the tumor in the bladder, risk of recurrence is low, and bladder function is not substantially compromised
   - Involves a maximal TURBT + chemotherapy + radiation

9. **How is node positive/metastatic bladder cancer treated?**
   - Platinum (cisplatin or carboplatin in cisplatin-ineligible patients) containing combination chemotherapy
   - Phase III study comparing MVAC to gemcitabine + cisplatin demonstrated similar OS benefit (15.2 vs. 14 months) with less toxicity in the gemcitabine + cisplatin arm
   - For platinum refractory metastatic bladder cancer, atezolizumab, an anti-PDL1 antibody has recently been Food and Drug Administration (FDA) approved

10. **What is the surveillance after treatment of muscle-invasive bladder cancer?**
    - Exam, urine cytology, and comprehensive metabolic panel every 3 to 6 months for 2 years, then every 6 months for 3 years, then annually
    - CXR, CT A/P, CT urogram every 3 to 6 months for 2 years, then as clinically indicated
    - If neobladder: B12 level annually

- If bladder preservation: cystoscopy every 3 to 6 months for 2 years, then as indicated

QUESTIONS

1. A 71-year-old is referred to a urologist for new onset hematuria. A staging cystoscopy reveals a large, sessile bladder tumor. Pathology from the transurethral resection shows high-grade urothelial carcinoma invading the lamina propria but no muscle is included in the sample. Which therapy would you recommend?
   A. Cystectomy
   B. Radiation therapy
   C. Repeat staging with transurethral resection of bladder tumor (TURBT)
   D. Intravesical bacillus Calmette–Guérin (BCG)
   E. Watchful waiting

2. A 69-year-old male with hypertension develops hematuria. Cystoscopy shows a sessile bladder tumor and a palpable mass is detected on exam under anesthesia (EUA) after a complete transurethral resection of bladder tumor (TURBT). Pathology shows a high-grade muscle-invasive urothelial carcinoma. CT scan shows some perivesical stranding but no lymphadenopathy. Which treatment option would you recommend?
   A. Cystoprostatectomy + pelvic lymph node dissection
   B. TURBT followed by chemotherapy and radiation
   C. Neoadjuvant cisplatin-based chemotherapy followed by local therapy
   D. Cystoprostatectomy followed by adjuvant chemotherapy
   E. Chemoradiation

3. A 70-year-old male with a history of pT2bN0 urothelial carcinoma who is s/p cystectomy/pelvic lymph node dissection 2 years ago is found to have several new enlarged retroperitoneal lymph nodes on surveillance imaging. Fine needle aspiration (FNA) of one node confirmed urothelial carcinoma. He is asymptomatic and in good health. Which treatment option would you recommend?
   A. Retroperitoneal lymph node dissection (RPLND) since the disease is localized
   B. Cisplatin-based chemotherapy
   C. Non-cisplatin-based chemotherapy
   D. Radiation

4. A 65-year-old male is found to have microscopic hematuria on a urinalysis done for a work physical. A follow-up cystoscopy shows a low-grade Ta bladder tumor. What is the appropriate treatment?
   A. Observation with urine cytology every 6 months
   B. Observation with yearly cystoscopy as it is a low-grade tumor
   C. Transurethral resection of bladder tumor (TURBT)
   D. TURBT followed by intravesical mitomycin
   E. TURBT followed by intravesical bacillus Calmette–Guérin (BCG) with maintenance BCG

5. **Bladder cancer is associated with which of the following risk factors?**
   A. Alcohol
   B. HPV
   C. Smoking
   D. Obesity

6. **A 78-year-old male is found to have muscle-invasive bladder cancer but he refuses cystectomy. What is the optimal treatment for his bladder cancer?**
   A. Single agent gemcitabine
   B. MVAC
   C. Transurethral resection of bladder tumor (TURBT)
   D. Chemoradiation
   E. TURBT + MVAC
   F. TURBT followed by chemoradiation

ANSWERS

1. **C. Repeat staging with transurethral resection of bladder tumor (TURBT).** There was no muscle included in the sample and treatment depends on whether invasion into the muscularis propria is present or not.

2. **C. Neoadjuvant cisplatin-based chemotherapy followed by local therapy.** This is the preferred approach to patients with muscle-invasive bladder cancer with no evidence of metastatic disease.

3. **B. Cisplatin-based chemotherapy.** Cisplatin-based chemotherapy has improved survival compared to non-cisplatin-based regimens. Repeat local therapy is not sufficient for disease control in this case.

4. **D. TURBT followed by intravesical mitomycin.** Although it is a low-grade tumor, it still requires resection. However, a single dose of intravesical chemotherapy should be sufficient to reduce recurrence.

5. **C. Smoking.** Smokers have a 3× higher risk of bladder cancer than non-smokers.

6. **F. TURBT followed by chemoradiation.** Cystectomy is the preferred local therapy but for patients who are not surgical candidates, chemoradiation can be used.

20 | Prostate Cancer

Zachery R. Reichert, Megan E. V. Caram, and Kathleen Ann Cooney

EPIDEMIOLOGY

1. **What are the most common noncutaneous cancers in U.S. men?**
   - Prostate cancer is the most commonly diagnosed noncutaneous malignancy in U.S. men.
   - Between 2010 and 2012, the Surveillance Epidemiology and End Results (SEER) database estimates a man's lifetime risk of being diagnosed with prostate cancer at 14%.
   - There are estimated to be 180,890 new cases of prostate cancer diagnosed in the United States in 2016.

2. **True or false: While prostate cancer is one of the most common cancers, it does not account for many cancer deaths.**
   - False. Prostate cancer is the second leading cause of cancer-related mortality in men behind lung/bronchus.
   - Between 2010 and 2012, the SEER database estimates a man's risk of dying from prostate cancer at 2.6%.
   - 26,120 men are estimated to die from prostate cancer in 2016.

ETIOLOGY AND RISK FACTORS

1. **True or false: Similar to breast cancer, the mortality from prostate cancer is highest in African American men, but the incidence is less than in Whites.**
   - False. Both incidence and mortality from prostate cancer are highest in the African American population compared to Whites and Asians.
   - African American men are more likely to develop a prostate-specific antigen (PSA) recurrence after definitive local therapy, to present with advanced disease, and have a greater than twofold risk of death from the disease.

2. **What are the three well-established risk factors for prostate cancer?**
   - Age, race, and family history (genetic risk) are the three variables known to be significantly associated with the risk of prostate cancer.
   - Age:
     ○ A man's risk of developing prostate cancer increases steadily with his age. Sixty percent of prostate cancer cases are diagnosed in men older than 65 years.
     ○ Ten percent of all prostate cancer cases are diagnosed in men less than 56 years of age (some data suggest that prostate cancer diagnosed in younger men is more aggressive).

- Race: The incidence of prostate cancer in the United States is highest in the African American population and lowest in Asian men.
- Family history:
  - The risk of developing prostate cancer increases with the number of family members affected and also increases if the family members diagnosed were younger at diagnosis.
  - A man's risk of developing prostate cancer is twice as high if he has a first-degree relative diagnosed with prostate cancer and fivefold higher if he has two affected first-degree relatives.
  - Having a brother affected with prostate cancer carries a greater risk for developing prostate cancer than having an affected father.
  - Although there are nearly 100 common genetic polymorphisms that are consistently associated with the risk for prostate cancer, there is no clinical role for testing at this time. Prostate cancer is associated with germline mutations in several cancer predisposition genes (*BRCA1, BRCA2, DNA mismatch repair, HOXB13*, etc.).

3. Is diet a risk factor for prostate cancer?

- The answer to this is unknown, but there are reports of high-fat diets increasing the risk for prostate cancer, while lycopene-rich diets may be protective.

SCREENING

1. Who should be screened for prostate cancer?

- Screening should be discussed with patients as 40% of cancers are "overdiagnosed" and there is a significant amount of morbidity from overdiagnosis.
- The United States Preventive Service Task Force (USPSTF) recommends against routine screening in the average risk population. However, if a patient or provider feels screening may be beneficial, an informed discussion regarding risks and benefits should ensue before testing. Note that many insurance companies will not pay for PSA tests done specifically for early detection or screening given the recommendation of the USPSTF.
- In families with a high preponderance of lethal prostate cancer or known inherited risk factors of prostate cancer, screening may be considered since the potential benefit may be higher in that population of patients.

PREVENTION

1. Are there any agents that can prevent prostate cancer in men at high risk?

- Compared to placebo, finasteride was shown to decrease the risk of developing low-grade prostate cancer over 7 years in asymptomatic men more than 50 years old with a normal digital rectal examination (DRE) and PSA <30 ng/mL (1). However, there was concern that finasteride may increase the number of high-grade cancers. Overall survival was not impacted, so treating men with finasteride in an attempt to prevent prostate cancer is not recommended.
- Selenium and vitamin E have been studied in prostate cancer prevention trials and do not prevent prostate cancer.

PATHOLOGY

1. **What are the histologic subtypes in prostate cancer?**
   - Ninety-five percent of prostate cancers are adenocarcinomas.
   - Other potential histologic variants include: sarcoma, lymphoma, and small cell or neuroendocrine cancer.

2. **How is prostate cancer graded?**
   - Gleason grade is a grading system ranging from 1 to 5 that describes a cancer cell's morphologic differentiation from normal prostatic glands (grade 1 refers to tissue that is glandular appearing, grade 5 refers to tissue that has lost all glandular features).
     - ○ Primary Gleason grade denotes the dominant histologic pattern, while the secondary grade denotes the next most common histologic pattern. Occasionally a tertiary pattern is noted in some cases.
     - ○ The Gleason score is the sum of the primary and secondary Gleason grades.
     - ○ Scores less than 6 are generally not considered to be prostate cancer.
     - ○ Scores of 8 to 10 are poorly differentiated and represent high-risk disease.
   - Gleason score is the strongest predictor of clinical outcome.
   - Gleason score may change from biopsy to radical prostatectomy; 20% of scores upgraded and 10% downgraded.

3. **Are there premalignant lesions for prostate cancer?**
   - Yes. High-grade prostatic intraepithelial neoplasia (PIN) is considered a precursor lesion to prostate cancer.

SIGNS AND SYMPTOMS

1. **What are the symptoms of localized prostate cancer?**
   - Despite changes in screening practices since the USPSTF's recommendations, many men are still diagnosed with prostate cancer through early detection methods (abnormal DRE and/or elevated PSA), and therefore are asymptomatic at diagnosis.
   - Obstructive urinary symptoms (urinary frequency, nocturia, hesitancy) from an enlarged prostate can be the presenting symptoms from locally advanced disease.
   - Hematuria or hematospermia may be present if there is local invasion.

2. **What are common signs/symptoms of advanced prostate cancer?**
   - Weight loss, fatigue
   - Anemia from bone marrow replacement
   - Disseminated intravascular coagulation (DIC) with a tendency toward bleeding
   - Bone pain at sites of metastatic bone disease
   - Spinal cord compression from metastatic bone disease

DIAGNOSIS

1. **When should a prostate biopsy be done to evaluate for malignancy?**

- Men should be informed about the risks and benefits of diagnosing prostate cancer and of the potential treatments before proceeding with a prostate biopsy.
  - The decision to biopsy should be individualized based on the magnitude as well as the rate of rise of the PSA value.
- Rapidly rising PSAs are strongly associated with a diagnosis of prostate cancer.
- Age-adjusted cutoffs have been developed to try to improve specificity for PSA screening: PSA <2.5 ng/mL is considered normal for men 40 to 49, <3.5 ng/mL for men 50 to 59, <4.5 ng/mL for men 60 to 69, and <6.5 ng/mL for men 70 to 79 years old.
  - Other causes of PSA elevation include benign prostatic hyperplasia (BPH) and prostatitis.
  - A palpable hard nodule on DRE is an indication for prostate biopsy, even in the setting of a low PSA.

2. **How many biopsies are done to diagnose prostate cancer?**
- Since prostate cancer is multifocal, 12 cores are generally recommended to ensure adequate sampling of the gland. The highest score found in the gland is used regardless of the volume.
- A negative biopsy in a man in whom there is a high clinical suspicion should prompt reassessment in 6 months with a repeat biopsy.

STAGING

1. **Define the staging system of prostate cancer:**
- The current (seventh edition) American Joint Committee on Cancer (AJCC) staging system for prostate cancer includes Gleason score, PSA level, and the extent of disease based on tumor, node, and metastasis (TNM) criteria.
  - T1: tumor is not palpable or visible by imaging, usually detected by an elevated PSA or an incidental finding on transurethral resection of prostate (TURP) for BPH.
    - T1a: incidental finding in 5% or less of resected prostate tissue TURP
    - T1b: incidental finding in >5% of resected prostate tissue from TURP
    - T1c: detected by biopsy for an elevated PSA
  - T2: tumor confined to the prostate
    - T2a: involves half of one lobe or less
    - T2b: involves majority of one lobe
    - T2c: involves both lobes
  - T3: tumor extends through the prostatic capsule
    - T3a: extracapsular extension (unilateral or bilateral)
    - T3b: invasion of a seminal vesicle
  - T4: tumor is fixed or invades adjacent structures other than the seminal vesicle
  - N0: no lymph nodes involved
  - N1: regional lymph nodes involved
  - M0: no evidence of metastatic disease

○ M1: distant metastatic disease
  ■ M1a: nonregional lymph nodes
  ■ M1b: bone involvement
  ■ M1c: other

Stage	PSA (ng/mL)	Gleason Score	T	N	M
I	<10	6	T1, T2a	N0	M0
IIA	<10	6	T2b	N0	M0
	≥10 but <20	6	T1, T2a, T2b	N0	M0
	<20	7	T1, T2a, T2b	N0	M0
IIB	≥20	Any	T1, T2	N0	M0
	Any	8 or greater	T1, T2	N0	M0
	Any	Any	T2c	N0	M0
III	Any	Any	T3	N0	M0
IV	Any	Any	T4	N0 or N1	M0 or M1

- Note that invasion of any surrounding structures other than the seminal vesicles and any dissemination to the nodes or other organs all fall under the umbrella of stage IV disease.

2. **What is the appropriate method for staging a patient with newly diagnosed prostate cancer?**
   - Bone scan should be done prior to definitive local therapy if symptoms are suggestive of metastatic disease (eg, new bone pain), Gleason score ≥8, T3, T4 or T1 and PSA >20 ng/mL or T2 and PSA >10 ng/mL.
   - CT or MRI of the abdomen/pelvis should be done prior to definitive local therapy if T3, T4, or T1/T2 and nomogram predict a likelihood of lymph node involvement above 10%.
   - For stage III and IV disease, bone scan and CT or MRI of the abdomen and pelvis should be done for staging prior to definitive therapy.

3. **What are the three most important variables that affect a patient's risk for failing local therapy?**
   - Stage, Gleason grade, and PSA at diagnosis are the three most important prognostic variables that together define a patient's prostate cancer as very low-, low-, intermediate-, high- or very high-risk disease.
     ○ Very low-risk disease is defined as: T1c, PSA ≤10 ng/mL, Gleason score ≤6, fewer than three prostate biopsy cores positive, ≤50% cancer in any core, and PSA density <0.15 ng/mL/g.
     ○ Low-risk disease is defined as: T1–T2a, PSA <10 ng/mL, and Gleason score of ≤6.
     ○ Intermediate-risk disease is defined as one of the following: T2b–T2c disease, pretreatment PSA 10 to 20 ng/mL, or Gleason score of 7.

○ High-risk disease is defined as one of the following: T3a or greater disease, pretreatment PSA >20 ng/mL, or Gleason score 8 to 10.

○ Very high-risk disease is defined as one of the following: T3b–T4, primary Gleason pattern of 5, or >4 cores with Gleason score of 8 to 10.

INDICATIONS FOR TREATMENT

1. Do all prostate cancers need to be treated?

- Life expectancy should be considered when making treatment decisions for men with prostate cancer.

- Guidelines state that patients with very low-risk or low-risk prostate cancer with life expectancies under 10 years should be observed, while those with longer life expectancies consider active surveillance, or definitive local therapy.

- Men with intermediate- to very high-risk prostate cancer localized to the prostate, and who can tolerate therapy should consider definitive treatment (radiation or surgery).

- Men with metastatic disease who can tolerate therapy should be considered for systemic treatment since treatment has been shown to improve overall survival and quality of life.

2. What is active surveillance?

- Active surveillance can also be considered delayed intervention for low-stage/low-grade prostate cancer. Active surveillance involves monitoring the patient's PSA, DRE, and periodically rebiopsying the prostate gland as appropriate.

- Guidelines describing appropriate active surveillance strategies can be found in the National Comprehensive Cancer Network Guidelines.

PROGNOSTIC FACTORS

1. What factors affect prognosis in prostate cancer?

- High Gleason grade/Gleason score
- High percentage and volume of cores involved with cancer on biopsy
- High PSA level or rapidly rising PSA
- Short interval between definitive local therapy and PSA relapse
- Advanced stage

2. What is so important about PSA doubling time?

- PSA doubling time at diagnosis predicts prostate-cancer-specific mortality.

- Studies have shown that following definitive treatment, men with a PSA doubling time of <3 months had a significantly greater risk of dying of prostate cancer compared to patients who had a longer doubling time.

TREATMENT

Treating Localized Disease

1. What are surgical options for prostate cancer localized to the prostate?

- Different methods are used for radical prostatectomy that must be tailored to each individual patient: retropubic, perineal, and laparoscopic are the common methods. Laparoscopic is usually done with robotic assistance.

- Outcomes are dependent on the institution and the volume of procedures performed.
- Nerve-sparing prostatectomies to preserve sexual function should be considered when the cancer is not close to or invading the neurovascular bundles.
- Patients can expect to be in the hospital between 1 and 2 days with between 7 and 14 days of urethral catheterization.

2. **Should lymph node dissection be done during radical prostatectomy surgery?**
   - Pelvic lymph node dissection should be done in patients with regional lymph node involvement and no evidence of distant metastatic disease.
   - Pelvic lymph node dissection is controversial in patients without known lymph node involvement, but should be considered in patients with a possibility of positive nodes over 2% based on predictive nomograms.

3. **What are the complications of surgery?**
   - Immediate morbidity or mortality <1% of patients
   - Complete urinary incontinence with no urinary control occurs in approximately 2% of patients after 2 years, but up to 40% of patients report some issues with leakage and require protective garments after 2 years.
   - Urinary stricture can occur in up to 10% of patients who undergo prostatectomy.
   - Impotence rate is 35% to 60%. Medications for erectile dysfunction may still be helpful. Bilateral nerve-sparing technique is associated with 60% to 90% of patients recovering spontaneous erections. Unilateral nerve-sparing technique carries only a 10% to 50% chance of recovery of spontaneous erections.
   - The laparoscopic method of radical prostatectomy compared to the open method may be associated with a shorter time to recovery.

4. **What kind of radiation can be used?**
   - External beam radiation therapy targets the whole prostate and sometimes a margin of extraprostatic tissue, seminal vesicles, and pelvic lymph nodes.
   - Intensity-modulated radiation therapy (IMRT) is a type of three-dimensional (3D) conformal radiation therapy that conforms more precisely to the target. IMRT is typically used for both definitive, adjuvant, and salvage radiation therapy.
   - Higher radiation doses per fraction (3 Gy instead of 2 Gy), thereby shortening duration of therapy, is an area of active research but may carry higher local toxicities.
   - A total radiation dose between 70 and 78 Gy is typically recommended for definitive treatment.
   - Brachytherapy is a method that uses radioactive seeds to deliver higher doses of radiation directly to the prostate tissue. This method can be considered in patients with low-risk tumors, but it is not recommended for patients with intermediate- to high-risk tumors.

- There is no definitive evidence that combined external beam radiation and brachytherapy should be used for definitive therapy. However, a "brachytherapy boost" is sometimes used in patients undergoing definitive radiation for intermediate- to high-risk prostate cancer.

5. What are the complications of radiation?

- Acute complications include inflammation of the surrounding structures such as cystitis, proctitis, and enteritis.
- Fatigue can also be an acute complication.
- Mild cytopenias can occur due to radiation of the pelvic marrow.
- Chronic complications can include impotence, urethral stricture, cystitis, and hematuria.
- Diarrhea and proctitis can be acute or chronic complications of radiation.

6. Which primary treatment method is preferred: radiation or surgery?

- Overall survival is slightly improved in patients who undergo surgery versus definitive radiation over a long period of follow-up, likely due to an increased local relapse rate with radiation.
- The Prostate Cancer Outcomes Study found statistically significant differences in complication outcomes between groups undergoing radical prostatectomy versus radiation. Radical prostatectomy was associated with worse urinary incontinence, but better bowel function compared to radiation. Sexual dysfunction was similar between the two groups.

7. Is neoadjuvant treatment warranted prior to radical prostatectomy or radiation?

- Neoadjuvant androgen deprivation therapy (ADT) or chemotherapy is not indicated prior to surgery.
- Neoadjuvant and adjuvant ADT should be considered for patients undergoing definitive external beam radiation for intermediate- and high-risk prostate cancer.

8. In which circumstances is adjuvant ADT warranted?

- Adjuvant ADT starting before radiation and treating between 4 and 6 months should be used in patients with intermediate-risk prostate cancer who undergo definitive radiation therapy to improve disease-free survival.
- Adjuvant ADT for 2 to 3 years after definitive radiation therapy has been shown to improve overall survival in men with high-risk prostate cancer.
  - Based on data from Messing et al. (2) lifelong ADT may be considered for men after radical prostatectomy and the identification of node + disease.

9. Is adjuvant chemotherapy warranted and in which circumstances?

- Adjuvant chemotherapy is not recommended after radical prostatectomy or definitive radiation. While adjuvant ADT plays a role in certain circumstances, adjuvant chemotherapy has not been shown to benefit patients undergoing prostatectomy or definitive radiation.

10. Is adjuvant radiation warranted and in which circumstances?

- Adjuvant radiation to the prostatic bed after radical prostatectomy should be considered in patients with extracapsular extension of their prostate cancer or those with positive surgical margins.

- This approach has been shown to decrease the risk for local recurrence, but there are conflicting reports about whether it affects overall or metastasis-free survival.

11. What kind of surveillance should be done after definitive therapy is complete?

- PSA should be checked every 6 months for 5 years and then annually indefinitely.

- Annual DRE should be done to evaluate for local recurrence.

12. What can be done for local recurrence?

- In the setting of biochemical recurrence (a PSA rise after definitive local therapy), local recurrence is more likely if the PSA rise occurs more than 1 year after surgery or when the PSA rises slowly; for example, a PSA doubling time >10 months.

- Salvage radiation to the prostatic bed should be considered in patients who have a local recurrence after radical prostatectomy. A lower PSA level prior to salvage radiotherapy is associated with a better relapse-free outcome.

- Salvage radical prostatectomy for local recurrence after radiation therapy is very difficult and carries a high risk for complications and morbidity, but can be considered in select patients.

- Cryosurgery does not have a role in initial definitive therapy, but may be considered for local recurrence after definitive radiation.

Treating Biochemical Recurrence

1. What is a biochemical recurrence?

- According to the American Urological Association (AUA) guidelines, biochemical recurrence after radical prostatectomy is defined as serum PSA >0.2 ng/mL with a second confirmatory level >0.2 ng/mL.

- Biochemical recurrence after definitive radiation is defined using the "Phoenix definition" of PSA failure: PSA rise by 2 ng/mL or more above the postradiotherapy nadir. Of note, PSA usually nadirs within 1 year after completion of radiation therapy.

2. Has treatment for biochemical recurrence been shown to improve outcomes?

- Neither chemotherapy nor androgen deprivation has been shown to prolong overall survival when utilized in the setting of biochemical recurrence.

Primary Treatment for Metastatic Prostate Cancer

1. What is the best initial therapy for newly diagnosed metastatic prostate cancer?

- Most patients who present with metastatic prostate cancer will benefit from initial therapy with androgen suppression.
- Patients with severe bone pain or an acute presentation causing them to be hospitalized or acutely ill could be considered for aggressive and immediate-acting ADT such as degarelix (GNRH antagonist) or ketoconazole. Local radiation can also be considered to a painful metastatic lesion or a bony metastasis at risk for fracture.

2. **What is ADT?**
   - ADT is therapy that deprives the body of natural androgens. Androgens are normally produced by the testes and adrenal glands.
   - The majority of prostate cancers are driven by testosterone. Therefore, reducing a patient's natural ability to produce testosterone or blocking the androgen receptor from binding testosterone deprives the cancer cells of their fuel source.
   - Prior to the development of hormonal agents, surgical castration by removing both testes was the primary mode of ADT.
   - Currently, gonadotropin-releasing hormone (GnRH) agonists are used for androgen suppression.
     - Goserelin, leuprolide, triptorelin, and buserelin are different GnRH agonists that can be given as depot injections. There are different doses of depots available to last varying lengths of time.
     - The continuous exposure of the pituitary to GnRH causes a transient surge of luteinizing hormone and hence systemic testosterone before the pituitary downregulates its GnRH receptors resulting in an ultimate decline in testosterone production.
   - Antiandrogen receptor agents:
     - To avoid tumor flare when a GnRH agonist is initiated, an oral antiandrogen mediator (eg, bicalutamide) should be started at least 1 week prior to giving the GnRH agonist. This maneuver will block the androgen receptor from binding testosterone.
     - The long-term addition of an oral antiandrogen mediator to the GnRH agonist can be done, though the survival benefit with long-term use of an antiandrogen is very small and should be weighed against the increased risk of adverse effects.
     - In patients who have PSA progression on a GnRH agonist alone, the addition of an antiandrogen agent can decrease the PSA or provide symptomatic improvement in up to 40% of patients.
     - Antiandrogen agents should not be used alone for the treatment of prostate cancer.
     - Bicalutamide is the antiandrogen most commonly used. Flutamide and nilutamide are other antiandrogens that are available. Side effects include: diarrhea, nausea, breast tenderness, hepatotoxicity, loss of libido, and impotence.
   - Degarelix is a GnRH antagonist that is given monthly and can be considered in place of a GnRH agonist in a patient who needs immediate ADT and is unable to wait a week for the antiandrogen lead-in.

3. **Should chemotherapy be given in combination with ADT for initial hormone naïve disease?**
   - Docetaxel for six cycles in combination with initial ADT should be considered in men who present with high-volume metastatic disease (visceral disease or at least four bone metastases with one beyond the vertebral body/pelvis). This has an overall survival benefit of 10 to 17 months. Docetaxel may be started up to 120 days after starting ADT.

4. **Is there a role for intermittent ADT in metastatic prostate cancer?**
   - This is controversial. Intermittent ADT was compared to continuous ADT in a noninferiority trial (SWOG trial 9346) but the hazard ratio (HR) of death crossed the prespecified upper limit of 1.2 (HR 0.99, 90% confidence intervals [CIs; 0.99, 1.23]). There was some benefit with erectile function and mental health 3 months after stopping therapy. However, intermittent ADT should not routinely be recommended for men with metastatic disease.

5. **What should be done when a patient has a rising PSA on total androgen blockade (combination of a GnRH agonist and an antiandrogen agent)?**
   - It is important to check a serum testosterone in this setting to be sure the patient is truly castrate.
   - Discontinuing the antiandrogen (antiandrogen withdrawal) can cause a decrease in PSA and symptomatic improvement in about 25% of patients, but this usually has a short duration of response (<6 months).

Treatment of Castration-Resistant Prostate Cancer

1. **What is castration-resistant prostate cancer?**
   - Castration-resistant prostate cancer is cancer that has progressed despite androgen deprivation (testosterone must be under 50 ng/mL).
   - If given the time, all patients who have metastatic prostate cancer will eventually progress to develop castration-resistant disease.
   - Duration of response to ADT ranges generally from 18 to 24 months.
   - Twenty percent of patients will not develop castration resistance for at least 5 years while on ADT.

2. **Should a patient's ADT be discontinued if they are castration-resistant?**
   - ADT should be continued despite castration resistance as much of the prostate cancer is still driven by androgens.
   - Additional therapies should be added to continuous ADT.

3. **How does castration-resistant prostate cancer develop?**
   - Many different mechanisms exist for prostate cancer cells to grow in a low-testosterone environment. These include:
     - Upregulation of androgen receptor expression
     - Activation of the androgen receptor by other steroid hormones
     - Splice variants of the androgen receptor
     - Prostate cancer cells synthesize their own androgens, so the local tumor androgen environment is higher

4. **What are treatment options for patients with castration-resistant prostate cancer?**
   - Secondary hormonal therapy (abiraterone, enzalutamide)
   - Chemotherapy (docetaxel, cabazitaxel)
   - Vaccines (sipuleucel-T)
   - Radiopharmaceutical (radium-223)
   - Clinical trials
   - The optimal sequencing of these treatments is unknown

   In addition to one of the aforementioned options, bone-targeting agents can be considered for patients who have bone metastases to prevent skeletal-related complications.

5. **What is secondary hormonal therapy?**
   - The goal of further hormonal manipulation is to decrease/block androgen mediated signaling. This is achieved by blocking other sources of testosterone production in the body (testosterone produced from the adrenal glands and the tumor itself) or inhibiting androgen receptor signaling.
   - Testosterone biosynthesis reduction by inhibiting CYP17
     - Abiraterone improves median survival from 10.9 months to 14.8 months in patients who already received chemotherapy and has been shown to improve progression-free survival in men who have not received prior chemo-therapy. Patients should have their blood pressure, liver function tests, and potassium levels monitored regularly while on abiraterone. Prednisone 5 mg twice a day must be given with abiraterone. Abiraterone should be used with caution in patients with hypertension, heart failure, or arrhythmias.
   - Androgen receptor signaling inhibition
     - Enzalutamide is a second-generation antiandrogen that inhibits the binding of testosterone to the androgen receptor, while also decreasing the androgen receptor:testosterone translocation to the nucleus and the complexes' ability to bind DNA. It increases survival after chemotherapy (13.6 to 18.4 months) and improves the combination end point of radiographic progression-free survival/overall survival prior to chemotherapy. Enzalutamide should not be used in patients with a seizure disorder and fatigue is a main side effect.
     - Ketoconazole and hydrocortisone may also be considered, but this treatment has generally been replaced by the newer agents that have shown a survival benefit for treatment of men with castration-resistant prostate cancer.

6. **What nonhormonal first-line options are possible in castration-resistant prostate cancer?**
   - Sipuleucel-T is a vaccine approved for the treatment of men with castration-resistant prostate cancer and can be considered in asymptomatic patients with a good performance status and low-volume disease.
   - Docetaxel with prednisone, given once every 3 weeks, has an overall survival benefit of approximately 2 to 3 months and an improvement in quality of life for patients who can tolerate it.

- Radium-223 is a radioactive element that mimics calcium and tracks to bone. It emits alpha particles locally to treat bone metastases. It is used in bone-only metastatic disease. It treats and delays the onset of symptomatic bone metastases, while improving overall survival from 11.2 to 14 months. Since radium-223 can be toxic to the bone marrow, blood counts should be monitored during therapy.

7. **What are appropriate second-line options for castration-resistant prostate cancer?**
   - Changing to a different agent from the approved first-line therapy options is commonly done.
   - Cabazitaxel is a taxane that has been approved for the treatment of castration-resistant prostate cancer. Given with prednisone, cabazitaxel improves progression-free and overall survival compared to mitoxantrone + prednisone in men who progressed through docetaxel. Cabazitaxel has similar toxicities to docetaxel.
   - Mitoxantrone + prednisone has been shown to improve quality of life, but does not affect the disease-free/overall survival or PSA. Cardiac dysfunction is the main toxicity and must be monitored. Given the many new agents for treatment of castration-resistant prostate cancer, this treatment option should only be considered in patients who may benefit from chemotherapy and cannot tolerate taxanes.

8. **When should bone-targeting agents be used and what are they?**
   - Patients with castration-resistant prostate cancer metastatic to the bone should be considered for treatment with a bone-targeting agent as these agents reduce the time to skeletal events (pain, fracture).
   - Two different types of osteoclast inhibitors have shown benefit in patients with castration-resistant metastatic disease to the bone: bisphosphonates and the RANKL inhibitor denosumab.
   - Denosumab was shown to be noninferior to zoledronic acid in preventing or delaying time to first skeletal-related event in patients with bone metastases.
   - No difference in progression-free or overall survival was seen when denosumab was compared to zoledronic acid.
   - Both denosumab and zoledronic acid can cause osteonecrosis of the jaw and hypocalcemia, but denosumab was associated with higher rates of hypocalcemia compared to zoledronic acid.

9. **When should radiation be considered in metastatic disease?**
   - Focal radiation should be considered for bone metastases that are painful or at risk for pathologic fracture.
   - Radiation to vertebrae should be considered in lesions concerning for or causing spinal cord compression.
   - Eighty percent of patients will get significant palliation of pain when radiation is used for painful vertebral metastases.

10. **What other palliative agents are available?**

- Strontium-89 is a calcium analog. It is a radiopharmaceutical that relieves pain in about three quarters of patients with effects lasting for several months.
- Samarium-153 is another radiopharmaceutical that improves pain in two thirds of patients during the first month and provides complete relief in a third of patients. Samarium-153 has less marrow toxicity than strontium.
- With radium-223 carrying an indication earlier in disease therapy and a survival benefit, it is unclear how to integrate these other radiopharmaceuticals into practice.

11. **When should treatment in the castration-resistant metastatic setting be changed?**
    - In general, treatment should not be stopped in response to PSA rises alone as long as the patient is clinically benefiting (stable to improved pain, fatigue) and there is no radiographic evidence of progression.
    - Radiographic progression entails new (≥ 2) lesions arising on a bone scan or the interval growth of visceral or lymph node disease.

Complications of ADT

1. **What are the adverse effects of ADT?**
   - Hot flashes
   - Fatigue
   - Loss of libido, decline in sexual function
   - Increased risk for diabetes mellitus since ADT reduces insulin sensitivity.
   - Decreased muscle mass and increased truncal obesity can occur, but are usually early events and plateau after 18 months of treatment.
   - Increased cardiovascular risk since ADT can augment low-density lipoprotein (LDL), high-density lipoprotein (HDL), and triglyceride (TGL).
   - Gynecomastia is seen more often when antiandrogen inhibitors (ie, bicalutamide) are used as monotherapy, which is not standard. Painful gynecomastia can be prevented with external beam radiation to the breasts.
   - Osteoporosis; decreased bone mineral density has been seen in men on ADT after just 6 months of treatment. There is an increase in fractures in men on ADT compared to controls. Men who receive more doses of ADT have a greater risk of fracture.
   - ADT has also been associated with a small but increased risk of Alzheimer disease.

2. **What should be done for bone health in men on chronic ADT?**
   - A baseline bone density test should be done in men prior to initiating ADT. Bone density should be repeated every 2 years while on ADT to monitor if bone supportive therapy is necessary.
   - Unless medically contraindicated, men on ADT should take 1,200 mg of calcium daily and 800 IU of vitamin D daily.
   - Lifestyle modifications such as weight-bearing exercises and smoking cessation can reduce the risk of fracture.

- Oral bisphosphonate therapy should be considered in patients who already have osteopenia and are starting ADT.
  - There are studies showing men with baseline osteopenia or osteoporosis who were started on ADT had improved bone mineral density and decreased fracture rate in the bisphosphonate group compared to placebo.
  - Zoledronic acid improves bone mineral density given as infrequently as once a year.
  - Denosumab given once every 6 months improves bone mineral density and reduces the risk for fracture compared to placebo in men on ADT.

QUESTIONS

1. A 62-year-old patient returns to your office for continued management of his previously painful bone-only, castration-resistant metastatic prostate cancer. He is asymptomatic and has been maintained on continuous leuprolide while zoledronic acid and abiraterone + prednisone were added 6 months ago when he became castration-resistant. The addition of abiraterone + prednisone decreased his prostate-specific antigen (PSA) from 87 ng/mL to 65 ng/mL after 3 months and his pain improved. The PSA has risen today to 74 ng/mL. A CT of the chest/abdomen/pelvis was obtained, which did not show any metastatic disease outside the bones. His bone scan described more intense uptake in three different lesions that were previously seen and no new lesions noted. What is the best next step?
   A. Continue the current therapy
   B. Continue abiraterone but change zoledronic acid to denosumab
   C. Discontinue abiraterone and start enzalutamide
   D. Brain MRI

2. A healthy 68-year-old man comes to your medical oncology office 6 months after completing an 8-week course of external beam radiotherapy for his T1c Gleason score 3 + 4 = 7 prostate cancer. His preradiation prostate-specific antigen (PSA) was 6 ng/mL and today it is 1.2 ng/mL. He has no rectal bleeding or dysuria. He is concerned about residual cancer with his PSA still being measurable and inquires what further therapy is needed.
   A. Salvage radical prostatectomy
   B. Continued surveillance with a repeat PSA in 6 months
   C. Total androgen blockade for 6 months
   D. Sipuleucel-T

3. A 64-year-old man with diabetes and a myocardial infarction 7 years ago is diagnosed with T1c Gleason grade 3 + 3 prostate cancer after a screening prostate-specific antigen (PSA) was 8.3 ng/mL. He walks 2 miles a day and can do a flight of stairs without problem. He is on baby aspirin, lisinopril, metformin, and metoprolol. What is the next step in his treatment?
   A. Radical prostatectomy
   B. External beam radiation

C. Active surveillance

D. Any of the above

4. A 57-year-old man presents to his local emergency room with bone pains and constipation. On imaging he is found to have multiple lytic lesions involving two ribs, three vertebrae, and his left humerus. He has no spinal cord compression on MRI but CT of the abdomen and pelvis shows an enlarged prostate with external compression of the rectum causing complete obstruction. Prostate-specific antigen (PSA) is 180 ng/mL. He is otherwise healthy. Which of these options is the best step for him?

A. Biopsy of a malignant bone lesion

B. Radium-223

C. Bicalutamide for 1 week and then leuprolide injection

D. Abiraterone + prednisone

E. Degarelix

5. A 78-year-old man without comorbid conditions, but with metastatic prostate cancer to the bone and liver, is coming to your office for regular follow-up. He was treated with external beam radiation therapy (EBRT) 10 years ago. He developed recurrence with bone metastases 3 years ago and was started on androgen deprivation therapy (ADT) with a good response. After 18 months of continuous ADT, he became castration-resistant when a liver lesion arose, which was biopsy confirmed as prostate adenocarcinoma. He has been receiving abiraterone + prednisone and zoledronic acid for 6 months but is now demonstrating prostate-specific antigen (PSA) progression and radiographic progression in the liver. What is the best next step for him?

A. Radium-223

B. Best supportive care

C. Increase the abiraterone dose to 1,500 mg a day

D. Enzalutamide

E. Docetaxel + prednisone

6. A 64-year-old man is diagnosed with metastatic prostate cancer when an x-ray for persistent lumbar back pain showed a sclerotic lesion in L4. Subsequent workup revealed a prostate-specific antigen (PSA) of 107 ng/mL. A CT with enlarged pelvic lymph nodes and prostate, and bone scan showed sclerotic lesions in L4, T4, left 12 rib, and right scapula. He is otherwise healthy. He has been on bicalutamide for 2 weeks that was prescribed by his urologist. What is the best treatment plan?

A. Add leuprolide

B. Add high-dose finasteride

C. Add leuprolide and radium-223

D. Add leuprolide and six cycles of docetaxel

E. Add leuprolide and definitive radiation to the prostate

ANSWERS

1. **A. Continue the current therapy.** The patient has castration-resistant metastatic prostate cancer. He is clinically benefiting from treatment based on pain response and shows no drug-related toxicity. Therapy should not be changed based on PSA rise, nor change in uptake intensity of known bone lesions. A change in therapy should occur when the patient is having progressive symptoms, visceral or lymph node progression, or new bone lesions arising.

2. **B. Continued surveillance with a repeat PSA in 6 months.** This patient has had a normal response to radiation. The PSA nadir may not occur for a year and may not be undetectable after radiation. Concurrent/adjuvant androgen deprivation therapy (ADT) could have been considered up front for his intermediate risk (based on Gleason score of 7) but plays no role this late after his treatment.

3. **D. Any of the above.** Despite his comorbidities, he appears functional and without an immediate life-limiting comorbidity. A shared decision-making strategy between the patient and his providers regarding his goals of treatment and personally acceptable risks is necessary.

4. **E. Degarelix.** He likely has hormone naïve metastatic prostate cancer. A biopsy is desired, but should not delay therapy. Note that pathological confirmation of disease would generally be required for a patient to participate in a clinical trial in the future. Surgery is also likely needed. The flare from leuprolide may worsen his situation and waiting a week to allow bicalutamide to take effect also places him at significant risk. As a GnRH antagonist, degarelix is immediate acting and does not carry the risk of flare. Hence it is preferred.

5. **E. Docetaxel + prednisone.** He has progressive metastatic castration-resistant prostate cancer involving both the bone and liver. Docetaxel and enzalutamide are both options in this setting, but the progression of disease in his liver is very concerning for aggressive disease that may no longer be sensitive to secondary hormonal agents. Therefore, chemotherapy is the next best option if he is a candidate.

6. **D. Add leuprolide and six cycles of docetaxel.** He has high-volume (defined as visceral disease or at least four bone metastases with one beyond vertebral body/pelvis) de novo metastatic prostate cancer. This chemohormonal strategy by adding six cycles of docetaxel to traditional androgen deprivation therapy improved overall survival by 10 months.

REFERENCES

1. Thompson IM Jr, Goodman PJ, Tangen CM, et al. Long-term survival of participants in the prostate cancer prevention trial. *N Engl J Med.* 2013;369(7):603–610. doi:10.1056/NEJMoa1215932
2. Messing, EM, Manola J, Sarosdy M, et al. Immediate hormonal therapy compared with observation after radical prostatectomy and pelvic lymphadenectomy in men with node-positive prostate cancer. *N Engl J Med.* 1999;341(24):1781–1788. doi:10.1056/NEJM199912093412401

Testicular Cancer

Zachery R. Reichert and David C. Smith

EPIDEMIOLOGY

1. **What are the main epidemiological features of testis cancer?**
   - One percent of all cancers in men
   - 8,430 new cases with 380 deaths estimated in the United States in 2015
   - Most common solid tumor in men 20 to 34 years of age
   - Incidence has increased by 60% in the last 40 years and is more common in Whites
   - It can occur in extragonadal sites (5%, most commonly retroperitoneum or mediastinum)
   - Referral to an experienced cancer center is recommended

RISK FACTORS

1. **What are the known risk factors for developing testis cancer?**
   - Personal history (1%–5% bilateral synchronous, 1%–2% contralateral metachronous)
   - Family history (fourfold increased risk with an affected brother, twofold increase with affected father)
   - Germ-cell neoplasia in situ (GCNIS) is a premalignant condition with a 50% risk of 5-year progression. The rationale to screen and treat GCNIS in high-risk populations or during surveillance is unclear.
   - Cryptorchidism (10% of all testicular tumors are associated with cryptorchidism, but ~20% of those cases are in the normal descended testicle)
   - Testicular dysgenesis
   - Down syndrome
   - Klinefelter syndrome (mediastinal tumors)
   - Peutz–Jeghers syndrome or Carney complex (Sertoli cell tumors)

2. **What are common tumor genomic events within testis cancer?**
   - Seminoma, nonseminoma: gain of 12p sequences or creation of an isochromosome 12p (i12p)
   - Seminoma: KIT mutations
   - Spermatocytic seminoma: chromosome 9 gain
   - Most infantile yolk sac tumors and teratomas: no chromosomal changes

3. **Is there a role for screening or prophylactic surgery in testicular cancer?**
   - There is no role for screening the general population for testicular cancer and no consensus on screening high-risk populations.
   - Undescended testicles should be surgically removed or relocated to the scrotum prior to puberty to decrease (but does not negate) the risk of testicular cancer.

PATHOLOGY

1. **What are the histological types of testis cancer?**
   - Germ-cell histologies account for 95% of all cancer
     - One third of germ-cell tumors contain multiple histologies in the same mass. If any nonseminoma component is present that is used for treatment decisions.
   - Germ cell; seminoma histologies:
     - Classical seminoma ("fried-egg" appearance, pure histology, 40%–50% of all testicular germ-cell tumors, 50% have i12p)
     - Spermatocytic tumor (elderly with indolent course—rare)
   - Germ cell; nonseminoma histologies (more aggressive; 50%–60% of all tumors; i12p 80%)
     - Embryonal cell (most undifferentiated subtype)
     - Choriocarcinoma (most aggressive subtype, increased beta-human chorionic gonadotropin [beta-HCG])
     - Yolk sac (increased alpha-fetoprotein [AFP])
     - Teratoma (mature or immature)
     - Stroma tumors (Sertoli cell, Leydig cell, primitive gonadal structures; 1%–2% of tumors)

2. **What are the associated serum tumor markers used in testicular cancer?**
   - Lactate dehydrogenase (LDH): noncancer type specific
   - AFP: yolk sac, embryonal (never in seminoma); liver and gastrointestinal (GI) tract carcinomas; $t_{\frac{1}{2}}$ 5 to 7 days
   - beta-HCG: nonseminoma (choriocarcinoma) or seminoma (15%); $t_{\frac{1}{2}}$ 1 to 2 days

SIGNS AND SYMPTOMS

1. **What are the most common signs and symptoms of testis cancer?**
   - Painless testicular mass (most common)
   - Testicular discomfort, heaviness, dullness, and swelling (not resolved with antibiotics)
   - Cough, shortness of breath, hemoptysis, chest pain, and superior vena cava (SVC) syndrome (mediastinal)
   - Back or bone pain (retroperitoneal or bone)
   - Neurologic symptoms (brain metastasis)—rare

- Systemic symptoms (fever, weight loss, sweats) in advanced disease
- Gynecomastia (beta-HCG)—rare

DIAGNOSTIC WORKUP

1. What are the main diagnostic and staging tests used in testis cancer?

- History, physical exam, comprehensive metabolic panel, and complete blood count (CBC)
- Testicular ultrasound
- Serum markers (LDH, AFP, beta-HCG)
- CT abdomen/pelvis and chest x-ray (CXR)
- CT chest if CXR abnormal or retroperitoneal adenopathy on CT abdomen/pelvis
- Radical inguinal orchiectomy; consider open inguinal biopsy of the contralateral testis if cryptorchid, marked atrophy, hypoechoic mass, or macrocalcifications
- Consider CT contrast or MRI brain and bone scan if pertinent symptoms/signs
- Pathology
- Consider fertility consultation and sperm banking prior to chemotherapy, retroperitoneal lymph node dissection (RPLND), or radiation therapy (RT)

STAGING

1. How is testis cancer staged?

- Testicular cancer uses the American Joint Committee on Cancer (AJCC) staging system (tumor, node, and metastasis [TNM] and serum markers after orchiectomy)

pT0	No evidence of primary tumor (eg, histologic scar in testis)
pTis	Germ-cell neoplasia in situ
pT1	Tumor limited to the testis and epididymis without vascular/lymphatic invasion; tumor may invade into tunica albuginea, but not the tunica vaginalis
pT2	Tumor limited to the testis and epididymis with vascular/lymphatic invasion, or tumor extending through tunica albuginea involving the tunica vaginalis
pT3	Tumor invades the spermatic cord with or without vascular/lymphatic invasion
pT4	Tumor invades the scrotum with or without vascular/lymphatic invasion
N0	No regional LN metastasis
N1, pN1	≤5 LN and all LNs ≤2 cm in greatest dimension on imaging and measured on pathology

(continued)

(continued)

N2, pN2	>5 LN *or* any LN between 2–5 cm in greatest dimension on imaging or measured on pathology
N3, pN3	LN >5 cm in greatest dimension on imaging or pathology
M0	No distant metastasis
M1a	Nonregional nodal *or* lung metastasis
M1b	Distant metastasis other than nonregional nodal/lung
S0	LDH beta-human chorionic gonadotropin (bHCG), alpha-fetoprotein (AFP) within normal limits
S1	LDH <1.5 × normal, *and* bHCG <5,000 mIU/mL *and* AFP <1,000 ng/mL
S2	LDH 1.5–10 × normal, *or* bHCG 5,000–50,000 mIU/mL *or* AFP 1,000–10,000 ng/mL
S3	LDH >10 × normal, *or* bHCG >50,000 mIU/mL, *or* AFP >10,000 ng/mL

LDH, lactate dehydrogenase; LN, lymph node.

PROGNOSTIC FACTORS, BASED ON THE INTERNATIONAL GERM CELL CANCER COLLABORATIVE GROUP (IGCCCG)

1. **What are the main prognostic factors in testis cancer?**
   - Seminoma
     - ○ Good risk: absence of extrapulmonary visceral metastasis (90%)
     - ○ Intermediate risk: presence of extrapulmonary visceral metastasis (10%)
   - Nonseminoma
     - ○ Good risk: testis/retroperitoneal primary, S0–S1, absence of extrapulmonary visceral metastasis (60%)
     - ○ Intermediate risk: testis/retroperitoneal primary, S2, absence of extrapulmonary visceral metastasis (20%–30%)
     - ○ Poor risk: mediastinal primary, S3, or nonpulmonary visceral metastases (10%–20%)

TREATMENT

1. **What are the parameters that affect management decisions in testis cancer?**
   - Histologic type, serum markers, stage, and patient clinical factors (pulmonary and renal status)

2. **What is the goal of treatment?**
   - Treatment with curative intent (even in metastatic cases) should be pursued if the patient can tolerate therapy.

3. **What chemotherapy regimens are used in testis cancer (all are 21-day cycles)?**

- EP: etoposide/cisplatin
- BEP: bleomycin/etoposide/cisplatin
- VIP: etoposide/ifosfamide/cisplatin
- TIP: paclitaxel/ifosfamide/cisplatin
- VeIP: vinblastine/ifosfamide/cisplatin

4. **How is seminoma treated?**
   - Stage IA/B (pT1–4N0M0S0): inguinal orchiectomy and one of the following:
     - Surveillance (pT1/pT2) is preferred if the patient is compliant (15%–20% relapse rate, median time of relapse 1 year, may occur later).
     - Single agent carboplatin (AUC 7) for one or two cycles.
     - RT: infradiaphragmatic (20 Gy) including para-aortic lymph node (LN) (inclusion of ipsilateral iliac LN could be considered on special occasions). Avoid RT if prior RT in the intended field, horseshoe/pelvic kidney, inflammatory bowel disease.
   - Stage IS (T-anyN0M0S1–3): inguinal orchiectomy and further therapy dictated by extent of disease on imaging.
     - Persistent elevation is rare and other causes of LDH, AFP, beta-HCG elevation must be ruled out.
   - Stage IIA/B (T-anyN1/2M0S0–1): inguinal orchiectomy and one of the following:
     - RT: infradiaphragmatic (30–36 Gy) including para-aortic LN and ipsilateral iliac LN
     - Chemotherapy for multiple LN in selected IIA and IIB cases (EP × four cycles or BEP × three cycles)
   - Stage IIC (T-anyN3M0S0–1); stage III (T-anyN-anyM1a/b/S-any or T-anyN1–3M0S2–3): inguinal orchiectomy and risk adapted chemotherapy
     - Good risk: chemotherapy (EP × four cycles or BEP × three cycles); intermediate risk: chemotherapy (BEP × four cycles)
   - Chemotherapy can be done prior to orchiectomy in patients with visceral disease, supradiaphragmatic adenopathy, N3 (bulky retroperitoneal tumor), tumor-related back pain, elevated tumor markers, or mediastinal primary. Orchiectomy should be completed after therapy.
   - For stage II and above, treatment response should be confirmed by tumor markers and CT postchemotherapy:
     - If markers are normal and mass is ≤3 cm, standard surveillance per national guidelines.
     - If markers are normal but residual tumor >3 cm, PET scan should be done at least 6 weeks after therapy completion. If it is negative, then begin surveillance. If it is positive, then second-line chemotherapy or RT or LN resection.
     - If markers are persistently elevated, or a residual mass is growing, then second-line chemotherapy.
   - If radiation is planned during therapy, it should start within 7 weeks after orchiectomy when the wound has healed and should occur 5 days per week.

5. **What is the surveillance after completion of initial therapies for seminoma?**
   - History, physical exam, serum markers, CXR, and CT abdomen/pelvis (interval between visits and tests as well as duration of surveillance depend on stage and treatment, according to guidelines, eg, National Comprehensive Cancer Network [NCCN]).

6. **How is nonseminoma treated?**
   - Stage IA (T1N0M0S0): inguinal orchiectomy and one of the following:
     - Surveillance is preferred if the patient is compliant (20%–25% relapse rate, relapse usually within 2 years but may occur later)
     - Open nerve-sparing RPLND (within 4 weeks from CT and 7–10 days from serum markers)
   - Stage IB (T2–4N0M0S0): inguinal orchiectomy and one of the following:
     - Open nerve-sparing RPLND (within 4 weeks from CT and 7–10 days from serum markers)
     - Chemotherapy (BEP × one or two cycles) *and* open nerve-sparing RPLND (if residual mass ≥1 cm or noncompliance) *or* surveillance
     - Surveillance (pT2 only), if the patient is compliant and pathology without lymphovascular invasion
       - 50% relapse rate if lymphovascular invasion, high embryonal component
       - Absence of yolk sac, high tumor size, and high Ki67 increase relapse risk
   - Stage IS (T-anyN0M0S1–3): this is advanced disease and treated with EP × four cycles or BEP × three cycles:
     - Care must be taken to consider other reasons for marker elevation (hepatobiliary disease, marijuana use, and hypogonadism).
   - Stage IIA (T-anyN1M0S0-1); stage IIB (T-anyN2M0S0-1) (lymphatic drainage sites only, asymptomatic): inguinal orchiectomy and one of the following:
     - Modified bilateral (nerve-sparing if possible) RPLND (within 4 weeks from CT and 7–10 days from serum markers)
     - Chemotherapy (EP × four cycles or BEP × three cycles) *and* either open nerve-sparing RPLND (if residual mass ≥1 cm or noncompliance) *or* surveillance
   - Stage IIB (T-anyN2M0S0-1) (multifocal, aberrant lymphatic drainage, symptomatic): inguinal orchiectomy and one of the following:
     - Chemotherapy (EP × four cycles or BEP × three cycles) *and* either open nerve-sparing RPLND (if residual mass ≥1 cm or noncompliance) *or* surveillance.
     - Chemotherapy can be done prior to orchiectomy in patients with pain from psoas invasion, bilateral retroperitoneal involvement, suprahilar or retrocrural adenopathy. Orchiectomy should be completed after therapy.
   - After RPLND for stage I/II (N0–2, S0): surveillance for pN0; surveillance (if compliant patient) or adjuvant chemotherapy (EP or BEP × two cycles) for pN1; adjuvant chemotherapy (EP or BEP × two cycles) for pN2, adjuvant chemotherapy (BEP × three cycles or EP × four cycles) for pN3

- Advanced disease treatment (based on prognostic categories):
  - Good risk advanced: stage IS, stage II (S1 or N3); stage IIIA (M1a/S0–1)
    - Inguinal orchiectomy and chemotherapy (EP × four cycles or BEP × three cycles) (90% cure)
  - Intermediate risk advanced: stage IIIB (T-anyN1–3/M0/S2 or T-anyN-anyM1a/S2)
    - Inguinal orchiectomy and chemotherapy (BEP × four cycles) (70% cure)
  - Poor risk advanced: stage IIIC (T-anyN1–3/M0/S3 or T-anyN-anyM1a/S3 or T-anyN-anyM1b)
    - Inguinal orchiectomy and chemotherapy (BEP × four cycles or VIP × four cycles if the patient cannot tolerate bleomycin) (50% cure)
  - Brain metastases: primary chemotherapy +/− RT +/− surgery

7. **What is the management for advanced nonseminoma postchemotherapy (based on response)?**
   - Complete response, S0: open bilateral RPLND *or* surveillance
   - Partial response, S0: resection of residual masses *and* either surveillance for teratoma (40% of patients) or necrosis (45% of patients) *or* chemotherapy (EP or TIP or VIP/VeIP × two cycles) if residual disease is other cancer histology (15% of patients)
   - Incomplete response or persistently elevated markers: clinical trial, second-line chemotherapy (resection of solitary mass would rarely be considered <5%).

8. **How is refractory/recurrent disease treated (20%–30% of all patients)?**
   - Favorable (low markers, low volume, complete response on first-line therapy, testis primary):
     - Clinical trial, chemotherapy (TIP or VeIP) or high-dose chemotherapy with autologous stem cell rescue
   - Unfavorable (high markers, high volume, incomplete response, extratesticular primary): one of the following:
     - Clinical trial (preferable)
     - Chemotherapy with TIP or VeIP or high-dose chemotherapy with autologous stem cell rescue
     - Surgical salvage (solitary site)
   - Late relapse (>2 years): consider surgical salvage (preferred), chemotherapy, or high-dose chemotherapy with autologous stem cell rescue.
   - Advanced relapsed/refractory nonseminoma: palliative chemotherapy (gemcitabine/oxaliplatin, gemcitabine/paclitaxel, oral etoposide, gemcitabine/paclitaxel/oxaliplatin) and/or RT can be used.

9. **What is the surveillance after the initial treatment of nonseminoma?**
   - History, physical exam, serum markers, CXR, and CT abdomen/pelvis (interval between visits and tests as well as duration of surveillance depend on stage and treatment, according to guidelines, eg, NCCN).

SPECIAL CONSIDERATIONS

1. Are there any cancers associated with testis cancer?

- Teratoma can transform to several malignant histologic types.
- The exact frequency of treatment (radiation and chemotherapy) related secondary malignancies is unclear but has typically been higher in testicular cancer survivors than age-matched controls (especially hematologic malignancies, nonmelanoma skin cancer). With the current trend of de-escalating therapy, it is unclear how much a role this will play in the future but long-term clinical exam and awareness must be maintained.
- Minority of patients with cancer of unknown primary origin can respond to cisplatin-based chemotherapy (young men with midline tumors, high serum markers, i12p).

2. What are noncancer medical complications from the management of testis cancer?

- Cardiovascular, neurologic, pulmonary, renal, infertility, hypothyroidism

3. Should doses be adjusted or cycle extended for neutropenia during chemotherapy?

- Chemotherapy doses should not be reduced or delayed. Growth factor support can be carefully utilized as per NCCN guidelines.

4. What are some complications from RPLND (up to 20% of patients have complications with salvage RPLND after radiation)?

- Sexual dysfunction, infertility, retrograde ejaculation, bowel perforation, ascites, lymphocele, vascular injury, and pancreatitis

QUESTIONS

1. A 36-year-old man underwent a right inguinal orchiectomy 7 days ago for a pT1 pure embryonal histology germ-cell tumor with original markers of a normal lactate dehydrogenase/beta-human chorionic gonadotropin (LDH/beta-HCG) and alpha-fetoprotein (AFP) of 4,139 ng/mL. Markers were drawn today and show a persistently elevated AFP of 2,276 ng/mL while the others remain normal. What is the best next step?
   A. PET scan
   B. Brain MRI
   C. Four cycles of EP
   D. Repeat markers in 2 weeks

2. A 28-year-old man arrives in your office 4 weeks after undergoing a left orchiectomy with pathology showing dysmorphic cells with a "fried-egg" appearance. The tumor involved the tunica vaginalis, but imaging last week revealed no enlarged lymph nodes in the chest, abdomen, pelvis, or masses within other organs suggestive of metastases. Pre- and postorchiectomy tumor markers were negative. What is the preferred next step?
   A. Surveillance
   B. Carboplatin one to two cycles of AUC 7

C. Infradiaphragmatic radiation
D. EP (etoposide/cisplatin) × two cycles

3. A 21-year-old man presents to the emergency room with shortness of breath. A chest x-ray shows multiple lung masses and a left-lower lobe postobstructive consolidation. Cross-sectional imaging reveals bilateral pulmonary masses up to 4.8 cm with distal consolidation, and thoracic/retroperitoneal adenopathy. Tumor markers reveal lactate dehydrogenase (LDH) 2.5× the upper limit of normal, beta-human chorionic gonadotropin (beta-HCG) 2,128 mIU/mL, and alpha-fetoprotein (AFP) 11,680 ng/mL. Testicular ultrasound is normal. He underwent bronchoscopic biopsy of one of the lung lesions, which revealed a mixed germ-cell tumor of seminoma and yolk sac components. He has normal renal function and is on 2 L by nasal cannula. What is the best treatment option?
   A. EP (etoposide/cisplatin) × three cycles
   B. EP × four cycles
   C. BEP (bleomycin/etoposide/cisplatin) × four cycles
   D. Radiation to obstructing pulmonary mass

4. A 38-year-old man transfers his care to your office. He underwent a right orchiectomy and EP (etoposide/cisplatin) × four cycles for his stage III seminoma because of pulmonary involvement. His posttreatment imaging showed resolution of his disease and he has remained without evidence of disease since. He is 3 years out and the last imaging with CT of the chest, abdomen, and pelvis was 1 year ago, which was negative. He is asymptomatic, exam is normal, and tumor markers today are normal. What should his follow-up be for the subsequent year?
   A. CT of the chest, abdomen, and pelvis now, physical/tumor markers in 6 and 12 months
   B. Chest x-ray (CXR) now and in 12 months, and physical/tumor markers in 6 and 12 months
   C. CXR now and in 6 and 12 months, physical/tumor markers in 6 and 12 months
   D. Physical/tumor markers in 6 and 12 months

5. A 33-year-old man is seen 4 weeks after completing four cycles of BEP (bleomycin/etoposide/cisplatin) for a mixed germ-cell tumor involving both seminoma and choriocarcinoma on original orchiectomy. Disease originally involved the retroperitoneum and two solitary lung metastases. A new CT of his chest, abdomen, and pelvis reveals a residual conglomerate of lymph nodes in the retroperitoneal space measuring 5 × 3.5 cm (original size of 8 × 6.0 cm). Tumor markers are normal. He underwent retroperitoneal lymph node dissection (RPLND) and pathology showed necrosis and a 3.3 × 2.6 cm teratoma. What is the next step?
   A. Begin surveillance
   B. Radiation to the surgical bed of resected tissue
   C. Two cycles of TIP (etoposide/ifosfamide/cisplatin)
   D. Prophylactic whole-brain radiotherapy

ANSWERS

1. **D. Repeat markers in 2 weeks.** The tumor markers should be repeated in 2 weeks to confirm this normal decline. The half-life of AFP is between 5 and 7 days, so postorchiectomy changes need to be assessed within that context.

2. **A. Surveillance.** This is a pT2N0M0 seminoma. Although surveillance, carboplatin, or radiation therapy (RT) are acceptable treatments, the preferred option is surveillance. For patients who do relapse, the salvage cure rate is high.

3. **C. BEP (bleomycin/etoposide/cisplatin) × four cycles.** This is an advanced disease mixed germ-cell tumor with nonseminomatous components. He is poor risk based on the AFP elevation and standard would be BEP × 4. His hypoxia is disease related from the obstructing mass and should be reversible with chemotherapy, thereby allowing for bleomycin use.

4. **B. Chest x-ray (CXR) now and in 12 months, and physical/tumor markers in 6 and 12 months.** He is 3 years out from definitive treatment and the likelihood of relapse is low. Pulmonary relapse is the most common and an annual CXR is appropriate. He does not require abdominal imaging without clinical suspicion.

5. **A. Begin surveillance.** Teratoma is often chemotherapy resistant and requires surgical resection. As no seminoma, embryonal, yolk sac, or choriocarcinoma tissue was found, it is presumed all nonteratoma cancer was eradicated.

Renal Cell Carcinoma

Benjamin Y. Scheier and Bruce Redman

EPIDEMIOLOGY

1. **What is the most common type of malignant renal tumor?**
   - Ninety percent of malignant renal tumors are renal cell carcinoma (RCC) and 80% of RCC are clear cell tumors. Papillary, chromophobe, and collecting duct type are the less common histologic subtypes.

2. **What is the 5-year survival rate in patients with RCC?**
   - The estimated average 5-year survival rates in RCC are over 80% for patients presenting with stage I, over 70% for stage II, 50% to 70% for stage III, and under 10% for stage IV disease.

3. **What is the most common stage at which RCC is diagnosed?**
   - Fifty percent of patients with RCC present with localized disease, 25% with locally advanced disease, and 25% to 30% with distant metastatic disease.

4. **What are the common sites of metastatic spread?**
   - Lung (70%–75%), lymph nodes (30%–40%), bone (20%–25%), and central nervous system (CNS)

ETIOLOGY AND RISK FACTORS

1. **What is the etiology of RCC?**
   - The exact etiology of sporadic RCC has not been determined.

2. **What are the risk factors for RCC?**
   - Smoking and obesity are associated with increased incidence.
   - Toxic/occupational exposures to petroleum products, asbestos, and heavy metals are associated risk factors for RCC.
   - Acquired cystic disease of the kidney associated with long-term dialysis has a 30 times higher risk of developing RCC.
   - There is noted to be an increased incidence of RCC in patients with non-Hodgkin lymphoma (NHL) and sickle cell trait (medullary histology, in particular).

3. **What are the various familial syndromes associated with RCC?**
   - Von Hippel–Lindau (VHL) disease predisposes to clear cell carcinoma. This autosomal dominant syndrome is associated with a mutation in the *VHL* gene on chromosome 3, which inactivates one copy of the *VHL* gene in all cells. For tumors to develop there has to be a loss of second allele via somatic mutation or deletion or promoter hypermethylation.

- Hereditary papillary renal carcinoma (HPRC) predisposes to type 1 papillary RCC. HPRC is a highly penetrant autosomal dominant condition associated with activating germline mutation in the c-MET proto-oncogene on chromosome 7 accompanied by nonrandom duplication of aberrant chromosome 7.
- Birt–Hogg–Dube (BHD) syndrome is associated with chromophobe (34%), hybrid chromophobe–oncocytomas (50%), and oncocytomas. It is caused by the mutation in the folliculin gene localized to chromosome 17.
- Hereditary leiomyomatosis and RCC (HLRCC) predisposes to papillary type 2 RCC, multiple cutaneous and uterine leiomyomas, and is associated with a defect in (autosomal dominant inheritance) Krebs cycle enzyme, fumarate hydratase located on chromosome 1.
- Hereditary paraganglioma and pheochromocytoma (HPP) predisposes to clear cell and chromophobe RCC. It is an autosomal dominant condition characterized by paragangliomas and caused by mutation in genes encoding succinate dehydrogenase (involved in the Krebs cycle).
- Tuberous sclerosis complex is associated with an increased risk for angiomyolipomas and only infrequently (<5%) with RCC.

4. **What are the various tumors associated with VHL syndrome?**
- Up to 65% of all patients with VHL will develop RCC by age 60. RCCs are more likely bilateral, multicentric, and only clear cell type. Also associated are pheochromocytoma, pancreatic cyst, islet cell tumors, retinal angiomas, hemangioblastomas, inner ear tumors, and epididymal cystadenoma. Renal cell cancer and renal failure are the leading causes of death in VHL syndrome.

STAGING

1. **How do we stage RCC?**

Stage	Description
I	Tumor <7 cm in greatest dimension, limited to the kidney
II	Tumor >7 cm in greatest dimension, limited to the kidney
III	Tumor limited to kidney with regional lymph node involvement
	or
	Tumor extends into major veins or perinephric tissues but not into the ipsilateral adrenal gland and not beyond the Gerota's fascia with or without regional lymph node involvement
IV	Tumor involves ipsilateral adrenal gland and/or extends beyond Gerota's fascia
	or
	Presence of distant metastasis

SIGNS AND SYMPTOMS

1. **What is the most common presentation of renal cancer?**
- A majority of RCC is diagnosed via incidental tumor detection.

- Renal cancer presents with the triad of hematuria, flank mass, and flank pain in <10% of cases.
- Other presentations include fever, weight loss, anemia, or a varicocele.
- Few patients may present with hypercalcemia from parathyroid-related protein (PTHrp), polycythemia from increased erythropoietin, and/or Stauffer syndrome (nonmetastatic hepatic dysfunction that improves with removal of primary tumor).
- Patient with advanced disease can present with symptoms pertaining to metastases.

DIAGNOSTIC CRITERIA

1. How do we work up a patient with a kidney mass, suspected RCC?

- History, physical exam, routine blood tests—complete blood count (CBC) and comprehensive metabolic panel, urine analysis, and CT scan of the abdomen and pelvis with contrast are indicated.
- On CT scan, thickened irregular walls or septa and enhancement after contrast injection are suggestive of malignancy.
- If there is a concern for renal vein or inferior vena cava (IVC) involvement, MRI of the abdomen is recommended.
- MRI is also valuable in assessing the extent of collecting system involvement.
- Chest x-ray (CXR) is routinely done, but if abnormal or if large primary tumor or symptoms such as cough/chest pain are noted, chest CT is recommended.
- Bone scan and MRI of the brain are done only if clinically indicated.
- If urothelial carcinoma suspected (central mass), get urine cytology, ureteroscopy.

PROGNOSTIC FACTORS

1. What are the predictors for poor prognosis in metastatic RCC in the context of cytokine use?

- The following confer a poor prognosis:
  - Lactate dehydrogenase level more than 1.5 times upper limit of normal
  - Hemoglobin level less than the lower limit of normal
  - Corrected serum calcium level >10 mg/dL (2.5 mmol/L)
  - Karnofsky performance score <80
  - Absence of prior nephrectomy
- Favorable risk group (1–2 risk factors) and poor risk group (>3 risk factors)
- Survival at 1 year for favorable, intermediate-risk, and poor risk patients are 71%, 42%, and 12%, respectively.
- Long interval between nephrectomy and the appearance of distant metastases, a single site of metastatic disease, and the absence of retroperitoneal adenopathy predict a longer survival.

TREATMENT

1. When should we pursue surgical resection for RCC?

- Surgical resection is the only effective therapy for clinically localized RCC, with options being radical nephrectomy and nephron-sparing surgery.

- Radical nephrectomy is the preferred treatment for larger tumors (>7 cm) and/or if the tumor extends into the IVC.
- Patients in stable medical condition should undergo resection for stage I to III tumors.
- Stage IV patients with a solitary resectable metastasis can be managed surgically with nephrectomy and metastasectomy.
- Solitary recurrence after nephrectomy may be managed by metastasectomy.
- Palliative nephrectomy can be considered for symptom relief in patients with significant pain, hematuria, hypercalcemia, malaise, or erythrocytosis if they are good surgical candidates.

2. **Is lymph node dissection routinely recommended with radical nephrectomy?**
   - In the absence of preoperative evidence of lymph node involvement, lymphadenectomy does not improve disease-free survival or overall survival in patients with localized disease.
   - If there is suspected lymph node involvement preoperatively or intraoperatively, extended lymph node dissection is recommended, which can be potentially curative.

3. **Is nephron-sparing surgery comparable to radical nephrectomy in outcomes?**
   - For tumors <7 cm, nephron-sparing surgery gives results that are comparable with those after a radical nephrectomy, and is preferred if surgically feasible.

4. **Is there a role for any adjuvant treatment in completely resected stage I–III tumors?**
   - There is no role for adjuvant treatment after complete surgical resection outside of a clinical trial. Observation is the standard of care.

5. **What are the medical treatment options for advanced/stage IV, previously untreated renal clear cell carcinoma?**
   - If eligible, participation in a clinical trial is recommended.
   - In appropriate candidates (excellent performance status and normal organ function) with metastatic clear cell carcinoma, high-dose interleukin-2 (IL-2) is the only potentially curative therapy, although in a small minority of patients.
   - Sunitinib, pazopanib, or combination of interferon (IFN) and bevacizumab are all first-line treatments in patients with metastatic clear cell RCC and good to intermediate prognosis who are not candidates for high-dose IL-2.
   - Temsirolimus can be considered as first-line therapy in patients with clear cell carcinoma with poor risk features.

6. **Which subgroup of patients benefit from a trial of IL-2 based therapy?**
   - Patients with clear cell histology, good performance status (0–1), and minimal disease burden demonstrate a more favorable response to high-dose IL-2, which is the only treatment that may result in long-term disease remission.

7. **What are the treatment options for stage IV RCC of non-clear-cell histology?**
   - Participation in clinical trial for eligible patients is recommended.
   - Temsirolimus has shown survival benefit compared to IFN in patients with previously untreated RCC of all histologic types and poor prognostic features.
   - Though not specifically evaluated in non-clear-cell carcinoma, vascular endothelial growth factor (VEGF)-targeted therapies are also appropriate.

8. **What are the treatment options for patients with RCC refractory to VEGF-targeted therapy?**
   - Participation in clinical trials for eligible patients is recommended.
   - Cabozantinib, a small molecule TKI targeting VEGF, AXL, and MET, has shown improved progression-free survival, response rate, and overall survival compared to everolimus in patients previously treated with anti-angiogenic therapy. It is FDA approved for this indication.
   - Nivolumab, an antiprogrammed death-1 antibody, has demonstrated prolonged overall survival compared to everolimus as a second-line therapy after progression on an initial vascular endothelial growth factor tyrosine kinase inhibitor (VEGF TKI) and recently received Food and Drug Administration (FDA) approval for this indication.
   - Axitinib has also shown an improved progression-free survival (PFS) compared to sorafenib in patients with prior treatment with a cytokine or sunitinib.

9. **When would you consider cytoreductive nephrectomy in the setting of metastatic RCC?**
   - Cytoreductive nephrectomy was associated with improved survival when tested in conjunction with IFN. There is no evidence for benefit from cytoreductive nephrectomy in the current era of tyrosine kinase inhibitor use, and trials are ongoing.
   - It may be considered for patients with a good performance status, resectable primary tumor that represents the majority of total tumor burden, no evidence of rapidly progressing extrarenal disease, and no prohibitive medical comorbidities.

10. **When would you consider metastasectomy in RCC patients?**
    - This can be considered in patients with radiographically limited, usually solitary metastasis.

11. **Is there any role for chemotherapy in treatment of metastatic disease?**
    - A modest response rate in the realm of 5.5% to 6% has been reported with use of chemotherapy and is therefore not recommended.
    - In poorly differentiated kidney cancer with high degree of sarcomatoid changes, palliative chemotherapy may be considered.

QUESTIONS

1. **All of the following are risk factors associated with renal cell carcinoma (RCC), except for:**
   A. Smoking
   B. Obesity

    C. Acquired cystic disease of the kidneys
    D. Asbestos exposure
    E. Prior radiation

2. A 70-year-old woman underwent a radical nephrectomy for a right kidney mass 2 years ago, initially identified by CT scan during a workup by her primary care physician for painless hematuria. Pathology revealed a 9 cm renal cell carcinoma (RCC), clear cell histology, with 4 of 10 lymph nodes involved by neoplasm. She was observed clinically after the operation.

She is referred to you now after a CT obtained for right-sided abdominal pain showed five liver lesions measuring 2 cm each, and scattered noncalcified pulmonary nodules in both lungs. CT-guided core biopsy of one of the liver lesions showed clear cell carcinoma consistent with the histopathology of the primary kidney tumor removed 2 years ago. She has a history of coronary artery disease and well-controlled hypertension and takes a thiazide diuretic as well as aspirin.

Her abdominal pain is well controlled with oral analgesics and she is otherwise asymptomatic. Her Eastern Cooperative Oncology Group (ECOG) performance status is 0.

What would you recommend next?
    A. Nivolumab
    B. Staged resections of liver metastases and lung metastases
    C. Temsirolimus
    D. Pazopanib
    E. High-dose interleukin-2 (IL-2)
    F. Cisplatin and gemcitabine

3. Which of the following is true regarding renal cell carcinoma (RCC)?
    A. There is no role for nephrectomy in stage IV RCC
    B. Chemotherapy is a preferred first-line treatment due to high response rates across all histologies
    C. Sarcomatoid differentiation is a poor risk feature in RCC
    D. Interferon-alpha therapy improves survival compared to surveillance following resection of a primary RCC

4. A 61-year-old man is diagnosed with a 9 cm right kidney mass seen on CT scan of the abdomen and pelvis with intravenous contrast during a workup for gross hematuria. A right radical nephrectomy is planned. Preoperative lab evaluation reveals an alanine aminotransferase (ALT) of 200 U/L and an aspartate aminotransferase (AST) of 190 U/L. An MRI of the liver is normal. A radical right nephrectomy is performed revealing clear cell carcinoma. He is sent to your office 6 weeks later for evaluation and you note that the ALT and AST elevations have resolved.

What do you suspect is the cause of this lab abnormality?
    A. Occult liver metastases
    B. Stauffer syndrome
    C. Contrast induced liver injury
    D. Nonalcoholic steatohepatitis

ANSWERS

1. **E. Prior radiation.** In addition to A through D, chronic dialysis, hypertension, and occupational exposures to cadmium, trichloroethylene have been identified as risk factors for RCC.

2. **D. Pazopanib.** This patient has metastatic RCC, clear cell type. Pazopanib, a vascular endothelial growth factor tyrosine kinase inhibitor (VEGF TKI), is an effective frontline therapy for metastatic RCC of clear cell type. It has superior progression-free survival compared to placebo, but no overall survival benefit has been seen in phase 3 randomized trials. Nivolumab, an antiprogrammed death-1 antibody, has demonstrated prolonged overall survival compared to everolimus as a second-line therapy after progression on an initial VEGF TKI and is now Food and Drug Administration (FDA) approved in the second line. Temsirolimus is reserved for patients with RCC with poor prognostic features. High-dose IL-2 can induce durable remissions in a minority of patients with metastatic RCC; however, the patient's age, medical history, and volume of metastases make her a poor IL-2 candidate. Her volume and distribution of disease make metastasectomy a poor option. Cytotoxic chemotherapy is considered ineffective in metastatic kidney cancer.

3. **C. Sarcomatoid differentiation is a poor risk feature in RCC.** Palliative nephrectomy can be considered for symptom relief in patients with significant pain, hematuria, hypercalcemia, malaise, or erythrocytosis if they are good surgical candidates. Chemotherapy has a poor response rate (<10%) in RCC, so its use is not recommended. Adjuvant therapy trials comparing interferon alpha to surveillance for RCC have not shown a survival benefit.

4. **B. Stauffer syndrome.** Stauffer syndrome is a cytokine-mediated paraneoplastic phenomenon manifested by nonmetastatic hepatic dysfunction, which resolves after resection of the primary renal cell tumor.

VI

GASTROINTESTINAL MALIGNANCIES

Esophageal Cancer

23

Raymond M. Esper, Paul L. Swiecicki, and James A. Hayman

ETIOLOGY AND RISK FACTORS

1. **What are the risk factors?**
   - Squamous cell carcinoma
     - Smoking and alcohol
     - Previous ionizing radiation exposure
     - Anatomic abnormalities (esophageal webs, achalasia, and Zenker's diverticulum)
     - Familial tylosis (nonepidermolytic palmoplantar keratoderma)
   - Adenocarcinoma
     - Obesity
     - Gastroesophageal reflux disease (GERD)
     - Barrett's esophagus (intestinal metaplasia); rate of transformation is 0.5% per year
     - High-grade dysplasia (stage 0); rate of transformation is 10% to 15% per year

STAGING

1. **What are the tumor, node, and metastasis (TNM) staging definitions?**

	TNM	Description
Primary tumor (T)	Tis	High-grade dysplasia
	T1a	Tumor invades lamina propria or muscularis mucosae
	T1b	
	T2	Tumor invades submucosa
		Tumor invades muscularis propria
	T3	Tumor invades adventitia
	T4a	Tumor invades adjacent structures (pleura, pericardium, or diaphragm), resectable
	T4b	Tumor invades adjacent structures (aorta, vertebral body, trachea, etc.), unresectable

(continued)

1. **What are the tumor, node, and metastasis (TNM) staging definitions?**
   (*continued*)

	TNM	Description
Regional lymph nodes (N)	Nx	Regional lymph nodes cannot be assessed
	N0	No regional lymph node metastasis
	N1	Metastasis in 1–2 regional lymph nodes
	N2	Metastasis in 3–6 regional lymph nodes
	N3	Metastasis in 7 or more regional lymph nodes
Distant metastases	M0	No distant metastases
	M1	Distant metastases

2. **How is esophageal cancer staged?**
   - The staging system was updated in 2010, and there are now separate stage groups for adenocarcinoma and squamous cell carcinoma that use TNM, histologic grade, and, for squamous cell carcinoma, location in the esophagus.
   - Presence of tumor in one to three lymph nodes increases the stage to at least stage IIB for both adenocarcinoma and squamous cell carcinoma.
   - Presence of distant metastasis increases the stage to stage IV.

3. **What percentage are resectable at the time of diagnosis?**
   - Fifty percent are resectable.

SIGNS AND SYMPTOMS

1. **What are the symptoms and signs?**
   - Symptoms include dysphagia (75%, solids > liquids), weight loss (50%), gastroesophageal reflux (25%). Patients may also complain of dyspepsia, odynophagia, epigastric or retrosternal pain, anorexia, malaise, hematemesis, cough, or hoarseness.
   - Late signs on physical exam include
     o Horner syndrome, supraclavicular lymphadenopathy (Virchow's node)

WORKUP AND DIAGNOSIS

1. **What tests should be ordered?**
   - History and physical, routine lab work (complete blood count [CBC], comprehensive metabolic profile).
   - Endoscopy with biopsy is diagnostic. Endoscopic ultrasound (EUS) adds T and N staging information.
   - CT or PET/CT scan of the chest, abdomen, and pelvis to assess for distant metastases; esophageal cancer frequently spreads to the liver and lung.

2. **What is the pathology?**
   - Adenocarcinoma (65%)
   - Squamous cell carcinoma (35%)

3. **Where are tumors located?**
   - Fifty percent of tumors arise from the lower third of the esophagus, 25% from the midesophagus, and 25% from the upper third of the esophagus.
   - Adenocarcinomas are typically in the lower third of the esophagus or at the gastroesophageal junction.
   - Squamous cell carcinomas usually occur in the upper half of the esophagus.

PROGNOSTIC FACTORS

1. **What determines prognosis?**
   - Prognosis is largely determined by stage and ability to tolerate treatment.
   - Adenocarcinomas and squamous cell carcinomas have similar outcomes.

2. **What is the overall 5-year survival rate?**
   - All stages combined—18.4%
   - Early stage—60% to 80%

TREATMENT—FIRST LINE

1. **What is the treatment of patients with high-grade dysplasia (stage 0)?**
   - Endoscopic mucosal resection (EMR), mucosal ablation, or esophagectomy
   - The transformation rate of high-grade dysplasia to invasive cancer is 10% to 15% per year.

2. **What is the treatment of patients with early-stage, node-negative disease (stage I)?**
   - Esophagectomy alone
     - Either the transhiatal or transthoracic approach is acceptable.
   - Tumors in the cervical esophagus
     - These tumors are less amenable to surgery due to the need for pharyngo-laryngo-esophagectomy.
     - Tumors above the aortic arch are generally not resectable.
     - Generally these tumors are treated with definitive chemoradiation.

3. **What are the treatment options for patients with locally advanced, resectable disease?**
   - Definitive chemoradiation
     - Preferred approach for cervical tumors
     - Preferred in patients with squamous cell carcinomas of the esophagus
     - Weekly carboplatin and paclitaxel with daily radiation (50–50.4 Gy lasting 5–5.5 weeks) is the standard of care.
   - Preoperative chemoradiation, followed by esophagectomy (trimodality therapy)
     - Weekly carboplatin and paclitaxel with daily radiation for 5 to 5.5 weeks is standard.

○ For preoperative nutritional support, prefer nasogastric feeding tube or J-tube over percutaneous endoscopic gastrostomy (PEG) due to the need to use the stomach to create a conduit following removal of the esophagus.

● Adjuvant chemotherapy or adjuvant radiation has no role as sole postoperative therapy. Perioperative chemotherapy alone, without radiation, does not have any benefit for patients with nonmetastatic disease (adjuvant therapy following surgery with 4 months of oral capecitabine and 1 month of radiation is sometimes used but is *not* considered the standard of care).

4. **What is the treatment for patients with locally advanced, unresectable disease?**

   ● T4b esophageal cancer is unresectable.

   ● Chemoradiation is preferred; however, radiation alone is also an option for patients who are not candidates for treatment with chemotherapy.

5. **What is the treatment for patients with stage IV disease?**

   ● Palliative chemotherapy

   ○ Trastuzumab should be added to chemotherapy for patients with HER2/neu-positive adenocarcinomas.

   ○ Combination chemotherapy using a platinum agent paired with 5-FU, a taxane, or irinotecan is an acceptable treatment option.

   ● Palliative radiation for dysphagia or pain

   ○ Brachytherapy or external beam

   ● Photodynamic therapy (PDT)

   ● Best supportive care

   ○ Including esophageal stenting

6. **What are treatment options for elderly patients with poor performance status?**

   ● For stage 0 and stage I patients who are not surgical candidates, EMR, mucosal ablation, or PDT may be considered.

   ● For patients with locally advanced tumors who are not surgical candidates, definitive chemoradiation is an option.

   ● For patients with locally advanced tumors who are not chemotherapy candidates, radiation therapy alone can be utilized.

   ● Best supportive care.

7. **How should patients who have received therapy for locoregional disease be monitored?**

   ● History and physical examination with routine blood work every 3 to 6 months for 1 to 2 years, then every 6 to 12 months for 3 to 5 years, then annually.

   ● Imaging (PET–CT or CT chest/abdomen) may be considered every 6 to 12 months for the first 3 years, and then as clinically indicated.

TREATMENT—RECURRENT DISEASE

1. **How is recurrent disease treated?**

- Trastuzumab should be added to chemotherapy for patients with HER2/neu-positive adenocarcinomas.
- Similarly to metastatic or unresectable disease, use platinum-based combination chemotherapy and/or palliative radiation therapy.
- Ramucirumab with or without paclitaxel in the second-line setting.
- Patients with localized recurrences who have not previously received radiation therapy in the region of the recurrence could be treated with concurrent chemoradiation.
- Best supportive care.

SPECIAL CONSIDERATIONS

1. Who should be screened?
- Screening for the general population is not indicated in the United States.
- Patients with Barrett's esophagus are at higher risk of esophageal cancer.
  - Rate of transformation to esophageal cancer is 0.5% per year.
  - Consider screening esophagogastroduodenoscopy (EGD) every 3 to 5 years.

2. What are some life-threatening complications?
- Esophageal-airway fistula
  - Presents with cough, aspiration, and fever, frequently leading to pneumonia
  - Treated with a coated, expandable metal stent to seal the fistula

QUESTIONS

1. Which of the following is an appropriate initial treatment option for a 50-year-old man with stage III esophageal adenocarcinoma with HER2 overexpression?
   A. Ivor Lewis esophagectomy followed by adjuvant chemotherapy and concurrent radiation
   B. Neoadjuvant chemotherapy consisting of carboplatin and paclitaxel with concurrent radiation
   C. Neoadjuvant chemotherapy consisting of carboplatin, paclitaxel, and trastuzumab with concurrent radiation
   D. Perioperative chemotherapy with epirubicin, cisplatin, and fluorouracil.

2. Which of the following is a risk factor for esophageal adenocarcinoma?
   A. Smoking
   B. Obesity
   C. Ionizing radiation
   D. *Helicobacter pylori* infection

3. Which of the following would be an appropriate first-line treatment option for a 70-year-old man with poorly controlled hypertension and stage IV esophageal adenocarcinoma with immunohistochemistry for HER2 showing 3+?
   A. Ramucirumab plus paclitaxel
   B. FOLFOX plus bevacizumab

C. FOLFOX plus trastuzumab
D. Capecitabine plus lapatinib

4. **Which of the following is *true* about esophageal cancer?**
    A. First-line treatment of stage I esophageal squamous cell carcinoma of the cervical esophagus includes transhiatal resection followed by adjuvant capecitabine and radiation
    B. Percutaneous endoscopic gastrostomy (PEG) tubes should be empirically placed for preoperative nutritional support in patients being treated with trimodality
    C. Invasion of the trachea is a contraindication to esophagectomy
    D. Brachytherapy is a first-line treatment option in patients with locally advanced, unresectable esophageal cancer

5. **Which of the following is *true* about the management of esophageal cancer in patients with poor performance status?**
    A. Endoscopic mucosal resection (EMR) is an option for patients with early-stage esophageal cancer
    B. For patients with locally advanced tumors who are not chemotherapy candidates, radiation alone is not recommended
    C. Empiric esophageal stenting should be considered to help the patients get through therapy
    D. In elderly patients with localized disease, single-agent chemotherapy with capecitabine is an option

6. **Which of the following has been shown to be an effective screening strategy for the detection of esophageal cancer in the United States?**
    A. An EGD at age 50, and then every 10 years
    B. An endoscopic ultrasound (EUS) at age 50, and then every 10 years
    C. Annual assessment of serum carcinoembryonic antigen (CEA) and Ca19-9
    D. Regular screening for esophageal cancer is not recommended in the United States

7. **Which of the following chemoprevention agents has been shown to significantly reduce the risk of esophageal cancer?**
    A. A proton pump inhibitor daily for at least 10 years
    B. High-dose vitamin C daily for at least 10 years
    C. 81 mg aspirin daily for at least 10 years
    D. None of the above

ANSWERS

1. **B. Neoadjuvant chemotherapy consisting of carboplatin and paclitaxel with concurrent radiation.** The current standard of care for advanced but resectable esophageal cancer is 5 weeks of neoadjuvant carboplatin and paclitaxel and concurrent radiation followed by transhiatal resection based on the CROSS trial. Trastuzumab is not given concurrently with radiation. Rather, it is approved for HER2-positive esophageal and gastroesophageal junction (GEJ) cancer in the metastatic setting.

2. **B. Obesity.** Significant risk factors for the development of esophageal adenocarcinoma are obesity, gastroesophageal reflux disease (GERD), and Barrett's esophagus. Smoking, alcohol, and ionizing radiation are risk factors of the development of esophageal squamous cell carcinoma. Unlike gastric cancer, *H. pylori* is associated with a lower incidence of esophageal adenocarcinoma.

3. **C. FOLFOX plus trastuzumab.** The ToGA trial showed a survival advantage with the addition of trastuzumab to chemotherapy (platinum and fluoropyrimidine) in HER2-overexpressing esophageal adenocarcinoma. Ramucirumab (with or without paclitaxel) is approved in the second-line treatment of stage IV gastroesophageal junction (GEJ) adenocarcinoma. Uncontrolled hypertension is a relative contraindication to ramucirumab. Bevacizumab and lapatinib were both studied in esophageal cancer, with negative results.

4. **C. Invasion of the trachea is a contraindication to esophagectomy.** Invasion into local structures including the trachea defines T4b disease, which is considered to be unresectable. In the absence of metastatic disease, these patients are treated with radiation (+/− concomitant chemotherapy). Esophageal cancer of the cervical esophagus is less amenable to surgery given the need to perform an extensive surgery (pharyngo-laryngo-esophagectomy). Hence these are generally treated with definitive chemoradiation. Preoperative nutritional support is an important consideration in the treatment in patients with resectable esophageal cancer. However, PEG tubes are avoided given the need to use the stomach to create a conduit. Brachytherapy is a treatment option reserved for the palliative setting to relieve dysphagia or pain.

5. **A. Endoscopic mucosal resection (EMR) is an option for patients with early-stage esophageal cancer.** In patients with early-stage esophageal cancer and poor performance status, several nonsurgical options can be considered for local control including EMR. In patients with locally advanced tumors who are not chemotherapy candidates, definitive radiation is an option. There is no role for empiric esophageal stenting; this should be reserved for supportive care in the setting of symptomatic esophageal lesions. Similarly, there is no role for single-modality therapy using chemotherapy in localized disease. Chemotherapy should be reserved for use in combination with radiation or for the metastatic setting.

6. **D. Regular screening for esophageal cancer is not recommended in the United States.** Although screening for esophageal cancer is standard in some countries such as Japan where the incidence is high, there are no data to support regular screening of the general population in the United States. No circulating tumor markers have been shown to correlate with the presence of esophageal cancer.

7. **D. None of the above.** Some data suggest that regular use of aspirin/nonsteroidal anti-inflammatory drugs (NSAIDs) or a proton pump inhibitor may be associated with a lower incidence of esophageal cancer; causality has not been proven. Consumption of citrus fruits has been associated with a reduced incidence of gastroesophageal malignancies, but supplemental vitamin C has not.

Gastric Cancer

David B. Zhen and Mark M. Zalupski

EPIDEMIOLOGY

1. **What is the median age at diagnosis?**
   - Seventy years

2. **What is the incidence of gastric cancer?**
   - There is a wide global variation in incidence of gastric cancer.
   - The incidence of gastric cancer has steadily decreased in the United States and Western European countries during the last three decades likely related to changes in diet, food preparation and storage, and treatment of *Helicobacter pylori* infection. Over the past 80 years, gastric cancer incidence and mortality have decreased by almost 90%.
   - At the same time, the incidence of tumors of the gastroesophageal junction (GEJ) among young White individuals has increased in Western countries secondary to the increase in the rates of obesity and reflux disease.

ETIOLOGY AND RISK FACTORS

1. **What are the risk factors for gastric cancer?**
   - Risk factors:
     - *H. pylori* infection:
       - High-salt diet
       - Presence of nitrates in cured foods
       - Tobacco and alcohol exposure
       - Gastroesophageal reflux, obesity
       - Chronic gastritis
     - Protective factors:
       - Diet rich in fruit and vegetables
       - Refrigeration of food
       - Exposure to vitamin C and other carotenoids
     - Genetic predisposition:
       - Lynch syndrome, deficiencies of mismatch repair genes (*MLH1*, *MSH2*, *MSH6*, *PMS2* autosomal dominant)
       - Hereditary diffuse gastric cancer (HDGC), germline truncating mutations in *CDH1,* which encodes for the protein E-cadherin (autosomal dominant). Prophylactic gastrectomy recommended for patients aged 18 to 40.

- Juvenile polyposis syndrome (JPS) (*SMAD4, BMPR1A*; autosomal dominant)
- Peutz–Jeghers syndrome (*STK11*; autosomal dominant)
- Familial adenomatous polyposis (*APC*; autosomal dominant)
- These hereditary syndromes have implications with regard to screening endoscopies

SIGNS AND SYMPTOMS

1. How do gastric cancers present?

- Twenty-three percent of the patients present with localized tumor (5-year survival of 62%), 32% with locally advanced disease (5-year survival of 27%), and 34% with distant metastasis (5-year survival of 3%).

STAGING

1. What is required in the staging workup for gastric cancer?

- Esophagogastroduodenoscopy (EGD) is critical to visualize the tumor, evaluate its location and extent, and obtain tissue biopsy.
- Endoscopic ultrasound (EUS) is helpful in determining the depth of tumor invasion, the proximal and distal extent of the tumor, and regional nodal status.
- CT scans of the chest/abdomen and pelvis provide staging, which determines treatment and prognosis.
- In clinical settings, the classification most used is based on the potential for resection and evidence for extent of disease, thus dividing patients into resectable, locally advanced unresectable, and metastatic gastric cancer (Figure 24.1; Table 24.1).
- HER2 status: HER2 is overexpressed and/or amplified in 13% to 22% of gastric cancer. Overexpression may be determined using immunohistochemistry (IHC)

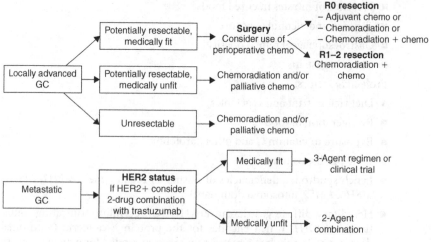

FIGURE 24.1 ■ Schematic algorithm for the treatment of gastric cancer.
Chemo, chemotherapy; GC, gastric cancer; +, positive.

TABLE 24.1 ■ Staging Classification for Gastric Cancer

Primary Tumor (T)

Tis	Carcinoma in situ: intraepithelial tumor without invasion of the lamina propria
T1	Tumor invades lamina propria, muscularis mucosae, or submucosa
T2	Tumor invades muscularis propria
T3	Tumor penetrates subserosal connective tissue without invasion of visceral peritoneum or adjacent structures
T4	Tumor invades serosa (visceral peritoneum) or adjacent structures

Regional Lymph Nodes (N)

N1	Metastasis in one to two regional lymph nodes
N2	Metastasis in three to six regional lymph nodes
N3	Metastasis in seven or more regional lymph nodes

Distant Metastasis (M)

M0	No distant metastasis
M1	Distant metastasis

Source: Adapted from Edge S, Byrd DR, Compton CC, et al. eds. *AJCC Cancer Staging Handbook: From the AJCC Cancer Staging Manual.* 7th ed. New York, NY: Springer-Verlag; 2010.

with a monoclonal antibody (HercepTest) and amplification using fluorescence in situ hybridization (FISH) following the same procedures as in breast cancer.

- HER2 overexpression is associated with the intestinal subtype and GEJ tumors. HER2 targeting is an important component of therapy in advanced disease.

DIAGNOSIS

1. **How is the pathology of gastric cancer described?**
   - Classification of the disease (see the table in the following question)
     - Based on the *anatomic location* in the stomach
       - *Cardiac:* involves the GEJ.
       - *Noncardiac:* located in the corporal or the antral area.
   - Based on *Lauren classification* of the histological pattern
     - *Intestinal:* this subtype forms rudimentary glands, usually arises from a background of intestinal metaplasia, and follows a stepwise progression from chronic gastritis to intestinal metaplasia, increasing grades of dysplasia, and invasive carcinoma.
     - *Diffuse:* cells fail to form any recognizable structures and resemble glands with the classical appearance of signet ring cells. Sometimes small amounts of interstitial mucin are observed.

2. **What are the characteristics of gastric cancer based on tumor subtypes?**

	Cardiac GEJ	Noncardiac Intestinal	Noncardiac Diffuse
Epidemiology	Incidence increasing in Western countries	Incidence decreasing worldwide	Incidence stable
Biology	Possible link with HER2 biology	Lynch syndrome related	*CDH1* mutations, Loss of E-cadherin
Clinical features	• GERD • Obesity	• *Helicobacter pylori* infection • Tobacco/alcohol • Salt intake • Poor fruit/vegetable diet	No clear relation to classical risk factors
Pathology		Stepwise progression model: • Chronic gastritis • Intestinal metaplasia • Dysplasia	No stepwise progression No precursor lesion Signet ring cells Interstitial mucin
HER2 status	32% GEJ	18% gastric cancer 32% intestinal	6% diffuse

GEJ, gastroesophageal junction; GERD, gastroesophageal reflux disease.

TREATMENT

1. **What is the treatment for resectable gastric cancer?**
   - Surgical treatment
     ○ Attempt at curative resection is often the initial treatment for gastric cancer, although complete resection is sometimes not possible.
     ○ Extent of luminal resection
       ■ Tumors located distally: gastrectomy or a distal subtotal gastrectomy
       ■ Tumors located more proximally
         • Proximal subtotal gastrectomy for well or moderately differentiated tumors that arise within the GE junction
         • Total gastrectomy with some extent of esophagectomy and a Roux-en-Y reconstruction for poorly differentiated tumors, those associated with Barrett's esophagus, and those extending into the esophagus
       ■ Extent of the lymph node dissection continues to be debated.
       ■ Lymph node dissection categories
         • D1: perigastric lymph nodes along greater and lesser omentum

- D2: D1 dissection plus more distal lymph nodes of the celiac axis
  - Generally, it is believed that D2 dissections offer a survival advantage over D1 dissections.
  - In Western countries the standard is a modified D2 dissection, achieving the goal of removing at least 15 lymph nodes.

2. **What are the adjunctive therapies for resectable gastric cancer?**
   - Perioperative chemotherapy (preoperative and postoperative treatment)
     - Studied in the MAGIC Phase 3 trial
       - Compared six cycles of epirubicin, cisplatin, 5-fluorouracil (ECF) versus surgery alone
       - Survival benefit noted with ECF
   - Adjuvant chemotherapy (for patients who did not receive preoperative therapy)
     - Adjuvant Chemotherapy Trial of S-1 for Gastric Cancer (ACTS-GC) study
       - Japanese study
       - Adjuvant S1 $\times$ 1 year versus observation alone following D2 dissection
       - Three-year survival rate improved with S1
     - Questions remain as to the benefit of adjuvant chemotherapy with S1 in Western population.
     - Meta-analysis data in resected gastric cancer show adjuvant chemotherapy is associated with a statistically significant benefit in terms of overall survival and disease-free survival over observation.
     - In the United States, adjuvant therapy often includes fluoropyrimidine-based chemoradiotherapy.
   - Chemoradiation
     - Intergroup 0116 Study
       - North American study
       - Compared adjuvant 5-fluorouracil (5-FU)/leucovorin + radiation versus surgery alone
       - Five-year survival rate improved with adjuvant treatment

3. **How is locally advanced unresectable and metastatic gastric cancer treated?**
   - Palliative chemotherapy is the primary therapy for advanced gastric cancer.

4. **Is chemotherapy better than best supportive care (BSC)?**
   - The most recent update of these series of meta-analysis from the Cochrane Collaboration published in 2010 showed a significant benefit in survival rate for chemotherapy and quality-adjusted survival versus BSC.

5. **Is combination chemotherapy superior to single-agent therapy?**
   - Combination chemotherapy is superior to single-agent treatment in terms of overall survival, progression-free survival, and response rate.
   - A classical two-drug regimen is cisplatin and 5-FU and often serves as a comparator.

6. **How many drugs should be incorporated into combination chemo-therapy regimens?**
   - Two-drug regimens are typically preferred due to lower toxicity.
   - Three-drug regimens can be considered in those patients with high performance status.

7. **Which drugs should be incorporated into combination chemotherapy regimens for gastric cancer?**
   - ECF
     - First treatment established for advanced gastric cancer
     - Based on phase 3 trial comparing ECF versus FAMTX (5-FU/doxorubicin/methotrexate)
     - ECF resulted in improved median survival rate (8.9 months vs. 5.7 months)
   - DCF (docetaxel, 5-FU, and cisplatin)
     - Based on phase 2/3 V325 trial comparing DCF to CF (cisplatin + 5-FU)
     - DCF associated with improved time to progression (32% risk reduction) and survival (23% risk reduction)
     - DCF limited by toxicities, particularly grade 3/4 neutropenia including febrile neutropenia
   - Oxaliplatin (O) = cisplatin (C) and capecitabine (X) = infusional 5-FU (F)
     - Based on the REAL-2 study
     - Median survival: ECF (9.9 months) versus EOF (9.3 months) versus ECX (9.9 months) versus EOX (11.2 months)
   - Cisplatin/S-1 = cisplatin/infusional 5-FU
     - Based on two Japanese studies showing noninferiority
   - Based on these studies, acceptable two-drug regimens often include fluoropyrimidines + platinums (eg, FOLFOX)

8. **What targeted therapies can be used for metastatic gastric cancer?**
   - Trastuzumab for HER2-positive metastatic gastric cancers
     - Based on phase 3 ToGA trial comparing cisplatin/fluoropyrimidine +/− trastuzumab in advanced untreated HER2-positive advanced gastric cancers
     - Improved survival rate with use of trastuzumab, leading to Food and Drug Administration (FDA) approval in this setting
   - No benefit of adding bevacizumab
     - Based on phase 3 trial data comparing cisplatin/capecitabine +/− bevacizumab showing no survival benefit

9. **What is the standard second-line treatment of metastatic gastric cancer?**
   - There is no standard second-line therapy for advanced gastric cancer, and choice depends on prior therapy and performance status of the patient.
   - Preferred options based on available evidence include:

○ Ramucirumab + paclitaxel (RAINBOW, phase 3 trial)

○ Ramucirumab alone (REGARD, phase 3 trial)

○ Taxanes alone (paclitaxel, docetaxel)

○ Irinotecan alone

QUESTIONS

1. A 30-year-old man with no significant past medical history seeks genetic counseling for a family history of multiple malignancies. His father was diagnosed with metastatic gastric cancer at age 42, and his paternal grandfather had localized gastric cancer diagnosed at age 45. His paternal aunt was also diagnosed with lobular breast cancer at age 35. The patient undergoes multigene panel testing and is found to have a germline truncating mutation in *CDH1*. In addition to routine age-appropriate screening, which of the following would you also recommend to the patient?
   A. CT abdomen/pelvis yearly
   B. Check carcinoembryonic tumor marker and then follow every 3 months
   C. Diagnostic laparoscopy
   D. Prophylactic gastrectomy
   E. Surveillance esophagogastroduodenoscopy (EGD) at age 35 and then every 5 years

2. A 58-year-old otherwise healthy man has a 6-month progressive course of episodic upper abdominal pain, weight loss, and early satiety prompting an esophagogastroduodenoscopy (EGD), which identifies a gastric cardiac mass that is biopsied and confirms adenocarcinoma. Staging endoscopic ultrasound (EUS) reveals a uT3 lesion, and PET scan shows no evidence for systemic disease. You are considering perioperative chemotherapy as initial treatment. Which of the following would you recommend in completing the patient's workup?
   A. MRI abdomen/pelvis
   B. Diagnostic laparoscopy
   C. Check carcinoembryonic antigen (CEA) level
   D. Colonoscopy
   E. Upper barium esophagogram

3. The patient in Question 2 has a diagnostic laparoscopy, which shows no evidence for peritoneal metastases. Which of the following are considered reasonable options for treatment of this patient's malignancy?
   A. Gastrectomy followed by adjuvant chemotherapy +/− radiation
   B. Perioperative chemotherapy + gastrectomy
   C. Radiation alone to the mass
   D. A and B
   E. Endoscopic resection of the mass

4. A 62-year-old woman presents with a large gastric body mass and evidence of peritoneal metastases and ascites on CT imaging. An

esophagogastroduodenoscopy (EGD) with biopsy of the gastric mass was performed and confirmed adenocarcinoma. Her history is only significant for hypertension and arthritis. There is no family history of malignancy. She has had a 10 lb weight loss over the past month from early satiety, but she is holding foods down. She has minimal abdominal discomfort. She remains active performing her routine housework. She presents to you to discuss further management and treatment. Which of the following would you recommend?

A. No further testing/procedures are recommended and proceed with palliative chemotherapy
B. HER2/neu testing on the biopsied tissue
C. Diagnostic paracentesis
D. Duodenal stent placement
E. Placement of an abdominal drain for her ascites

5. The patient in Question 4 is found to have a HER2/neu-positive gastric cancer. Which of the following treatment regimens would be appropriate for this patient?

A. Epirubicin, cisplatin, 5-fluorouracil (5-FU) (ECF) + trastuzumab
B. ECF
C. Cisplatin, 5-FU, trastuzumab
D. Infusional 5-FU alone
E. Cisplatin, 5-FU + trastuzumab and pertuzumab

6. A 55-year-old man with metastatic gastric cancer (HER2/neu-negative) was treated with 4 months of FOLFOX. Imaging reevaluation shows evidence of disease progression. He has otherwise tolerated therapy well. Which of the following are options for second-line management of this patient?

A. Ramucirumab + paclitaxel
B. Ramucirumab alone
C. Paclitaxel alone
D. Irinotecan-based therapy
E. All of the above

ANSWERS

1. **D. Prophylactic gastrectomy.** This patient's family history along with germline truncating mutation in *CDH1* is consistent with hereditary diffuse gastric cancer (HDGC) syndrome. Prophylactic gastrectomy is recommended given the patient's high risk for developing diffuse gastric cancer (lifetime risk by age 80 for males, 67%, and for females, 83%), which often involves the stomach lining rather than presenting with visible ulcer/tumor. Baseline esophagogastroduodenoscopy (EGD) with multiple random biopsies is recommended prior to prophylactic gastrectomy and also every 6 to 12 months in those patients who decide not to undergo prophylactic gastrectomy. The other choices are not indicated.

2. **B. Diagnostic laparoscopy.** Diagnostic laparoscopy with peritoneal biopsies would be indicated in this patient to rule out subclinical peritoneal metastases that would have implications in determining if this patient has localized disease that is amenable to surgical resection versus metastatic disease for which surgery would not be beneficial. CEA can be elevated in gastric cancer but is not sensitive or specific enough to formally diagnose metastases. The other modalities would have no role in the initial workup.

3. **D. A and B.** Gastrectomy with multimodality therapy given perioperatively or in the adjuvant setting are considered acceptable options. If the patient was unfit for surgery, definitive chemoradiation could be considered, but radiation alone to the mass would be insufficient. Endoscopic resection is not an option for this stage of malignancy.

4. **B. HER2/neu testing on the biopsied tissue.** HER2/neu testing through immunohistochemistry (IHC) and fluorescence in situ hybridization (FISH), if IHC equivocal, is indicated in this patient with metastatic gastric cancer. A positive test result would allow for the use of trastuzumab, which results in improved survival based on the ToGA trial. The other procedures would not be of benefit based on the patient's current clinical situation.

5. **C. Cisplatin, 5-FU, trastuzumab.** Based on phase 3 data, ECF is certainly an available option, and trastuzumab would be recommended in this patient given the HER2/neu positive status of her tumor. However, combination of epirubicin (an anthracycline) + trastuzumab would come at the risk of increased cardiotoxicity. In this case, omission of epirubicin would be recommended. Unlike breast cancer, there is no evidence for use of combination HER2-directed therapies in metastatic gastric cancer.

6. **E. All of the above.** All of the choices are appropriate second-line treatment options. Therapy choice ultimately depends on the anticipated toxicities and patient preferences.

25 Colorectal Cancer

Maryann Shango and John C. Krauss

EPIDEMIOLOGY

1. **Among all cancers, where does colorectal cancer (CRC) rank in terms of incidence and death?**
   - CRC is the second most common cause of cancer-related deaths, accounting for 8.4% of all cancer deaths.
   - Lifetime incidence of CRC is about 5%.

2. **What is the median overall survival of CRC?**
   - Overall, approximately one third of patients diagnosed with colon cancer will die from the disease.
   - Median survival: 48 months.
   - Five-year survival for all CRC patients (all stages and sites) is 61%.

ETIOLOGY AND RISK FACTORS

1. **What is the typical cytopathological pattern of colon cancer development?**
   - The majority of colon cancers develop through an orderly sequence of histologic stages beginning with the *normal colonic epithelium*, which advances to the *adenoma*, and culminates in the *carcinoma* driven by the development of progressive genetic mutations. This process evolves over 10 years in patients without inherited genetic defects.

2. **What are the major molecular pathways of CRC development, and what molecular alterations do they involve?**
   - There are three primary pathways, which are as follows:
     - *Chromosomal instability pathway:*
       - Present in 75% to 80% of sporadic colon cancers
       - Contributes to the development of a number of inherited CRCs such as familial adenomatous polyposis (FAP) (adenomatous polyposis coli [APC])
       - Characterized by the sequential accumulation of mutations in the *APC*, *KRAS*, *SMAD*, and *p53* genes, among others
     - *CpG island methylator phenotype (CIMP) pathway:*
       - Present in 15% of sporadic colon cancer
       - Involves the methylation and, therefore, the inactivation of the promoter regions of various tumor suppressor genes such as *CDKN2A* and *THBS1*

○ *Microsatellite instability (MSI) high pathway:*

- Inherited mutations in DNA repair enzymes (*MLH1, MSH2, MSH6, and PMS2, and EPCAM*)
- These genetic defects are responsible for Lynch syndrome, also known as hereditary nonpolyposis colorectal cancer (HNPCC)

3. What are the major risk factors associated with CRC?

Factors that impact CRC screening recommendations:

- Personal history of colon cancer or advanced adenomas (>1 cm, villous or tubulovillous histology and high-grade dysplasia).
- Inflammatory bowel disease, particularly in patients with pancolitis. Risk increases with degree of extent, duration, and inflammatory activity. Proctitis or proctosigmoiditis alone does not increase risk of CRC.
- First-degree relative(s) with colon cancer or advanced adenoma.
- Hereditary CRC syndromes:
  ○ HNPCC: About 3% of CRC, autosomal dominant mutation in DNA mismatch repair genes (*hMLH1, hMSH2, hMSH6, PMS2*). Lynch syndrome reserved for classification of families with germline mutation in mismatch repair gene.
  ○ FAP: About 1% of CRC. Germline mutation in *APC* gene.
  ○ MUTYH-associated polyposis (MAP): Autosomal recessive syndrome secondary to biallelic germline mutation in base excision repair gene mutY homolog *(MUTYH)* with variable clinical presentations. Can be associated with polyposis phenotype, usually <500 adenomas, and has a high incidence of somatic *APC* mutations.
  ○ Cowden syndrome, Bannayan–Riley–Ruvalcaba syndrome (PTEN hamartoma syndrome): autosomal dominant inheritance, usually from mutations in the *PTEN* gene, but also can result from mutations in the *SDHB, SDHD,* or *KLLN* gene.
- Abdominal and pelvic radiation: higher risk of CRC 10 years after treatment with at least 30 Gy to the abdomen.
- Increased age. Over 90% of CRCs occur after age 50 years.

Factors that do not impact CRC screening recommendations:

- Excessive alcohol use
- Cigarette smoking
- Obesity
- Race, although incidence and mortality is higher in African Americans
- Gender, although CRC is more common in men than women

SCREENING

1. Screening for CRC is recommended to begin at what age?

- For the average-risk patient: Start screening at age 50 years.
- Family history of CRC or advanced adenoma: Colonoscopy 10 years prior to the age of earliest occurrence, or beginning at age 40 years (whichever comes

first), if an affected first-degree relative is <60 years old at diagnosis or if CRC or advanced adenomas are present in more than two first-degree relatives.

2. **For patients who develop CRC before age 50 what clinical workup is recommended?**
   - Clinical genetic consultation with testing for MSI (microsatellite instability), with germline mutational assessment of DNA mismatch repair genes (*MLH1, MSH2, MSH6, and PMS2*) if their tumor is MSI high
   - Additional germline mutational assessment, for example, of the *APC* or *MYH* genes if the family history or patient's clinical presentation is suggestive for these mutations

3. **Until what age is screening recommended?**
   - Screening is recommended to be continued up to 10 years prior to a patient's life expectancy.

4. **What are the acceptable tests for screening and at what intervals should they be performed?**
   - Colonoscopy every 10 years
   - Flexible sigmoidoscopy every 5 years
   - CT scan of the colon (virtual colonoscopy) every 5 years
   - Double contrast barium enema every 5 years
   - Fecal occult blood testing each year
   - Fecal immunochemical testing each year
   - Fecal DNA testing every 1 to 2 years

PREVENTION

1. **What lifestyle modifications and interventions reduce the risk of CRC?**
   - Daily use of aspirin and nonsteroidal anti-inflammatory medications
   - Postmenopausal estrogen and progesterone hormone replacement therapy
   - Reduced intake of fat and meat
   - Diets rich in folate, fiber, calcium, vitamin D, magnesium, garlic, and omega-3 fatty acids
   - Polypectomy with adenoma removal
   - Increased physical activity

PATHOLOGY

1. **What are the major subtypes of CRC?**
   - Majority are carcinomas, with >90% adenocarcinomas
     - CK20 (cytokeratin 20) and CDX2 (caudal-type homeobox 2) positivity are the sensitive and specific markers of adenocarcinoma of colorectal origin (with exception of medullary carcinomas due to high microsatellite instability).
     - Mucinous carcinomas: produce extracellular mucin that comprises ≥50% of tumor mass and dissects through tumor wall, increasing risk of local spread. Associated with one or more mismatch repair gene deficiencies.

○ Non-gland-forming carcinomas:

■ Signet ring cell carcinoma: ≥50% of tumor made up of cells with intracellular mucin that displaces the nucleus. They are aggressive tumors with high risk of intramural spread and peritoneal carcinomatosis.

■ Medullary carcinoma: large eosinophilic, polygonal cells growing in solid sheets with heavy infiltration of small lymphocytes. These tumors are characterized by high degree of microsatellite instability.

- Other non-adenocarcinoma CRC are adenosquamous carcinoma, squamous cell carcinoma, spindle cell, undifferentiated carcinomas, non-Hodgkin lymphomas, particularly mantle cell lymphoma, and neuroendocrine tumors (NETs)

2. How is CRC graded?

- Based on degree of well-formed glands. Tumors are low grade (grade 1 or 2) if >50% of the tumor has well-formed glands and high grade (grade 3) if less.

3. How are appendiceal tumors classified?

- About 50% of appendiceal tumors will be low-grade NETs.
- "Goblet cell carcinoids" are adenocarcinomas with some neuroendocrine differentiation. Considerable disagreement exists about this histologic type, but in general they should be treated like adenocarcinomas.
- Adenocarcinoma
- Signet ring carcinomas
- Appendiceal mucinous neoplasms are rare, and do not have an agreed upon classification.

SIGNS AND SYMPTOMS

1. What are some of the most common clinical presentations of CRC?

- Gross or occult blood in stool
- Alterations in bowel habits, including constipation, cramping, or diarrhea
- Abdominal pain or discomfort
- Obstruction
- Decreased appetite, early satiety, weight loss, and fatigue
- Iron-deficiency anaemia secondary to blood loss

DIAGNOSTIC WORKUP

1. What is the most accurate mode of diagnosis of CRC?

- Colonoscopy is the most accurate mode of diagnosis since it permits direct visualization and biopsy of a suspected lesion.

PROGNOSTIC AND RISK FACTORS

1. What are the poor prognostic factors related to CRC?

- Depth of tumor invasion through the colorectal wall
- Presence of one or more lymph node metastases
- Degree of tumor regression after preoperative treatment for rectal carcinomas

- Presence of distant metastases
- Positive surgical margins (ie, circumferential/radial margin)
- Less than 12 lymph nodes resected with surgical removal of CRC
- Irregular tumor border
- Elevated carcinoembryonic antigen (CEA)
- Absence of microsatellite instability
- Poor histologic differentiation
- Lymphovascular invasion, perineural invasion
- Bowel perforation or obstruction
- The presence of KRAS or BRAF mutations

STAGING

Stage	Description
0	Carcinoma in situ; disease restricted to the intraepithelial glandular basement membrane or the intramucosal lamina propria without nodal or distal metastases
I	Tumor restricted to the submucosa or muscularis propria without nodal or distal metastases
II	Tumor penetrates beyond the muscularis propria to the pericolorectal tissue, to the surface of the visceral peritoneum or directly to other organs or structures without nodal or distal metastases
III	Any tumor with nodal metastases, or extranodal tumor deposits in fat, but without distant metastases
IV	Any tumor associated with distant metastases

GENERAL TREATMENT PRINCIPLES

1. **What are the general principles of treatment of locoregional CRC?**
   - Locoregional disease is managed surgically with curative intent (stages I–III).
   - Neoadjuvant/adjuvant chemotherapy with FOLFOX is recommended for all stage III patients (regional nodal disease) and some "high-risk" stage II patients.

2. **What are the general principles of the treatment of metastatic CRC?**
   - In some stage IV patients with oligometastatic disease, particularly with liver metastases, long-term survival can be achieved with metastasectomy, in combination with preoperative or postoperative chemotherapy.
   - For patients with inoperable CRC, chemotherapy is palliative with treatment objectives limited to improving overall survival and quality of life. Combination chemotherapy is recommended for fit patients as first-line therapy in metastatic CRC as it helps obtain sufficient disease control to permit a prolonged treatment course.

3. **What are the frequently employed chemotherapy agents and regimens for the treatment of CRC?**

- 5-fluorouracil (5-FU)/leucovorin (folinic acid)
- Capecitabine
- Oxaliplatin
- Irinotecan
- Trifluridine–tipiracil (TAS-102). Tipiracil is an inhibitor of thymidine phosphorylase, preventing the degradation of trifluridine, a nucleoside analog that inhibits thymidylate synthase. Approved for third- or fourth-line metastatic CRC
- FOLFOX (combination 5-FU/leucovorin/oxaliplatin)
- FOLFIRI (combination 5-FU/leucovorin/irinotecan)
- FOLFOXIRI (combination 5-FU/leucovorin/oxaliplatin/irinotecan)
- CapeOX (combination capecitabine/oxaliplatin)

4. **What are the targeted agents that are currently employed in the treatment of CRC?**
   - Bevacizumab: a humanized monoclonal antibody that targets vascular endothelial growth factor A (VEGF-A). VEGF-A is the ligand for vascular endothelial growth factor receptor A and B. (VEGFR-1, VEGFR-2)
   - Ramucirumab: a human monoclonal antibody that is directed against vascular endothelial growth factor receptor 2 (VEGFR-2)
   - Cetuximab: a chimeric mouse/human antibody that targets the epidermal growth factor receptor (EGFR)
   - Panitumumab: a human monoclonal antibody that targets the EGFR
   - Aflibercept: an intravenous fusion protein with binding portions of VEGF-1 and VEGF-2 receptors linked to Fc portion of human IgG1, preventing VEGF-A,B and placenta growth factor (PGF) from binding to their respective receptors.
   - Regorafenib: an oral inhibitor of angiogenic tyrosine kinases.

5. **Prior to the use of cetuximab or panitumumab in any regimen, what testing must be performed?**
   - The tumor must be tested for mutations in exons 2 (codon 12 and 13), 3 (codons 59 and 61), and 4 (codons 117 and 146) in KRAS and NRAS, as they confer resistance to anti-EGFR therapy. Mutations in KRAS and NRAS are usually mutually exclusive.

6. **How are appendiceal tumors managed?**
   - If a low-grade NET of the appendix is less than or equal to 2 cm, and completely resected with negative margins, cure rate is 100%. If the tumor is greater than 2 cm, or positive margins, then consider a right hemicolectomy.
   - Goblet cell, adenocarcinoma, and signet ring histologies should be treated as colonic adenocarcinoma.

Principles of Colorectal Polyp Management

1. **Which polyp has the greatest malignant potential?**
   - Adenomatous sessile polyps

2. **What is the recommended therapy for a pedunculated or sessile polyp with pathological evidence of invasive cancer?**

   - Colonoscopy with complete assessment of colon and rectum with marking of the cancerous polyp site

   - For a *pedunculated polyp* that has favorable histological characteristics, is well defined, has clean margins and has been completely removed, surveillance is indicated. For cases of pedunculated polyps in which the margins are not well defined, the histological characteristics are unfavorable, including poor differentiation and stalk or lymphovascular invasion or incomplete polyp removal, stage-appropriate colon resection is appropriate.

   - For a *sessile polyp*, stage-appropriate resection should be considered because it is associated with an increased risk of incomplete resection and/or occult lymph node metastases.

Principles of Resectable Colorectal Cancer Management

Preoperative Workup for Resectable Disease

1. **What is the recommended preoperative workup for a resectable CRC?**

   - If not previously performed, a colonoscopy with complete assessment of the colon is recommended, together with laboratory studies (complete blood count [CBC], chemistries, and CEA) and a CT scan of the chest, abdomen, and pelvis.

   - For a rectal cancer, a rigid proctoscopy and an endorectal ultrasound or pelvic MRI are recommended in addition to the testing for colon cancer.

General Surgical Principles

1. **What is the general surgical approach for a patient with resectable colon cancer?**

   - A colectomy with resection of the primary tumor, adjoining mesentery and regional lymph nodes.

   - When the primary rectal tumor lies in the *distal one third of the rectum,* and exhibits invasion of the anal sphincter, an *abdominoperineal resection* (APR) with total mesorectal excision is performed by removal of the anus and rectum, resulting in the creation of a permanent colostomy. For selected low rectal tumors, a hand-sewn coloanal anastomosis, or creation of an ileal J-pouch, can be considered to avoid a permanent colostomy.

   - When the primary rectal tumor lies in the *proximal two thirds of the rectum,* a *low anterior resection* (LAR) is performed, sparing the anal sphincter.

   - For *distal small rectal tumors (T0, T1, or select T2 <3 cm), local excision of the primary tumor* may be considered without resection of the mesentery or lymph nodes.

General Principles of Neoadjuvant and Adjuvant Therapies in Operative Colorectal Cancer

1. **With regard to neoadjuvant and adjuvant therapies, which are considered for the management of CRC?**

   - Both neoadjuvant and adjuvant therapies may be employed in the management of locally advanced rectal cancer.

2. **What regimen is the standard of care for the neoadjuvant and adjuvant treatment of CRC?**
   - FOLFOX
   - CapeOX
   - Second-line therapies include single agent capecitabine or 5-FU/leucovorin for patients unable to receive oxaliplatin.

3. **Are targeted agents employed in adjuvant regimens?**
   - No. Targeted agents are reserved for treatment of advanced-stage metastatic disease and are *not* used in adjuvant regimens.

4. **Is irinotecan employed as part of an adjuvant regimen?**
   - No. Irinotecan is reserved for treatment of advanced-stage metastatic disease and is *not* used in adjuvant regimens.

TREATMENT BY STAGE

Colon Cancer

Early-Stage Localized Disease
1. **What is the appropriate management of stage 0 or stage I colon cancer?**
   - Resection followed by surveillance; no adjuvant therapy is employed.

Localized Disease
1. **What is the appropriate management of non-high-risk, early stage II disease in which the tumor extends to the pericolorectal tissues but not beyond (T3)?**
   - Resection followed by clinical trial, adjuvant capecitabine or 5-FU/leucovorin, or surveillance alone

2. **What is the appropriate management of high-risk, early stage II colon cancer and late stage II colon cancer (T4) in which tumor extends to the visceral peritoneum or other organs?**
   - Resection followed by clinical trial, adjuvant 5-FU/leucovorin or capecitabine with or without oxaliplatin, or surveillance are reasonable options. There is no official consensus on what defines "high-risk" stage II colon cancer, but factors considered to be high risk include T4 tumors, high-grade or poorly differentiated histology (including signet ring and mucinous histologies), close/indeterminate/positive surgical margins, high preoperative CEA, less than 12 regional lymph nodes assessed, perineural invasion, lymphovascular invasion, bowel obstruction, and bowel perforation.

3. **Do patients with non-high-risk stage II disease with MSI high disease require adjuvant therapy?**
   - No. Their prognosis is very good; one study suggested decreased survival of such patients treated with adjuvant 5-FU.

Stage III CRC
1. **What is the appropriate management of stage III colon cancer?**
   - Resection followed by adjuvant FOLFOX or CapeOx

Rectal Cancer

Early-Stage Localized Disease

1. What is the appropriate management of stage 0 or early stage I (*not T2*) rectal cancer with tumor not extending beyond the submucosa?

    ● Transanal excision, if feasible, followed by surveillance; no neoadjuvant or adjuvant therapies are indicated.

2. What is the appropriate management of stage I rectal cancer with high-risk features or tumor extending beyond the submucosa?

    ● APR or tumor-specific LAR followed by surveillance; no neoadjuvant or adjuvant therapies are indicated. The surgeon should perform a total mesorectal excision, and the pathology report should grade the quality of the total mesorectal excision.

Locally Advanced (Stage II and III Rectal Cancer)

1. What is the appropriate management of stage II, stage III, or potentially resectable locoregional rectal cancer?

    ● The three phases of therapy for locally advanced rectal cancer are concurrent chemotherapy and radiation therapy, surgery, and adjuvant chemotherapy. The order of therapies can be chemo/radiation therapy first, followed by surgical resection, followed by eight doses of FOLFOX or six doses of CapeOx, or neoadjuvant chemotherapy followed by chemoradiation, followed by surgery. The surgeon should perform a total mesorectal excision, and the pathology report should grade the quality of the total mesorectal excision. If an LAR is performed, sparing the anal sphincter, the surgeon should perform a tumor-specific total mesorectal excision, with 3 to 5 cm of distal rectal margin beyond the tumor.

Principles of Stage IV Colorectal Cancer Management

Therapeutic Options for Advanced-Stage Disease

1. What are the chemotherapeutic options for the treatment of advanced-stage CRC disease?

    ● First-line therapeutic options include FOLFOX, CapeOX, FOLFIRI, and 5-FU/leucovorin, Capecitabine or FOLFOXIRI, with or without bevacizumab. The authors only use FOLFOXIRI/bevacizumab for exceptionally good performance status patients with liver metastases only that are borderline resectable.

    ● Second-line treatment depends on the choice of first-line therapy, and the response to first-line therapy. The author's approach in 2016, for KRAS/NRAS mutant tumors, is to start with FOLFOX/bevacizumab, stop the oxaliplatin at the onset of neuropathy or maximal response (usually 6-12 doses), and then switch to FOLFIRI/bevacizumab at disease progression. For KRAS/NRAS wild-type tumors, cetuximab is used by the author as second or third line, depending on the tolerance or contraindications to bevacizumab.

    ● The addition of cetuximab or panitumumab to FOLFIRI or FOLFOX has been associated with improvement in progression-free survival in patients with *KRAS and NRAS wild-type tumors.*

    ● Ramucirumab and ziv-aflibercept can be used in place of bevacizumab in second-line therapy, but have not been demonstrated to be better than bevacizumab in this setting.

- Late-line therapy choices (after progression on oxaliplatin, irinotecan, 5-FU, bevacizumab, and cetuximab), if appropriate, include regorafenib or trifluridine/tipiracil. The authors typically use trifluridine/tipiracil before regorafenib due to the more favorable toxicity profile of trifluridine.

Approaches to the Assessment of Synchronous Metastatic Colorectal Cancer

1. What does the workup for synchronous metastatic CRC entail?

- CT scan of chest, abdomen, and pelvis
- Colonoscopy in the case of potentially resectable disease
- CBC and chemistries including CEA
- KRAS, NRAS, and BRAF mutational assessment
- Mismatch repair protein deficiency assessment
- PET/CT in the case of potentially resectable metastatic disease
- MRI of the liver, or three-phase CT scan of the liver in the setting of potentially resectable metastatic disease

Principles of Management of Synchronous Metastatic Colon Cancer

1. If a patient has resectable either hepatic or pulmonary only synchronous metastatic colon cancer, what is the appropriate management?

- Colectomy with simultaneous or later metastasectomy followed by 6 months of FOLFOX or CapeOX adjuvant therapy. Capecitabine or 5-FU/leucovorin can be considered in patients who cannot tolerate combination treatment; or
- Neoadjuvant FOLFIRI, FOLFOX, FOLFOXIRI, or CapeOx with or without a targeted agent followed by resection of primary and metastatic disease. A total of 6 months of perioperative chemotherapy is recommended; or
- Colectomy followed by FOLFIRI, FOLFOX, or CapeOx with or without a targeted agent followed by metastatectomy. A total of 6 months of chemotherapy is recommended.

2. If a patient has unresectable either hepatic or pulmonary only synchronous metastatic colon cancer, what is the appropriate management?

- Neoadjuvant FOLFOX, FOLFIRI, or CapeOx with or without a targeted agent followed by reassessment of resectability.
- If the metastatic disease remains unresectable, chemotherapy for advanced or metastatic disease is appropriate.
- If the metastatic disease becomes resectable, then colectomy with simultaneous or later metastatectomy followed by chemotherapy for advanced or metastatic disease is appropriate.

3. If a patient has synchronous abdominal or peritoneal colon cancer metastases, what is the appropriate management?

- If the metastases are not obstructing, therapy for advanced or metastatic disease is appropriate.
- If the metastases are obstructing, colectomy, stenting, colostomy, or bypass surgery is recommended to alleviate the obstruction, followed by therapy for advanced or metastatic disease.

Principles of Management of Synchronous Metastatic Rectal Cancer

1. **What is the appropriate management of advanced stage IV rectal cancer with resectable synchronous metastatic disease?**
   - FOLFIRI, FOLFOX, or CapeOX ± targeted agent, followed by radiation therapy plus 5-FU ± leucovorin *or* radiation therapy plus capecitabine, after which simultaneous or sequential primary tumor resection and metastasectomy is performed; or
   - Radiation therapy plus 5-FU ± leucovorin *or* radiation therapy plus capecitabine followed by simultaneous *or* sequential primary tumor resection and metastatectomy with adjuvant FOLFOX, FOLFIRI, CapeOX, capecitabine ± targeted agent; or
   - For a T1 or T2 primary tumor with metastatic disease, simultaneous or sequential tumor resection and metastasectomy followed by adjuvant therapy with 5-FU/leucovorin, FOLFOX, or capecitabine ± oxaliplatin

2. **What is the appropriate management of advanced stage IV rectal cancer with unresectable synchronous metastatic disease?**
   - If the primary tumor is causing obstructive symptoms, first consider palliative interventions to relieve symptoms such as colostomy, stent placement, palliative resection, or radiation therapy.
   - Neoadjuvant FOLFOX, FOLFIRI, or CapeOx with or without a targeted agent followed by reassessment of resectability.
   - If the metastatic disease remains unresectable, chemotherapy for advanced or metastatic disease is appropriate.
   - If the metastatic disease becomes resectable, then primary tumor resection with simultaneous or later metastasectomy followed by chemotherapy for advanced or metastatic disease is appropriate.

Principles of Recurrent Colorectal Cancer Management

Approaches to the Assessment of Recurrent Disease

1. **What are the features associated with a high risk of recurrence in CRC?**
   - Histologic grade 3 and 4 disease, positive or undefined surgical margins, bowel obstruction or perforation, perineural invasion, lymphatic or vascular invasion, and fewer than 12 lymph nodes assessed

2. **Following treatment for CRC, what is the recommended surveillance regimen?**
   - Clinical assessment every 3 to 6 months for the initial 24 months following treatment, and semiannually thereafter for an additional 36 months
   - For patients with tumor invading beyond the muscularis propria (ie, T2), CEA measurements at each interval of clinical assessment
   - For patients with a high risk of recurrence, CT scans of chest, abdomen, and pelvis each year for the first 36 to 60 months posttreatment.
   - Colonoscopy at 1 year; or at 3 to 6 months post-treatment if no preoperative colonoscopy was performed. Thereafter, colonoscopy should be repeated in

3 years followed by interval colonoscopies every 5 years. If the patient presented with an advanced adenoma at the time of diagnosis, repeat colonoscopy is recommended earlier at 1 year.

- If a patient has undergone an LAR for treatment of rectal cancer, a proctoscopy every 6 months for 60 months following treatment can be considered.

3. **If CEA levels suggest disease recurrence during surveillance, what is the indicated workup?**
   - Clinical assessment including physical exam, colonoscopy, and imaging studies with CT scan of chest, abdomen, and pelvis, MRI of the liver is useful in patients with hepatic steatosis, and PET/CT can be useful if other testing does not reveal cancer.

4. **If workup following elevation of CEA does not confirm disease recurrence, what further assessment is indicated?**
   - Continue to follow the CEA level, and if it remains elevated, repeat imaging studies in 3 months' time.

Principles of Management of Recurrent Rectal Cancer at an Anastomotic Site

1. **What is the appropriate management of resectable recurrent rectal cancer at an anastomotic site?**
   - Radiation therapy plus 5-FU followed by surgical resection if feasible *and* if no prior radiation therapy was administered

2. **What is the appropriate management of unresectable recurrent rectal cancer at an anastomotic site?**
   - Radiation therapy plus 5-FU-based chemotherapy if no prior radiation therapy, or systemic chemotherapy.

Principles of Management of Metachronous Metastatic Colorectal Cancer

1. **If a patient develops metachronous resectable metastatic CRC, what is the appropriate management?**
   - Resection followed by adjuvant 5-FU/leucovorin or capecitabine with or without oxaliplatin if the patient has not previously received chemotherapy, or consideration for other combinations if the patient has previously received a fluoropyrimidine, FOLFOX, or CapeOx; or
   - Neoadjuvant chemotherapy using a therapy for advanced or metastatic disease followed by resection

2. **What is the appropriate management of unresectable, metachronous metastatic CRC?**
   - If the patient *has* received FOLFOX within the previous 12 months, FOLFIRI ± a targeted agent is recommended followed by periodic reevaluation for resectability.
   - If the patient *has not* received FOLFOX within the previous 12 months, chemotherapy for advanced or metastatic colon cancer is appropriate followed by periodic reevaluation for resectability.
   - If the disease becomes resectable, resection is performed followed by additional chemotherapy for advanced or metastatic colon cancer.

QUESTIONS

1. A 35-year-old man admitted with melena was found to have a 4 cm adenocarcinoma invading the muscularis propria within his right colon. Staging scans were negative for metastatic disease, and he underwent complete surgical resection of the tumor along with 15 regional lymph nodes, which were all negative for metastatic disease. What is the next step in the management of his disease?
   A. Check for mismatch repair protein deficiency, and if deficient, recommend surveillance for stage II colon cancer
   B. Check for mismatch repair protein deficiency, and if deficient, recommend adjuvant fluoropyrimidine therapy for stage II colon cancer
   C. Recommend adjuvant therapy with FOLFOX for stage II colon cancer
   D. Recommend surveillance as he has stage II disease without "high-risk" features

2. A 65-year-old woman presents with a newly diagnosed adenocarcinoma of the anterior wall of her distal rectum after undergoing flexible sigmoidectomy for a several week history of hematochezia. MRI of the pelvis showed the tumor invades the bladder wall and is without evidence of lymphadenopathy. CT chest, abdomen, and pelvis are unremarkable for metastatic disease. She lives alone, and meets with friends for a 2 mile walk three times a week. How should her disease be treated?
   A. Chemoradiation, followed by surgery, followed by adjuvant FOLFOX
   B. FOLFOX, followed by chemoradiation, followed by surgery
   C. Chemoradiation followed by surgery
   D. A or B

3. A 60-year-old man with newly diagnosed metastatic adenocarcinoma of the sigmoid colon to his lungs and liver, presents to discuss starting therapy. He has a history of arterial thrombi with his last myocardial infarction (MI) about 2 months ago and an ischemic stroke approximately 2 years ago. He continues to exercise about three times a week and works full time as a professor at a local college. What regimen is most appropriate as first-line therapy?
   A. FOLFOX + bevacizumab
   B. FOLFOX + cetuximab
   C. FOLFIRI
   D. Regorafenib

4. A 55-year-old man who recently underwent resection of a stage III colon cancer presents to discuss the next step in his care. What adjuvant therapy would you recommend for him?
   A. FOLFIRI
   B. FOLFOX
   C. FOLFOX + bevacizumab
   D. FOLFOX + cetuximab

5. A 70-year-old man recently underwent colectomy of his stage I adenocarcinoma of the descending colon. He is doing well, with no complaints and his carcinoembryonic antigen (CEA) has become undetectable. His last colonoscopy was just prior to his diagnosis. What follow-up should he expect in the next year?
   A. History and physical every 3 to 6 months along with a CEA, and CT chest, abdomen, and pelvis every 6 months
   B. Colonoscopy in 1 year
   C. History and physical every 6 months along with CT chest, abdomen, and pelvis
   D. History and physical every 3 to 6 months along with a CEA, and PET/CT every 6 months

6. A 63-year-old woman presents with KRAS mutant metastatic colon cancer with a single metastatic lesion in the periphery of the right hepatic lobe measuring about 3 cm in diameter. What is the next step in management?
   A. Synchronous resection of primary colon tumor and en bloc resection of regional lymph nodes, along with metastasectomy of liver lesion followed by 6 months of adjuvant FOLFOX
   B. FOLFOX + bevacizumab until disease progression or intolerance
   C. Neoadjuvant FOLFOX + cetuximab, followed by resection of the liver lesion and primary colon tumor with en bloc resection of regional lymph nodes
   D. FOLFOX + cetuximab until disease progression or intolerance

ANSWERS

1. **A. Check for mismatch repair protein deficiency, and if deficient, recommend surveillance for stage II colon cancer.** All patients with stage II disease should undergo testing for mismatch repair protein deficiency, especially as its presence may identify those who will not benefit from adjuvant chemotherapy. This patient has stage II disease without any high-risk features. If his tumor tests positive for deficient mismatch repair proteins, he will not benefit from adjuvant 5-FU. The treatment of stage II microsatellite instability (MSI)-high patients with high-risk features is not clear at this time. Discussion regarding the risks and benefits of adjuvant therapy is recommended for stage II patients without MSI.

2. **D. A or B.** Locally advanced rectal cancer is treated with trimodal therapy: chemoradiation, chemotherapy, and surgery. Administering chemotherapy prior to chemoradiation, followed by surgery or chemoradiation, followed by surgery and then chemotherapy are both acceptable treatment options as per National Comprehensive Cancer Network (NCCN) guidelines. The benefit for the former schedule, however, is the increased likelihood of completing the entire course of chemotherapy. Less than half of patients who undergo chemotherapy after surgery receive full dose and/or course due to morbidity of the prior therapy and surgery.

3. **C. FOLFIRI.** The patient's recent MI is a relative contraindication to the use of bevacizumab given the increased risk of arterial thrombi with its use. We do not know the KRAS mutation status of the patient to recommend use of cetuximab. Usage of FOLFOX versus FOLFIRI is dependent on patient comorbidities and performance status. Regorafenib is not recommended as first-line chemotherapy for metastatic colon cancer, and is approved for patients who have failed first-line bevacizumab and FOLFOX or FOLFIRI.

4. **B. FOLFOX.** FOLFOX is the only approved adjuvant chemotherapy for stage III disease of the options provided. Targeted agents (ie, bevacizumab and cetuximab) and irinotecan have no role in adjuvant therapy for stage III disease, but are indicated in the treatment of advanced disease.

5. **B. Colonoscopy in 1 year.** As per National Comprehensive Cancer Network (NCCN) guidelines for surveillance after diagnosis and resection of stage I colon cancer, follow-up should entail a colonoscopy 1 year after preoperative colonoscopy. If this is negative, then a colonoscopy is repeated in 3 years.

6. **A. Synchronous resection of primary colon tumor and en bloc resection of regional lymph nodes, along with metastatectomy of liver lesion followed by 6 months of adjuvant FOLFOX.** This patient has a single metastatic lesion in her liver that is easily resectable as it is small, on the periphery, and localized to a single hepatic lobe. Therefore, the best management would be resection of both the metastatic liver lesion and her primary tumor, followed by adjuvant FOLFOX to target micrometastatic disease. Options B and D do not offer the possibility of resection of either the primary tumor or metastatic deposit, which would be inappropriate given the long-term survival benefit of metastasectomy. Furthermore, the patient is KRAS mutant and therefore would not benefit from therapy with Cetuximab.

Anal Cancer

Maryann Shango and John C. Krauss

EPIDEMIOLOGY

1. **How common is anal cancer?**
   - About 8,000 cases are diagnosed annually in the United States, making up around 2.5% of all gastrointestinal cancers.

ETIOLOGY AND RISK FACTORS

1. **What are the common risk factors for anal cancer?**
   - Seventy percent to 80% are associated with human papillomavirus (HPV), most commonly with HPV-16 and HPV-18.
   - Risk factors include history of receptive anal intercourse, history of sexually transmitted diseases, lifetime sexual partners, immunosuppression (such as immunosuppressive medication use after solid organ transplantation or for autoimmune disorders, HIV infection), history of cervical, vulvar, or vaginal cancer, and smoking.

SCREENING AND PREVENTION

1. **Who should be screened for anal cancer?**
   - There are no national guidelines, but some recommend screening HIV-positive men having sex with men, HIV-positive women with history of cervical or vulvar dysplasia, and anyone with history of anal or genital condyloma.
   - Screening is performed by rectal exam and a cytological smear of the anus (anal Pap smear). Optimal frequency of screening has not been defined. Abnormal cytology is followed up by high-resolution anoscopy with acetic acid application and biopsy if needed.

2. **What are the precursor lesions for anal cancer?**
   - Similar to cervical premalignant lesions.
   - Low-grade anal intraepithelial neoplasia (LG-AIN) may progress to high-grade anal intraepithelial neoplasia (HG-AIN).
   - HG-AIN is a truly premalignant lesion.

PATHOLOGY

1. **What are the common tumor histologies of anal cancer?**
   - The anus is anatomically defined as the anal verge distally to the dentate line proximally. Squamous mucosa merges with true epidermal tissue (containing apocrine and sweat glands, and hair follicles) of the perianal skin.
   - Four groups of tumors originate within the anal canal. First, transitional and squamous cell carcinomas behave similarly and are treated the same. Second,

perianal skin cancers are treated as primary skin squamous cell carcinomas if distinctly separated from the anal verge. Third are primary rectal squamous cell carcinomas, which are treated as primary anal squamous cell carcinoma. Finally, adenocarcinomas originate from anal glandular tissue and are treated according to the guidelines for rectal carcinomas.

2. **What is the most common anal carcinoma histology?**
   - Squamous cell carcinoma of the anal canal. For the remainder of this chapter, anal carcinoma or anal cancer will be referring to squamous cell carcinoma of the anus unless otherwise specified.

SIGNS AND SYMPTOMS

1. **What is the most common presentation of anal cancer?**
   - Bleeding (45%)
   - Rectal pain or sensation of a foreign body (30%)
   - Asymptomatic (20%)
   - Anorectal condyloma history is present in 50% of homosexual men and <30% in heterosexual men and women who develop squamous cell cancer (SCC) of the anus.

DIAGNOSTIC WORKUP

1. **What staging modalities/studies are indicated?**
   - Physical exam (including digital rectal examination [DRE], inguinal lymph node [LN] evaluation with consideration for biopsy if suspicious for involvement)
   - CT chest and abdomen
   - CT or MRI pelvis
   - Anoscopy with biopsy of the mass or fine needle aspiration (FNA)
   - PET/CT may be considered as many metastatic LNs are ≤5 mm
   - FNA of suspicious inguinal LNs to ascertain radiation field planning
   - HIV testing
   - Females: pelvic exam and cervical cancer screening

STAGING

1. **What are the anatomic boundaries of the anal canal?**
   - The histologically defined anal canal (lined by squamous mucosa) is limited by dentate line proximally and anal verge distally.

2. **Define the staging for anal cancer.**

AJCC UICC 2017 Stage	Definition
I	Primary tumor no more than 2 cm in greatest dimension and no LN involvement
IIA	Primary tumor >2 cm but ≤5 cm, without adjacent organ invasion (such as vagina, bladder, or urethra) and without LN involvement

(continued)

2. Define the staging for anal cancer. (*continued*)

AJCC UICC 2017 Stage	Definition
IIB	Primary tumor >5 cm without adjacent organ invasion (such as vagina, bladder, or urethra) and without lymph node involvement
IIIA	Primary tumor ≤5 cm without adjacent organ invasion (such as vagina, bladder, or urethra) and with inguinal, mesorectal or illiac LN involvement
IIIB	Primary tumor with adjacent organ invasion (such as vagina, bladder, or urethra) and without inguinal, mesorectal and illiac LN involvement
IIIC	Tumor >5 cm or invading adjacent organs with inguinal, mesorectal, external iliac, or internal iliac LN involvement
IV	Presence of distant metastatic disease

LN, lymph node.

GENERAL PRINCIPLES OF TREATMENT

1. **What treatment modalities are employed for all squamous cell carcinomas of the anus?**
   - Concurrent chemotherapy and radiation. Advanced-stage tumors (tumors >5 cm [T3] or invading adjacent organs [T4] and node positive disease) or residual T2 (tumors greater than 2, but less than 5 cm) disease after 45 Gy, receive an additional boost of 10 to 14 Gy.

2. **When is the response to first-line chemoradiotherapy assessed?**
   - In the United States, disease response is assessed at 8 to 12 weeks posttreatment, with decision to proceed with surgery for persistent disease at reassessment at 26 weeks.

3. **When is the role of surgery for treatment of anal carcinomas?**
   - Squamous cell carcinomas: surgery is only utilized in the setting of persistent disease at 26 weeks after first-line radiotherapy with concurrent 5-FU and mitomycin.
   - Adenocarcinoma of the anus is managed the same as rectal adenocarcinoma, with stage-specific combined modality treatment with chemotherapy, radiation therapy, and surgery.
   - Rectal squamous cell carcinoma is managed as anal squamous cell carcinoma with primary chemoradiotherapy.
   - Perianal SCCs, which originate distal to the anal verge, are excised as per guidelines for primary cutaneous skin squamous cell carcinoma.

TREATMENT BY STAGE

1. **How should precursor lesions for anal cancer be managed?**
   - LG-AIN: may progress to HG-AIN and therefore needs surveillance every 6 months. Can also consider treating with topical trichloroacetic acid or

bichloroacetic acid, topical 5-FU, intra-anal imiquimod, or anoscopy-guided electrocautery ablation.

- HG-AIN: a premalignant lesion. Treatment as mentioned previously or (less desirable) anoscopic surveillance every 3 to 4 months.

2. **What is the first-line treatment for anal cancer with no distant metastases (stages I–III)?**

- For stage I to IIIB anal cancer, chemoradiation (CRT) with concurrent 5-fluorouracil (5-FU) and mitomycin C is the standard of care.
  - A phase III EORTC trial: superior complete remission (CR) of 80% with CRT, superior colostomy-free survival, similar overall survival.
  - A phase III UKCCCR study (ACT I) also showed superior local control at 42 months median follow-up, which was confirmed at 13 years of follow-up.
  - A phase III intergroup trial confirmed superior colostomy-free and disease-free outcomes with 5-FU plus mitomycin C as part of CRT versus 5-FU alone based CRT.
- Stage I tumors can be treated with attenuated therapy, such as 5-FU with concurrent RT. This should be considered especially in older patients since morbidity of standard treatment may be very significant. Cisplatin in place of mitomycin C as part of CRT is not recommended (colostomy rate was higher in Radiation Therapy Oncology Group [RTOG] trial. Outcomes were equivalent in ACT II trial).
- Neoadjuvant or adjuvant chemotherapy in addition to concurrent CRT is not recommended.
- Treatment strategy is the same in HIV-positive patients, regardless of CD4 count.
- Salvage surgical resection can be performed in cases of CRT failure.
- Anal margin cancers at most 2 cm in size with negative LNs (ie, stage I) may be treated with wide local excision.

3. **How should surveillance be conducted following primary treatment?**

- DRE at 8 to 12 weeks following CRT.
- If CR, follow up every 3 to 6 months, including DRE, anoscopy, LN exam, for 5 years, and annual CT chest, abdomen, and pelvis for the first 3 years if primary tumor was over 5 cm or LNs were positive.
- If partial response or stable primary tumor after CRT, repeat exam in 1 month. If decreasing, follow up every 3 to 6 months, with DRE, anoscopy, LN exam for 5 years, and annual CT chest, abdomen, and pelvis for the first 3 years.
- Suspected progression on DRE should be confirmed by anoscopy with biopsies and restaging CT.

4. **How should locoregional failure after primary therapy be managed?**

- Locoregional failure rates after CRT are up to 30%.
- Abdominoperineal resection (APR) with very select cases being eligible for anal sphincter-sparing surgery.
- Recurrent or persistent disease in the LNs is managed primarily with inguinal lymphadenectomy if not candidates for additional radiation.

- Follow up with clinical exam, including LN exam, every 3 to 6 months for 5 years, and annual CT chest, abdomen, and pelvis for the first 3 years.

5. **What are the most common sites of distant metastatic disease?**
   - Liver, lungs, and extrapelvic LNs

6. **What is the only recommended first-line treatment for metastatic (stage IV) anal cancer?**
   - Cisplatin and 5-FU-based chemotherapy.

7. **What is the treatment for oligometastatic disease to the liver or para-aortic LN?**
   - Surgical resection of isolated liver metastases can be considered.
   - Chemoradiotherapy can be used to treat recurrent disease limited to the para-aortic LNs.

QUESTIONS

1. **A 56-year-old man with a history of anal condyloma presents with intermittent bright red blood per rectum for the past 3 months. He reports no other symptoms such as weight loss, fever, chills, change in bowel habits, and night sweats. What workup would you recommend in this gentleman?**
   A. Anoscopy with biopsy if a mass is seen
   B. A rectal exam with referral to gastrointestinal (GI) for hemorrhoid banding versus hemorrhoidectomy
   C. Colonoscopy to rule out a colonic lesion
   D. Digital rectal examination (DRE) and anoscopy with biopsy of any suspicious lesions in addition to inguinal lymph node exam

2. **A 45-year-old HIV-positive man presents with newly diagnosed stage II squamous cell carcinoma of the anus. He is not compliant with his antiretroviral medications, and his last CD4 count a month ago was less than 200. He is asymptomatic, with the anal cancer having been found incidentally on digital rectal examination (DRE) when he decided to reestablish care with his infectious disease physician. He has no history of opportunistic infections. What treatment would you recommend for him?**
   A. Concurrent 5-fluorouracil (5-FU), mitomycin, and radiation therapy without dose reduction, but with weekly monitoring of blood counts and close monitoring for treatment-related toxicity
   B. Concurrent 5-FU and radiation, omitting mitomycin due to concern for cytopenias
   C. Concurrent 5-FU, mitomycin, and radiation therapy with 25% dose reduction of mitomycin
   D. Radiation alone as he is too high risk for chemotherapy toxicity with his CD4 count <200

3. **A 65-year-old man presents with stage IIIB squamous cell carcinoma of the anus. What factors are most predictive of his prognosis?**

A. Nodal involvement and presence of angiolymphatic invasion
B. Tumor size, nodal involvement, and angiolymphatic invasion
C. Tumor size, nodal involvement, perineural and angiolymphatic invasion
D. Tumor size and nodal involvement

4. A 65-year-old man completed CRT for stage IIIB squamous cell carcinoma of the anus 12 months ago. He has since recovered and states his life has returned to normal. CT of his abdomen and pelvis today reveals a 2 cm tumor in his right hepatic lobe on the periphery. This was biopsied and pathology confirmed metastatic squamous cell carcinoma. He lives on his own, is able to shop for groceries, complete all of his household chores, and manage his finances. He continues to work full time as an office manager. How would you treat him?
   A. Refer to a surgeon for consideration of resection of a single small lesion within his liver once locoregional recurrence and chest metastases have been ruled out
   B. Start systemic chemotherapy with 5-fluorouracil (5-FU) and mitomycin
   C. Observe as he is asymptomatic and all therapy would be palliative in intent
   D. Start systemic chemotherapy with 5-FU and cisplatin

5. A 58-year-old man presents for follow-up 12 weeks after completing chemoradiotherapy (CRT) with 5-fluorouracil (5-FU) and mitomycin for stage III primary anal squamous cell carcinoma. His tumor is unchanged in size compared to evaluation immediately after CRT completion. He is very anxious, and asks whether this means he will have to undergo surgery. You tell him the following:
   A. The need for surgery cannot be determined at this time as tumor regression after CRT has been shown to continue for up to 26 weeks posttreatment completion
   B. The stable tumor size is concerning for persistent disease, and you will refer him to a surgeon for an abdominoperineal resection
   C. That you would like to biopsy the tumor to confirm that it is persistent disease
   D. You'll refer him to a surgeon for local resection

6. A 55-year-old man presented with a 3 week history of foreign object sensation in his anus. Anoscopy revealed an anal tumor and biopsy of the lesion confirmed squamous cell carcinoma. PET/CT revealed fluorodeoxyglucose (FDG) avid left-sided perirectal and inguinal lymph adenopathy, the largest measuring 1.5 cm. There was no evidence of distant metastases. How would you complete his staging workup?
   A. Biopsy a left inguinal lymph node to confirm metastatic disease
   B. No further workup is necessary
   C. Complete surgical staging with abdominoperineal resection with total mesorectal excision (TME)
   D. Biopsy perirectal lymph node

ANSWERS

1. **D. DRE and anoscopy with biopsy of any suspicious lesions in addition to inguinal lymph node exam.** Patients with a history of anal condyloma are at high risk for HPV+ squamous cell carcinoma of the anus. In a patient with this history presenting with rectal bleeding, which is the most common symptom of anal carcinoma, workup for a possible anal carcinoma should be initiated. This includes DRE, anoscopy with biopsy of any suspicious lesions, and inguinal lymph node exam. If cancer is confirmed, further diagnostic imaging should be done to complete staging.

2. **A. Concurrent 5-FU, mitomycin, and radiation therapy without dose reduction, but with weekly monitoring of blood counts and close monitoring for treatment-related toxicity.** Although this man has uncontrolled HIV, he is young, otherwise healthy, and has never had complications from his disease. A CD4 count <200 alone is not an indication for modification of standard of care of his disease with chemoradiotherapy with 5-FU and mitomycin.

3. **D. Tumor size and nodal involvement.** Tumor size and nodal involvement are the most important prognostic factors for anal carcinoma. Five-year overall survival ranges from 70% for stage I disease, to 59% for stage II, 41% for stage III, and 19% for stage IV disease. Perineural and angiolymphatic invasions are markers of high-risk histology, which is not part of the main prognostic factors for anal carcinoma.

4. **A. Refer to a surgeon for consideration of resection of a single small lesion within his liver once locoregional recurrence and chest metastases have been ruled out.** This patient has metastatic disease limited to a small lesion within his right liver periphery, along with a preserved performance status, making him a good surgical candidate. While there are no prospective data to determine the optimal management of a patient with single lesion or oligometastatic disease within the liver, a retrospective multicenter analysis suggests a subset of these patients may benefit from resection of isolated liver metastases.

5. **A. The need for surgery cannot be determined at this time as tumor regression after CRT has been shown to continue for up to 26 weeks posttreatment completion.** The ACT II trial, in which 940 patients were randomized first to 5-FU with mitomycin or cisplatin and concurrent radiation, then randomized again to maintenance chemotherapy, assessed local disease responses at 11, 18, and 26 weeks. Analysis showed that 29% of those who were not in complete clinical response at 11 weeks did demonstrate complete clinical response at 26 weeks, supporting the view that anal squamous cell carcinoma continues to regress up to 26 weeks postcompletion of chemoradiotherapy.

6. **A. Biopsy a left inguinal lymph node to confirm metastatic disease.** Confirmation of metastatic disease within his lymph nodes should always be considered when it could result in upstaging a patient as it could impact prognosis and treatment. Since an inguinal lymph node is easily accessible for a needle biopsy, that would be the best next step in workup of his disease to complete his staging. Surgical staging has no role in anal squamous cell carcinoma.

Pancreatic and Biliary Cancers

David B. Zhen and Mark M. Zalupski

EPIDEMIOLOGY

1. **What are the typical features of pancreatic cancer at presentation?**
   - The majority of patients have unresectable or metastatic disease at diagnosis.
   - About two thirds of tumors are located in the head of the pancreas.

2. **How are biliary cancers classified?**
   - Extrahepatic cholangiocarcinoma including perihilar tumors (ie, Klatskin tumors)
   - Intrahepatic cholangiocarcinoma
   - Gallbladder cancer

ETIOLOGY AND RISK FACTORS

1. **What are the known risk factors for pancreatic cancer?**
   - Cigarette smoking
   - Diabetes
   - Chronic pancreatitis
   - Genetic risk factors include hereditary pancreatitis, Peutz–Jeghers syndrome, Lynch syndrome, familial atypical multiple-mole melanoma (FAMMM) syndrome, *BRCA* mutations (*BRCA2*>*BRCA1*), *PALB2* mutations, and ataxia–telangiectasia mutated (*ATM*) gene mutations

2. **What pancreatic lesions predispose one to developing invasive cancer?**
   - Intraductal papillary mucinous neoplasms and mucinous cystic neoplasms carry the potential for the development of malignant disease.
   - Pancreatic intraepithelial neoplasia (PanIN) is considered a precursor lesion to ductal adenocarcinoma.

3. **What factors predispose one to biliary cancers?**
   - Risk factors for gallbladder cancer include gallstones, porcelain gallbladder, previous *Salmonella* infection, and gallbladder polyps.
   - Primary sclerosing cholangitis is associated with a 10% to 15% lifetime risk of cholangiocarcinoma; other risk factors include Lynch syndrome, multiple biliary papillomatosis, congenital biliary tract abnormalities, hepatitis C, and liver fluke infections.

STAGING

1. Define tumor, node, and metastasis (TNM) staging for pancreatic cancer.

Primary Tumor (T)	
T0	No evidence of primary tumor
Tis	Carcinoma in situ (includes PanIN with severe dysplasia)
T1	Tumor limited to the pancreas, ≤2 cm
T2	Tumor limited to the pancreas, >2 cm
T3	Tumor extends beyond the pancreas without involvement of the celiac axis or superior mesenteric artery (SMA)
T4	Tumor involves the celiac axis or SMA

Regional Lymph Nodes (N)	
N0	No regional lymph node metastasis
N1	Regional lymph node metastasis

Distant Metastasis (M)	
M0	No distant metastasis
M1	Distant metastasis

Stage	Description		
0	Tis	N0	M0
IA	T1	N0	M0
IB	T2	N0	M0
IIA	T3	N0	M0
IIB	T1–3	N1	M0
III	T4	Any N	M0
IV	Any T	Any N	M1

Source: Adapted from Edge S, Byrd DR, Compton CC, et al. eds. *AJCC Cancer Staging Handbook: From the AJCC Cancer Staging Manual.* 7th ed. New York, NY: Springer-Verlag; 2010.

2. What are the important features for the staging of biliary malignancies?
- Gallbladder cancer is staged according to the AJCC TNM (I–IV) (preferred in both United States and Europe) or the Nevin (I–V) staging system.
- Intrahepatic, extrahepatic, and perihilar cholangiocarcinomas are staged according to separate TNM staging systems.

SIGNS AND SYMPTOMS

1. What are the common signs and symptoms of pancreatic cancer?
- Patients with lesions in the head of the pancreas may experience jaundice related to bile duct obstruction and pain related to extrapancreatic extension.

- Tumors in the body or tail are less likely to cause symptoms until the development of advanced disease.
- New onset or worsening diabetes, thrombophlebitis/venous thromboembolic event, or pancreatitis may precede the diagnosis.

2. **What clinical features are seen in biliary cancers at presentation?**
   - Gallbladder cancer is often asymptomatic and approximately half of the cases are found incidentally at the time of cholecystectomy.
   - Cholangiocarcinomas often present with symptoms of cholestasis due to biliary obstruction (especially extrahepatic tumors).

DIAGNOSTIC CRITERIA

1. **What are the histological subtypes of pancreatic cancer?**
   - Most cases arise from the ductal system of the exocrine pancreas and are classified as adenocarcinomas.
   - Pancreatic neuroendocrine tumors (ie, islet cell tumors) are much less common and may be associated with a variety of hormonal syndromes due to the secretion of insulin, glucagon, gastrin, and other neurohormonal substances.

2. **What is the role of cancer antigen (CA) 19-9 in pancreatic and biliary cancers?**
   - CA 19-9 is elevated in a large majority of patients and the level relates to the extent of disease.
   - Other malignancies and nonmalignant causes including cholangitis, cholelithiasis, and cirrhosis may also cause an elevated CA 19-9.

3. **What imaging studies are used to diagnose pancreatic cancer?**
   - Triphasic CT is useful for identifying the presence of metastatic disease and for determining eligibility for resection.
   - Endoscopic ultrasound (EUS) provides additional T and N staging, information on vascular invasion, and can be used to obtain a fine needle aspiration (FNA) for diagnosis.
   - MRI may be helpful in cases where CT is nondiagnostic (eg, isodense lesions)

4. **What features characterize unresectable pancreatic cancer?**
   - Distant metastasis, superior mesenteric or portal vein encasement or occlusion, or involvement of the SMA, hepatic artery, or celiac artery

5. **What are the diagnostic considerations for biliary cancers?**
   - Diagnosing cholangiocarcinoma can be challenging and is often based on clinical presentation, serology (ie, elevated CA 19-9), and radiographic findings (MRI is often useful).
   - Endoscopic retrograde cholangiopancreatography (ERCP) can provide both anatomical information and cytologic/histologic diagnosis.

PROGNOSTIC FACTORS

1. **What are unfavorable prognostic features?**

- Poor prognostic factors include advanced stage, poor performance status, and peritoneal disease.
- Cholangiocarcinoma prognostic factors include ≥T2 stage, lymph node positive status, and R1 resection.

TREATMENT

1. How is surgically resectable pancreatic cancer best managed?
- Only 10% to 20% of patients have resectable disease at diagnosis.
- A pancreaticoduodenectomy (Whipple procedure) involves removal of the pancreatic head along with the distal stomach, gallbladder, cystic and common bile ducts, duodenum, and proximal jejunum.
- Adjuvant therapy consists of either 5-fluorouracil (5-FU) or gemcitabine-based chemotherapy with or without radiation (based on results of CONKO-001 and ESPAC-3 trials).
- Neoadjuvant chemotherapy ± radiation can be used for patients with borderline resectable disease.
- No standard neoadjuvant chemotherapy regimen but FOLFIRINOX (5-FU, irinotecan, oxaliplatin) and gemcitabine + nab-paclitaxel are preferred combination regimens.

2. How are patients with unresectable pancreatic cancer treated?
- Palliative chemotherapy is used for locally advanced or metastatic disease.
- Preferred combination regimens for untreated patients with good performance status include FOLFIRINOX and gemcitabine + nab-paclitaxel.
- While gemcitabine + erlotinib is considered a treatment option, the absolute benefit of this regimen on survival is small.
- Other appropriate treatments include gemcitabine or fluoropyrimidines alone or in combination with other agents.
- Radiation concurrent with a fluoropyrimidine initially or following chemotherapy can be considered for locally advanced disease or for palliation in patients with metastatic disease with the benefit on overall survival unclear (LAP-07 trial)
- Supportive care for patients with poor performance status.

3. What is the optimal approach for localized biliary cancers?
- Complete surgical resection is the only curative option.
- Most patients found to have incidental cancer after cholecystectomy for presumed benign gallbladder disease should undergo additional surgery as many of these patients have residual disease in the liver and/or locoregional lymph nodes.
- Based on the Phase II SWOG S0809 trial, adjuvant therapy consisting of chemotherapy with gemcitabine + capecitabine followed by concurrent chemoradiation with capecitabine can be considered for resected extrahepatic cholangiocarcinoma or gallbladder carcinoma, especially for patients with high-risk disease features (≥T2, lymph node positive, R1 resection).

- Liver transplantation may be appropriate for highly selected patients with small central tumors.

4. **What are the treatment options for advanced biliary malignancies?**
   - Gemcitabine and cisplatin was shown to be superior to single agent gemcitabine in a phase 3 study of patients with advanced biliary cancers (ABC-02 trial).
   - Gemcitabine or fluoropyrimidines combined or with another agent are also acceptable based on the performance status of the patient and anticipated toxicities.
   - Regional therapies such as transarterial chemoembolization or radioembolization are options for some patients with intrahepatic cholangiocarcinoma.
   - Chemotherapy with external beam radiation for locally advanced disease improves symptoms and may prolong survival.

SPECIAL CONSIDERATIONS

1. **What are the common complications of pancreatic and biliary cancers?**
   - Venous thromboembolic disease is seen in 20% to 40% of patients with pancreatic cancer.
   - Biliary obstruction with episodic cholangitis is often seen with pancreatic head or extrahepatic tumors and is managed with biliary stent placement or palliative surgical intervention.
   - Malabsorption due to pancreatic exocrine insufficiency can be managed with pancreatic enzyme replacement.
   - Pain can be managed with opioid analgesics and celiac plexus neurolysis.

QUESTIONS

1. **A 60-year-old male with no comorbidities underwent a pancreatico-duodenectomy for stage IIB pancreatic adenocarcinoma without complication 8 weeks ago. He is recovering well and is doing all his usual activities. He returns in follow-up for further management. Which of the following would you recommend?**
   A. Observation alone
   B. Adjuvant gemcitabine +/− subsequent radiation
   C. Obtain CA19-9 level to aid in deciding need for further therapy
   D. FOLFIRINOX
   E. Radiation therapy alone

2. **A 69-year-old male with stage III chronic kidney disease and long-standing type 2 diabetes mellitus complicated by peripheral neuropathy is referred to your clinic with newly diagnosed stage IV pancreatic adenocarcinoma with a large pancreatic head mass and numerous liver and lung lesions. He has had a 40 lb weight loss over the past couple of months and becomes dyspneic with just walking a few feet and is spending more than half of the day in bed. He now requires much assistance from his family for his activities of daily living (ADL).**

He comes in a wheelchair accompanied by multiple family members regarding treatment options. He has not had any abdominal pain. Which of the following would you recommend?

A. Gemcitabine alone

B. Gemcitabine + nab-paclitaxel

C. 5-fluorouracil (5-FU) alone

D. Radiation alone to the pancreatic mass

E. Hospice referral

3. A 55-year-old male undergoes CT imaging for abdominal pain and is found to have a 5.0 cm pancreatic head mass encasing >180 degrees of the superior mesenteric artery (SMA). He is considered to have unresectable disease. There is no evidence for any other systemic disease. CA19-9 is significantly elevated (1000s). Decision is made to proceed with chemotherapy with gemcitabine + nab-paclitaxel and initiation of opioids for pain control. After 3 months of therapy, he has restaging imaging, which shows no change in the size of the pancreatic mass. There is no evidence for occult metastatic disease, and his CA19-9 is improving (700s). While opioids have helped, the patient continues to experience episodes of abdominal discomfort. He otherwise has tolerated therapy fine. What could be recommended at this time?

A. Change to an alternative chemotherapy regimen

B. Continue gemcitabine + nab-paclitaxel and plan for restaging imaging after a couple of more treatment cycles

C. Consider concurrent chemoradiosensitizer + radiation therapy to the pancreatic mass

D. Either B or C

E. Recommend hospice as patient has not had significant regression of his mass on imaging and is unlikely to benefit from further chemotherapy

4. A 58-year-old male underwent resection of a T3N1 gallbladder adenocarcinoma about 8 weeks ago. Final pathology shows that the surgical margins were negative. Patient is doing well postoperatively and has returned to work. Which of the following are options for management of this patient?

A. Observation

B. Adjuvant stereotactic body radiation therapy (SBRT) to the tumor bed only

C. Adjuvant chemotherapy followed by concurrent chemoradiation to the tumor bed and regional lymphatics

D. All of the above

E. A or C

5. A 65-year-old female presents with obstructive jaundice (total bilirubin 5.0) and is found to have a mass within the right lobe of the liver. CT of the chest, abdomen, and pelvis is obtained and reveals several other satellite lesions in the liver and concerning pulmonary nodules. Endoscopic retrograde cholangiopancreatography (ERCP) reveals compression of the right biliary system by the mass, and a metallic biliary

stent is placed successfully, which appropriately relieves her obstruction. A biopsy of the mass is also obtained at the time of ERCP and shows adenocarcinoma, consistent with a biliary primary. The patient has no comorbidities and has an excellent performance status (Eastern Cooperative Oncology Group [ECOG] 0). Which of the following would you recommend as initial treatment?

A. Gemcitabine + cisplatin
B. 5-Fluorouracil (5-FU) alone
C. Transarterial radioembolization (TARE) to the right lobe mass
D. Transarterial chemoembolization (TACE) to the right lobe mass
E. Stereotactic body radiation therapy (SBRT) to the right lobe mass

6. A 45-year-old female is diagnosed with metastatic pancreatic cancer. She has no comorbidities and has otherwise been healthy. She has a mother diagnosed with ovarian cancer at age 55 and a maternal grandfather with prostate cancer diagnosed at age 57. You are concerned for a familial cancer syndrome. Which of the following genes is the most likely found to be altered in this patient?

A. *BRCA1*
B. *BRCA2*
C. *TP53*
D. *MSH1*
E. *STK11*

ANSWERS

1. **B. Adjuvant gemcitabine +/– subsequent radiation.** Adjuvant therapy is recommended in all patients who recover from operation and have an adequate performance status due to high risk of relapse with any stage of resected, invasive pancreatic cancer. Observation could be considered if the patient declines adjuvant therapy. Radiation therapy alone would not reduce risk for systemic relapse, which is common in patients with pancreatic cancer.

2. **E. Hospice referral.** Best supportive care with hospice would be most appropriate in this patient with a poor performance status whose anticipated benefits from systemic therapy are low and risks of toxicity from treatment are high. Radiation therapy for palliation could be considered if patient was symptomatic from his pancreatic lesion.

3. **D. Either B or C.** Chemotherapy is considered the main treatment for locally advanced, unresectable pancreatic cancer. The role of concurrent chemoradiation in improving overall survival is unclear based on available literature but can be used to achieve further local control in this patient who continues to have symptoms from his mass. Alternative chemotherapy would be needed if there were evidence of progression, and stable disease is common in patients being treated for metastatic disease.

4. **E. A or C.** The absolute risk for recurrence in this patient is unclear but is considered high given his high grade tumor and positive nodal status based on 2-year recurrence rates noted in patients who had received adjuvant therapy on the SWOG S0809 clinical trial (there was no control arm in this study). As such, it is reasonable to consider adjuvant therapy or observation based on the patient's preferences. Radiation to the tumor bed alone would be insufficient in reducing risk of systemic relapse.

5. **A. Gemcitabine + cisplatin.** Systemic chemotherapy is the preferred therapy in this fit patient with metastatic cholangiocarcinoma. Gemcitabine + cisplatin is an option based on the phase 3 ABC-02 trial. Combination therapies are more effective than single agents alone and so preferred in those with good performance status. The last three choices allude to liver-directed therapies and could be options if the predominant disease was in the liver. In the patient's case with multiorgan involvement, systemic chemotherapy would be recommended initially.

6. **B. *BRCA2*.** Hereditary and ovarian breast cancer (HOBC) syndrome is raised based on the patient's family history and the patient's early onset pancreatic cancer. *BRCA2* has a higher association in patients with early onset pancreatic cancer. The other genes are implicated in other hereditary familial syndromes (*TP53*—Li–Fraumeni syndrome; *MSH1*—Lynch syndrome; *STK11*—Peutz–Jeghers syndrome), and are considerations but less likely based on the available family history.

Hepatocellular Carcinoma

Paul M. Corsello and Neehar D. Parikh

EPIDEMIOLOGY

Etiology and Risk Factors

1. **What is the etiology of hepatocellular carcinoma (HCC)?**
   - Prevalence parallels geographic distribution of hepatitis B virus (HBV) and hepatitis C virus (HCV); primarily seen in Southeast Asia and sub-Saharan Africa, although rates are increasing in the United States and Europe
   - Primarily epithelial in origin, and typically (but not exclusively) occurs in the setting of chronic hepatocyte injury

2. **What are the common risk factors for HCC?**
   - Toxins
     - Aflatoxin: mostly in patients with HBV
   - Chronic liver disease
     - Chronic hepatitis infection: HBV, HCV. In the United States, HCV is the driving force for increase in incidence, although fatty liver disease is emerging
     - Alcohol
     - Hereditary hemochromatosis
     - Alpha-1 antitrypsin deficiency
     - Primary biliary cirrhosis
     - Nonalcoholic fatty liver disease related disease, including noncirrhotic fatty liver with HCC

3. **What variant of HCC is more common in women, occurs at younger age, and is associated with a better prognosis?**
   - Fibrolamellar variant

STAGING

1. **What is the staging for HCC?**
   - The tumor, node, and metastasis (TNM) staging system is not routinely utilized as it does not accurately reflect prognosis and because few patients are eligible for surgical intervention. The factors that determine prognosis are performance status, hepatic function, and tumor burden, and these are best incorporated within the Barcelona staging classification (see Barcelona Clinic Liver Cancer [BCLC] algorithm listed under Prognostic Factors).

SIGNS AND SYMPTOMS

1. **What are the most common symptoms of HCC?**
   - Mostly asymptomatic in the early stage. However, for advanced stages, symptoms include:
     ○ Upper abdominal pain; weight loss; generalized weakness; anorexia and early satiety; emesis

2. **What are the most common signs of HCC?**
   - For early and intermediate stage there are no signs noted. For advanced stage:
     ○ Hepatic bruit; hepatomegaly; ascites; jaundice; splenomegaly

3. **What are the paraneoplastic syndromes associated with HCC?**
   - Extremely rare, but include:
     ○ Hypercalcemia
     ○ Hypoglycemia
     ○ Erythrocytosis
     ○ Hypercholesterolemia
     ○ Dysfibrinogenemia
     ○ Carcinoid syndrome/diarrhea
     ○ Sexual changes (gynecomastia, testicular atrophy, precocious puberty)
     ○ Porphyria cutanea tarda

DIAGNOSTIC CRITERIA

1. **What is the recommended algorithm for evaluating a liver nodule in a patient with risk factors for HCC?**
   - See Figure 28.1.

2. **What serum markers are useful in the diagnosis of HCC?**
   - Alpha-fetoprotein (AFP) can be helpful in diagnosis, as well as surveillance and assessing response to treatment. However, AFP in isolation is not diagnostic, as HCV itself can cause elevations in AFP.

3. **What imaging studies are useful for diagnosing HCC?**
   - Ultrasound for surveillance in patients at risk
   - Contrast-enhanced multidetector CT or MRI
     ○ Arterial phase: HCC enhances more than surrounding normal liver tissue
     ○ Venous phase: HCC enhances less than surrounding liver, "washout period"
     ○ Delayed phase: persistent washout noted
   - Approximately 15% of cases have atypical imaging appearance

4. **When should the diagnosis be confirmed with liver nodule biopsy?**
   - When cross-sectional imaging does not meet the classic criteria of arterial enhancement and washout.

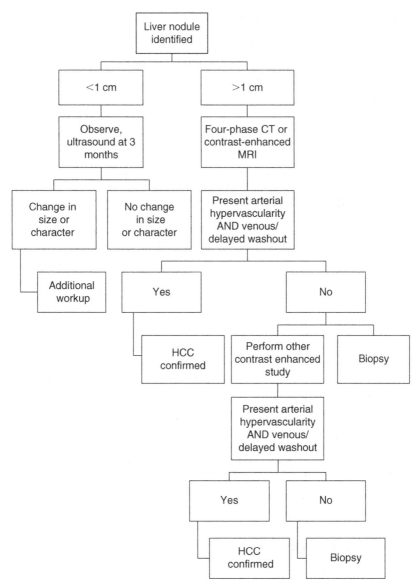

FIGURE 28.1 ■ Algorithm for evaluating a liver nodule in a patient with risk factors for hepatocellular carcinoma (HCC).

- Core biopsy preferred over fine needle aspiration (FNA).
- Risks of biopsy include bleeding (1%) and concern for needle tract seeding (<1%).
- Staining for CD34, CK7, glypican 3, HSP-70, and glutamine synthetase can help differentiate HCC from dysplastic lesions when HCC is not clear based on microscopy.

INDICATIONS FOR TREATMENT

1. What are the indications for therapy?

- A treatment modality is indicated in all cases that are not BCLC stage D

PROGNOSTIC FACTORS

1. What are prognostic factors for HCC?

- Tumor extent (number/size of lesions), underlying liver function as classified by Child–Pugh, and performance status (Eastern Cooperative Oncology Group [ECOG] score)
- While multiple staging systems exist, including TNM, CLIP score, Barcelona, Hong Kong Liver Cancer Criteria, ITA.LI.CA staging system, and the MESIAH score, the BCLC staging system is the most widely accepted.

2. What is the Child–Pugh classification of severity of liver disease?

- An assessment of hepatic function, which is critical for stratification of patients with HCC

	Number of Points Assigned		
Parameter	1	2	3
Ascites	Absent	Slight	Moderate
Bilirubin (mg/dL)	<2	2–3	>3
Albumin (g/dL)	>3.5	2.8–3.5	<2.8
Prothrombin time (sec)	<4	4–6	>6
International normalized ratio (INR)	<1.7	1.7–2.3	>2.3
Encephalopathy	None	Grades 1–2	Grades 3–4

Grade A: 5 to 6 points (early-stage cirrhosis).

Grade B: 7 to 9 points (intermediate-stage cirrhosis).

Grade C: 10 to 15 points (advanced-stage cirrhosis).

3. What is the BCLC algorithm?

See Figure 28.2.

4. What is the survival rate based on BCLC classification?

- Stage 0 and stage A: 5-year survival 50% to 70%
- Stage B and stage C: 3-year survival 20% to 40%
- Stage D: 1-year survival 0% to 15%

TREATMENT

1. What surgical therapies are available for treatment of HCC?

- *Surgical resection*
  - Potentially curative, optimal treatment for HCC
  - Assessment of hepatic reserve is paramount for appropriate patient selection.

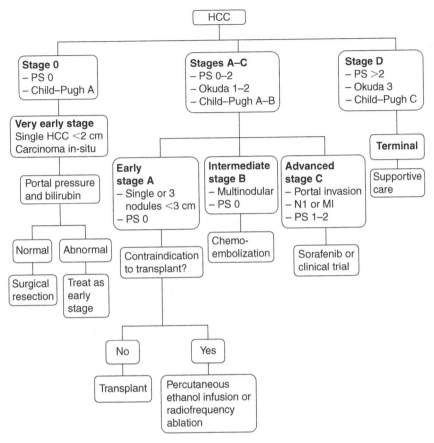

FIGURE 28.2 ■ The Barcelona Clinic Liver Cancer algorithm.

- ○ Ideal patient has solitary HCC confined to liver, no evidence of invasion into hepatic vasculature, no portal hypertension (platelet >100), and well-preserved hepatic function (bilirubin <1).
- • *Liver transplantation*
  - ○ Primarily for patients with unresectable disease, generally due to the degree of underlying liver dysfunction.
  - ○ Limited by organ availability. Patients must be otherwise candidates for liver transplantation.

2. **What liver-directed nonsurgical therapies are available for treatment of HCC (locoregional)?**
   - • *Radiofrequency ablation*
     - ○ For patients with disease confined to the liver who do not meet resectability criteria but are candidates for a liver-directed procedure, best outcomes are seen with tumors <3 cm in size.
     - ○ Needle electrode delivers high-frequency alternating current that leads to frictional heating and subsequent tissue necrosis.

- Transarterial chemoembolization (TACE)
  - Injection of chemotherapeutic agent or drug-eluting microspheres into hepatic artery
  - Commonly used as a bridging therapy prior to liver transplant, or as primary therapy for intermediate-stage HCC based on BCLC (about 60% of patients are at this stage)
- *External beam radiation*
  - No defined role and there are only case series to date. Although an emerging technology, there are no randomized controlled trials (RCTs) comparing to other locoregional therapies.
- *Radioembolization*
  - Focal radiation by delivering radioactive isotopes (iodine-131, Lipiodol, or yttrium-90-tagged glass microspheres or resin) to tumor via hepatic artery
  - Limited by lack of RCT data

3. **What systemic therapies are available for treatment of HCC?**
   - *Chemotherapy*: There are no data to support its use.
   - *Molecular targeted therapy*
     - Several studies have shown a role for targeting EGFR/EGF (HER1), VEGF, and MEK/ERK pathways.
     - Sorafenib, a tyrosine kinase inhibitor (targets RAF kinase and VEGFR), is the standard of care monotherapy for patients with unresectable HCC, based on SHARP trial (demonstrated overall survival benefit for sorafenib over supportive care alone).

QUESTIONS

1. **Which of the following patients would benefit from hepatocellular carcinoma (HCC) screening?**
   A. Hepatitis C virus (HCV) infected without cirrhosis
   B. HCV infected with Child–Pugh class A cirrhosis
   C. HCV Infected with Child–Pugh class C cirrhosis
   D. B and C
   E. All of the above

2. **A patient with three liver lesions concerning for hepatocellular carcinoma (HCC), size <3 cm, with platelets >100 and a bilirubin <1 and an Eastern Cooperative Oncology Group (ECOG) score of 0 would be considered what stage based on the Barcelona Clinic Liver Cancer (BCLC) criteria?**
   A. Stage 0
   B. Stage A
   C. Stage B
   D. Stage C
   E. Stage D

3. What is the classic enhancement pattern of hepatocellular carcinoma (HCC) on cross-sectional imaging with a venous, arterial, and delayed phase?
   A. Arterial: decreased, venous: decreased, delayed: persistent washout
   B. Arterial: decreased, venous: increased, delayed: no change
   C. Arterial: increased, venous: decreased, delayed: persistent washout
   D. Arterial: increased, venous: increased, delayed: persistent washout
   E. Arterial: increased, venous: increased, delayed: no change

4. A 54-year-old male presents for discussion of treatment options for his hepatocellular carcinoma (HCC). A 1.5 cm lesion consistent with HCC was seen on triple-phase CT. His platelet count is 156 and bilirubin is 0.9. He is otherwise in good health and has an Eastern Cooperative Oncology Group (ECOG) score of 0. What is the most appropriate treatment recommendation?
   A. Liver transplantation
   B. Local–regional therapy
   C. Sorafenib
   D. Surgical resection
   E. Supportive care

5. A 72-year-old female presents for discussion of treatment options for her hepatocellular carcinoma (HCC). Her albumin is 3, bilirubin 2.5, and international normalized ratio (INR) 1.5. Her Eastern Cooperative Oncology Group (ECOG) score is 1. She has no ascites, but does have hepatic encephalopathy controlled with lactulose. Imaging is consistent with primary HCC with portal invasion. What is the most appropriate treatment recommendation?
   A. Liver transplantation
   B. Local–regional therapy
   C. Sorafenib
   D. Surgical resection
   E. Supportive care

6. A 60-year-old female presents for discussion of treatment options for her hepatocellular carcinoma (HCC). Her albumin is 3, bilirubin 1.2, and international normalized ratio (INR) 1.5 with an Eastern Cooperative Oncology Group (ECOG) score of 1. She has no ascites or hepatic encephalopathy. The patient is actively drinking alcohol and smoking cigarettes and has poor social support. Triple-phase CT reveals two primary liver lesions, one 2.8 cm and the other 2.5 cm consistent with HCC. What is the most appropriate treatment recommendation?
   A. Liver transplantation
   B. Local–regional therapy
   C. Sorafenib
   D. Surgical resection
   E. Supportive care

ANSWERS

1. **D. B and C.** Cirrhosis is the most important risk factor for developing HCC in patients with chronic hepatitis C infection. The American Association for the Study of Liver Diseases (AASLD) practice guidelines recommend surveillance for HCC with abdominal ultrasound every 6 months in all patients with advanced fibrosis or cirrhosis.

2. **B. Stage A.** This patient has nonadvanced early stage disease given his three lesions <3 cm without evidence of portal hypertension or significant underlying liver disease using platelets and bilirubin as proxy measures.

3. **C. Arterial: increased, venous: decreased, delayed: persistent washout.** HCC classically has increased enhancement on arterial phase with decreased enhancement on venous phase (washout period). On delayed phase, persistent washout is seen. Fifteen percent of cases will have atypical imaging findings.

4. **D. Surgical resection.** This patient has very-early-stage disease, Barcelona Clinic Liver Cancer (BCLC) stage 0. Given his lack of underlying portal hypertension, primary resection is the best approach. Liver transplantation would not be appropriate given his otherwise nonadvanced underlying liver disease.

5. **C. Sorafenib.** This patient has Child–Pugh grade B cirrhosis, with imaging consistent with portal invasion. She would therefore not be a candidate for primary surgical resection or local–regional therapy. Sorafenib or a clinic trial would be most appropriate.

6. **B. Local–regional therapy.** This patient has Child–Pugh grade A cirrhosis. She has nonadvanced HCC given her two lesions that are <3 cm in size. She is actively drinking and has poor social support and would not currently be a liver transplant candidate. The best option is therefore local–regional therapy.

Neuroendocrine Tumors

29

Sarah Yentz and Vaibhav Sahai

Neuroendocrine malignancies are composed of a heterogeneous group of rare tumors arising from neuroendocrine cells throughout the body (including thorax, gastrointestinal tract, thyroid, adrenal glands, and others). These tumors have varying degrees of aggressiveness and are characterized by their ability to store and secrete different peptides and neuroamines. This review will focus on gastroenteropancreatic (GEP) neuroendocrine tumors (NETs).

EPIDEMIOLOGY

1. **What are the most common organs in which neuroendocrine tumors arise?**
   - Gastrointestinal (GI) tract 47% (small intestine 18%, large intestine 13%, rectum 12%, stomach 5%)
   - Lung 25%
   - Pancreas 4%

PATHOLOGY

1. **What pathologic characteristics are used to grade NETs?**
   - See Tables 29.1 and 29.2.

TABLE 29.1 ■ Pathological Characteristics of GEP NETs

Morphology	Mitotic Rate (count/10 hpf)	Ki-67 Index (%)
Well differentiated	<2	<3
Moderately differentiated	2–20	3–20
Poorly differentiated	>20	>20

GEP NETs, gastroenteropancreatic neuroendocrine tumors; hpf, high-power fields.

TABLE 29.2 ■ Grading System of GEP NETs

NETs	Grade 1	Well differentiated	AND	<2 mitotic rate	AND	<23% Ki-67
	Grade 2	Rest that do not fit grade 1 or grade 2 criteria				
NEC	Grade 3	Poorly differentiated	OR	>20 mitotic rate	OR	>20% Ki-67

GEP NETs, gastroenteropancreatic neuroendocrine tumors; NEC, neuroendocrine carcinoma; NETs, neuroendocrine tumors.

Neuroendocrine carcinomas (NEC) are a heterogeneous group of highly aggressive malignancies with a high propensity for distant metastases and an ominous prognosis. They are usually poorly differentiated (sometimes categorized as small or large cell subtypes), but may also rarely present as well-differentiated or moderately differentiated tumors with high Ki-67 index or mitotic rate.

SIGNS AND SYMPTOMS

1. **What is the difference between a "functional" NET and a "nonfunctional" NET?**
   - NETs store and secrete different peptides and neuroamines some of which may cause specific clinical syndromes and are termed "functional," while others may have elevated plasma or urine markers, but are without associated symptoms, and therefore "nonfunctional."

2. **What are the symptomatic manifestations of the functional GEP NET syndromes?**
   - See Table 29.3.

TABLE 29.3 ■ Clinical Presentations and Syndromes of GEP NETs

Hormonal Syndrome	Hormone	Signs and Symptoms
Serotoninoma or carcinoid syndrome	Serotonin	Flushing (usually without diaphoresis), secretory diarrhea, wheezing, and carcinoid heart disease (tricuspid valve and/or pulmonic valve regurgitation)
Insulinoma	Insulin	Hypoglycemia (with neuroglycopenic symptoms, including confusion, altered consciousness) and sweating (from sympathetic overdrive)
Gastrinoma or Zollinger–Ellison syndrome	Gastrin	Abdominal pain due to peptic ulcer disease, diarrhea and reflux esophagitis
Glucagonoma or 4D syndrome, or Sweet syndrome	Glucagon	4Ds include diarrhea, depression, deep venous thrombosis, and dermatitis (necrolytic migratory erythema). Also, glucose intolerance and weight loss can be seen.
VIPoma or Verner–Morrison syndrome	VIP	Watery diarrhea, hypokalemia, and achlorhydria
Somatostatinoma	Somatostatin	Malabsorptive diarrhea/steatorrhea, diabetes mellitus, hypochlorhydria, gallbladder disease

GEP NETs, gastroenteropancreatic neuroendocrine tumors; VIP, vasoactive intestinal peptide.

3. **What is the underlying etiology of the typical symptoms of a functional midgut NET, or carcinoid syndrome?**
   - Flushing: prostaglandins, kallikrein, and serotonin (5-HT)
   - Diarrhea: tachykinins release (persists with fasting in contrast to malabsorptive diarrhea)
   - Wheezing: substance P, histamine, or 5-HT
   - Carcinoid heart disease: 5-HT leading to fibrosis

4. **Which heart valves are involved in carcinoid heart disease?**
   - Tricuspid and/or pulmonic valve regurgitation

5. **What are the possible locations of primary NET in a patient with symptoms of carcinoid syndrome?**
   - Midgut or lung is most common.
   - Patients with pancreatic NET have also been uncommonly described in literature.
   - Majority of patients have liver metastases, which allow serotonin to bypass liver metabolism.

6. **What are the more common familial syndromes associated with GEP NETs?**
   - See Table 29.4.

DIAGNOSTIC WORK-UP

1. **A 32-year-old woman has been diagnosed with metastatic grade 1 GEP NET. What staging diagnostic workup should be completed before considering treatment?**
   - **Which imaging study or studies should be considered?**
     - **Functional imaging**
       - **Somatostatin receptor scintigraphy (also known as octreotide scan).** Recommended (usually in grade 1 and 2 NETs) to evaluate extent of disease and presence of somatostatin receptors. Sensitivity is between 80% and 90%. This test is only useful at the time of diagnosis and not follow-up during treatment evaluation.

TABLE 29.4 ■ Common Familial Syndromes in Patients with GEP NETs

Familial Syndrome	Gene	Incidence	Signs and Symptoms
MEN1	*MEN1*	1:20,000 to 1:40,000	Pancreatic NETs, hyperparathyroidism (high parathyroid hormone and hypercalcemia), pituitary tumor
VHL	*VHL*	1:36,000	Pancreatic NETs, renal cell cancer, pheochromocytoma, hemangioblastomas of central nervous system

GEP NETs, gastroenteropancreatic neuroendocrine tumors; MEN1, multiple endocrine neoplasia type 1; NET, neuroendocrine tumor; VHL, von Hippel–Lindau.

- ■ **⁶⁸Ga-DOTATATE PET/CT.** High sensitivity and specificity with much improved spatial resolution than octreotide scan.
- ■ **¹⁸F-FDG PET/CT.** Low sensitivity due to poor uptake of radiopharmaceuticals due to generally lower proliferative activity.
- ■ **Metaiodobenzylguanidine (MIBG) scan.** Low sensitivity but a positive scan may have implication for patient management with MIBG treatment.
- ○ **Anatomic imaging**
  - ■ **CT or MRI.** Recommended as the octreotide scan does not provide anatomical detail, unless the ⁶⁸Ga-DOTATATE PET with a diagnostic CT scan is performed. Scans should be a multiphasic contrast-enhanced study, specifically of the liver.
- ○ **Which laboratory tests should be considered?**
- ○ See Table 29.5.

TABLE 29.5 ■ Laboratory Investigations for GEP NETs

Test	NET	Specifics
Insulin	Pancreas	Fasting; also check fasting glucose, proinsulin, and C-peptide
Gastrin		Fasting (>1000 ng/L), consider gastric pH (<2.5), secretin provocation test
Glucagon		Levels between 500 and 1,000 pg/mL
Pancreatic polypeptide		Nonspecific marker for functional/nonfunctional NETs
Vasoactive intestinal polypeptide		Additionally, consider evaluation of electrolytes
Chromogranin A	GEP	Nonspecific marker for functional/nonfunctional NETs
		Correlates with treatment response, prognosis
		False-positive results may occur due to use of proton pump inhibitors, concurrent chronic atrophic gastritis, or impaired renal function
Somatostatin		Plasma SLI level
Neuron-specific enolase		Higher levels (>3x upper limit of normal) may correlate with worse overall survival
24-hour urine	Midgut	Not known to correlate with treatment response
5-HIAA		False-positive results may occur with ingestion of certain foods, including bananas, kiwis, avocado, tomatoes, eggplants, walnuts, and pineapple

There are additional tests that can be considered, including serum serotonin, pancreastatin, and neurokinin A.

5-HIAA, 5-hydroxyindole acetic acid; GEP, gastroenteropancreatic; GEP NETs, gastroenteropancreatic neuroendocrine tumors; NET, neuroendocrine tumor; SLI, somatostatin-like immunoreactivity.

TREATMENT

1. **What is the role of surgery in the management of NETs?**
   - Surgery is recommended for resectable NET.
   - For unresectable grade 1 (and low grade 2) NET, cytoreductive surgery can be considered if near complete resection can be achieved. Additionally, liver metastasectomy for oligometastatic disease can also be considered in this patient population. However, the supporting data for cytoreductive surgery are retrospective and sparse.

2. **What are treatment options for grade 3 NECs?**
   - Grade 3 NECs are treated similar to small and large cell cancers of the lung.
     - ○ Surgical metastasectomy is not recommended in the management of NEC.
     - ○ Locoregional unresectable tumors are treated with systemic chemotherapy and radiation.
     - ○ Metastatic tumors are treated with systemic chemotherapy such as platinum-based chemotherapy and etoposide, irinotecan/etoposide, cisplatin/irinotecan, and temozolomide with or without capecitabine.

3. **A 52-year-old male was recently diagnosed with a nonfunctional, grade 1 GEP NET. An octreotide scan revealed bilobar metastatic disease to the liver. What treatment options should be considered at this time?**
   - **Observation.** Close monitoring with no active treatment is a reasonable option to consider in an asymptomatic patient with low burden of disease.
   - **Somatostatin analogs such as octreotide long acting release (LAR) or lanreotide.** These agents are associated with a significant improvement in progression-free survival (PFS) compared to placebo.
     - ○ *Octreotide LAR.* In the phase 3B PROMID study, Rinke et al (1) prospectively randomized 85 patients with well-differentiated locally unresectable or metastatic midgut NET to either octreotide LAR 30 mg intramuscularly once every 4 weeks, or placebo. The median time to progression was 14.3 and 6 months (hazard ratio [HR], 0.34; P <.001) for patients in the octreotide and placebo groups, respectively. After 6 months of treatment, stable disease was observed in 67% of patients in the octreotide group versus 37% in the placebo group.
     - ○ *Lanreotide.* In the phase 3 CLARINET trial, Caplin et al (2) randomized 204 patients with well-differentiated or moderately differentiated, nonfunctioning, somatostatin-receptor-positive GEP NETs (grade 1 or 2) to either lanreotide 120 mg subcutaneously once every 4 weeks, or placebo. Patients on the lanreotide arm had a significantly prolonged median PFS compared to placebo (not reached versus 18 months; HR, 0.47; P <.001). Estimated PFS rate at 24 months was 65% in patients with lanreotide versus 33% with placebo. The median time to progression in the octreotide LAR arm was 14.3 months compared to 8 months in the placebo arm (HR, 0.34; 95% CIs [0.20, 0.59]; P <.001). The median PFS in the lanreotide arm was not reached versus 18 months in the placebo arm (HR, 0.47; 95% CIs [0.30, 0.73]; P <.001).

4. **The patient discussed above was noted to have disease progression after being on observation for 18 months. He subsequently started octreotide LAR 20 mg every 4 weeks with close monitoring with**

TABLE 29.6 ■ Biological Therapeutics in NETs

Study	Type of NET	Therapy	Progression-free survival (months)	HR; 95% CIs; P value
Yao et al (2011) (3)	Pancreatic	Everolimus	11.0	0.35; [0.27, 0.45]; P < .001
		Placebo	4.6	
Raymond et al (2011) (4)	Pancreatic	Sunitinib	11.4	0.42; [0.26, 0.66]; P < .001
		Placebo	5.5	
Yao et al (2016) (5)	Lung or gastrointestinal	Everolimus	11.0	0.48; [0.35, 0.67]; P < .001
		Placebo	3.9	

HR, hazard ratio; NET, neuroendocrine tumor.

chromogranin A. The biomarker started increasing after 2 years, and on repeat CT scan he was noted to have worsening liver metastasis. What treatment options should be considered?

- Biological or targeted therapeutics such as sunitinib and everolimus (see Table 29.6)
  - Everolimus is Food and Drug Administration (FDA) approved for both GI and pancreatic NETs, whereas sunitinib is FDA-approved only for pancreatic NETs.
- Cytotoxic chemotherapy such as temozolomide +/– capecitabine
  - The capecitabine plus temozolomide (CAPTEM) regimen was evaluated in a small, single-arm phase II trial with interim overall median PFS >20 months in all subtypes of NET.
- Liver-directed therapy including arterial-based (transarterial chemoembolization [TACE], transarterial or bland embolization [TAE], transarterial radioembolization [TARE]) or non-arterial-based (radiofrequency, microwave, or cryoablation) therapy.

QUESTIONS

1. A 47-year-old asymptomatic female presents with a hyperdense locally advanced pancreatic mass found on a routine CT scan. An endoscopic ultrasound (EUS) guided core biopsy is completed. Pathology report notes well-differentiated, small round cells with a mitotic count of 2 mitoses/10 high-power fields, and Ki-67 5%. What grade tumor does she have?
   A. Grade 1
   B. Grade 2
   C. Grade 3
   D. Grade 4

2. Which of the following imaging modalities would you consider in the staging of gastroenteropancreatic (GEP) neuroendocrine tumors for the patient in Q1?
   A. Metaiodobenzylguanidine (MIBG) scan
   B. Octreotide scan

C. MRI

D. ^{18}F FDG PET/CT

3. The octreotide scan for the patient in Q1 was positive for presence of somatostatin receptors. You elected to start the patient on octreotide long acting release (LAR) 20 mg IM every 4 weeks. Which of the following symptoms is NOT a side effect of octreotide LAR?

A. Diarrhea

B. Cholelithiais

C. Hyperglycemia

D. Hyperkalemia

4. The oncologist for the patient in Question 1 also decides to check blood tests including complete blood count, comprehensive metabolic panel, and chromogranin A. Which of the following patient attributes will not impact the chromogranin A level?

A. Chronic kidney disease, stage III

B. Use of proton pump inhibitor for reflux esophagitis

C. Fasting state

D. Chronic atrophic gastritis

E. Diet rich in avocadoes

5. A 65-year-old male was recently diagnosed with an esophageal neuroendocrine carcinoma (NEC) with innumerable metastases to the liver and lymph nodes. The tumor is poorly differentiated with a Ki-67 of 70% and a mitotic rate of 20 mitoses/10 high-power fields. Which of the following treatment options would you consider in his management?

A. Octreotide

B. Sunitinib

C. Cisplatin and etoposide

D. Everolimus

6. A 32-year-old female presents with newly diagnosed pancreatic neuroendocrine tumor (PNET). Which of the following familial syndromes has been associated with PNET?

A. Multiple endocrine neoplasia type 2 (MEN2A)

B. Von Hippel–Lindau (VHL)

C. Lynch

D. Li–Fraumeni

7. A 40-year-old gentleman with grade 1 metastatic pancreatic neuroendocrine tumor (PNET) has progression on octreotide LAR 30 mg IM every 4 weeks. He has diabetes mellitus type 2 and his A1C is 9.5. Which Food and Drug Administration (FDA) approved medication would you consider for further management?

A. Lanreotide

B. Temozolomide

C. Sunitinib

D. Everolimus

ANSWERS

1. **B. Grade 2.** Grade 1 NETs must be well-differentiated with a Ki-67 index <3% *and* a mitotic rate <2 mitoses/10 hpf (see table 29.2). Grade 3 tumors are poorly differentiated, have a Ki-67 rate >20% *or* have a mitotic count <20 mitoses/10 hpf. This tumor fits neither of these definitions, so is grade 2. There is no grade 4 NET.

2. **B. Octreotide scan.** Somatostatin receptor scintigraphy, or octreotide scan, has high sensitivity and has treatment implications. MIBG scan has lower sensitivity for GEP NETs. MRI is not required since the patient has had CT scan for anatomic assessment. PET scan also has low sensitivity for low and intermediate grade NETs.

3. **C. Hyperkalemia.** Somatostatin analogs can cause malabsorptive diarrhea/steatorrhea due to inhibition of pancreatic enzymes. They can also cause cholelithiasis over months to years of therapy due to decreased gallbladder contraction due to impaired postprandial cholecystokinin release. Somatostatin analogs can also cause hypoglycemia or hyperglycemia due to decreased secretion of glucagon and insulin. Octreotide LAR does not cause hyperkalemia.

4. **C and E. Fasting state and diet rich in avocadoes.** Chromogranin A is a plasma biomarker frequently used to follow the course of patient disease burden and can be elevated in both functional and nonfunctional gastroenteropancreatic neuroendocrine tumors (GEP NETs). The levels are not affected by fasting or change in diet. However, use of proton pump inhibitors, reduced glomerular filtration rate (GFR), or presence of chronic atrophic gastritis can result in falsely elevated levels. Gastrin and insulin levels are checked in a fasting state. Tryptophan-rich foods (avocadoes, pineapples, bananas, eggplant, tomatoes, and others) can lead to a falsely elevated level of the 24-hour urine 5-hydroxyindole acetic acid (5-HIAA) test.

5. **C. Cisplatin and etoposide.** This patient has a grade 3 NEC due to poor differentiation, and high Ki-67 and mitotic rates. Frontline treatment is systemic chemotherapy, such as cisplatin and etoposide, similar to the management of small cell lung cancer.

6. **B. VHL.** VHL is associated with PNETs, renal cell cancer, pheochromocytoma and hemangioblastomas of the central nervous system. MEN2A is characterized by medullary thyroid cancer, pheochromocytoma, and primary parathyroid hyperplasia. MEN1 is the familial syndrome characterized by PNETs, parathyroidism, and pituitary tumors.

7. **C. Sunitinib.** Both sunitinib and everolimus prolong progression-free survival (PFS) compared to placebo in patients with PNETs. However, everolimus can be associated with hyperglycemia (in 13% of patients) and therefore sunitinib would be a better choice in this patient with poorly controlled diabetes. The patient is already receiving a somatostatin

analog, so addition of lanreotide is incorrect. Moreover, lanreotide binds to the same somatostatin receptors (SSTR2 and SSTR5) as octreotide LAR, so a change of therapy is also not recommended. Temozolomide has been used alone and in combination with other agents such as capecitabine; however, it is not FDA-approved.

REFERENCES

1. Rinke A, Müller H-H, Schade-Brittinger C, et al. Placebo-controlled, double-blind, prospective, randomized study on the effect of octreotide LAR in the control of tumor growth in patients with metastatic neuroendocrine midgut tumors: A report from the PROMID Study Group. *J Clin Oncol*. 2009;27(28):4656–463.
2. Caplin ME, Pavel M, Ćwikła JB, et al. Lanreotide in metastatic enteropancreatic neuroendocrine tumors. *N Engl J Med*. 2014;371(3):224–233.
3. Yao JC, Shah MH, Ito T, et al. Everolimus for advanced pancreatic neuroendocrine tumors. *N Engl J Med*. 2011;364(6):514–523.
4. Raymond E, Dahan L, Raoul JL, et al. Sunitinib malate for the treatment of pancreatic neuroendocrine tumors. *N Engl J Med*. 2011;364(6):501–513.
5. Yao JC, Fazio N, Singh S, et al. Everolimus for the treatment of advanced, non-functional neuroendocrine tumours of the lung or gastrointestinal tract (RADIANT-4): a randomised, placebo-controlled, phase 3 study. *Lancet*. 2016;387(10022):968–977.

Sarcoma

Elizabeth J. Davis and Rashmi Chugh

30

EPIDEMIOLOGY

1. **How does sarcoma differ from carcinoma?**
   - Sarcoma is typically cancer arising from connective tissue of mesenchymal origin, while carcinoma is typically cancer arising from tissue of epithelial origin.

2. **What are the histologic subtypes of soft-tissue sarcoma (STS)?**
   - There are over 50 subtypes of sarcoma.
   - The more common STS subtypes:
     - Gastrointestinal stromal tumor (GIST)
     - Leiomyosarcoma
     - Liposarcoma
     - High-grade undifferentiated pleomorphic sarcoma
     - Synovial sarcoma
     - Fibrosarcoma
     - Malignant peripheral nerve sheath tumor (MPNST)
     - Angiosarcoma

3. **What are the different types of bone sarcomas and what age groups are most commonly affected?**
   - Osteosarcoma—most common sarcoma in bone
     - There are two age groups most affected by osteosarcoma: 60% occur in childhood with a peak incidence between 10 and 20 years and a smaller peak between 60 and 80 years.
     - Osteosarcoma in older patients (the second peak) often arises from preexisting Paget disease.
   - Chondrosarcoma—second most common bone sarcoma in adults.
     - Chondrosarcoma usually affects older patients (>60 years) and is rarely seen in children.
   - Ewing sarcoma—second most common osteogenic sarcoma in children, but can arise in bone or soft tissue.
     - Most patients are <18 years old and the peak incidence is between 10 and 15 years of age.

4. What about GISTs?

- What is the incidence of GIST in the United States?
  - In the United States, 3,300 to 6,000 adults are diagnosed annually, representing just under half of sarcoma diagnoses.
  - Many of these tumors may be considered "benign" with a low risk of metastasis.
- What is the median age at diagnosis?
  - Median age is 60 years at diagnosis
- Where do GISTs most commonly originate?
  - Stomach (60%)
  - Jejunum or ileum (30%)
  - Duodenum (5%)
  - Colon/rectum (<5%)
  - Esophagus (<1%)
  - Rarely, GISTs can originate in the omentum, mesentery, or retroperitoneum

5. Are males or females more affected by sarcoma?

- Osteosarcoma and Ewing sarcoma are more common in males than in females.
- Rhabdomyosarcoma has a male preponderance in children.

ETIOLOGY AND RISK FACTORS

1. Is age a risk factor for sarcoma as it is for other cancers?

- The incidence of certain sarcomas such as STS and chondrosarcoma increases with age.
- The risk for Ewing sarcoma and rhabdomyosarcoma is higher in children.
- Adults younger than 35 are at a greater risk of synovial sarcoma and desmoplastic small round cell tumors.
- Individuals older than 60 are at a greater risk of myxofibrosarcoma and undifferentiated pleomorphic sarcoma.

2. Is race a risk factor for sarcoma?

- Ewing sarcomas are more common in people of European ancestry than in people of African or Asian ancestry.

3. What genetic syndromes are associated with a greater risk for sarcoma?

- Li–Fraumeni syndrome (germline mutation in TP53)
  - Increased risk of STS and osteosarcoma
  - Often diagnosed at younger ages than sporadic sarcoma
  - Other associated malignancies include: breast cancer, adrenocortical cancer, brain cancer, leukemia, and lymphoma

- Neurofibromatosis type I (NF1 mutation)
  - NF1 patients have a 5% to 10% risk of developing an STS, most commonly MPNSTs.
- Familial retinoblastoma (RB) syndrome (germline mutation in the RB tumor suppressor)
  - Increased risk for STS, particularly leiomyosarcoma.
- Carney–Stratakis syndrome (autosomal dominant)
  - Increased risk for GIST, particularly a rare variant with loss-of-function mutations within the succinate dehydrogenase (*SDH*) gene.

4. **Do any environmental exposures increase the risk for sarcoma?**
- There is some evidence that vinyl chloride increases the risk for hepatic angiosarcoma.
- Some studies have linked dioxins, or phenoxyacetic acid herbicides such as Agent Orange to the development of sarcoma, but this remains controversial.

5. **Is there an increased risk of sarcoma after radiation?**
- Very small long-term risk of soft tissue or bone sarcoma after radiation therapy.
- Latency time of 10 to 30 years (median of 16 years).
- Mean radiation exposure in patients who subsequently develop radiation-induced sarcoma is 40 Gy.
- Most common previously treated cancers in patients found to have subsequent radiation-induced sarcoma: breast cancer, cervical cancer, and lymphoma.

6. **What are some other risk factors for sarcoma?**
- Chronic lymphedema is a risk factor for the development of lymphangiosarcoma (Stewart–Treves syndrome).
- Human herpes virus-8 (HHV-8) is associated with Kaposi sarcoma (KS).

7. **What are the cytogenetic and molecular abnormalities associated with the development of sarcoma?**
- Eighty percent of GISTs have a KIT mutation; 5% to 10% have a PDGFRA mutation.
- Thirty percent of non-GIST STSs are also associated with specific genetic alterations, which are thought to directly result in the pathogenesis of the sarcoma.

Sarcoma Subtype	Molecular Abnormalities Associated With Selected Sarcomas
Gastrointestinal stromal tumor (GIST)	KIT (CD117) mutation, exon 9 or 11 PDGF receptor alpha (PDGFRA) mutations
Well-differentiated/dedifferentiated liposarcoma	Giant or ring chromosomes (CDK4, MDM2 amplification) concurrently have aneuploidy

(continued)

(*continued*)

Sarcoma Subtype	Molecular Abnormalities Associated With Selected Sarcomas
Synovial sarcoma	t(X;18)(p11:q11) SS18-SSX1 or SS18-SSX2
Alveolar soft-part sarcoma	t(X;17)(p11.2;q25) ASPL-TFE3
Myxoid/round cell liposarcoma	t(12;16)(q13;p11) FUS-CHOP(DDIT3) t(12;22) EWSR1-CHOP(DDIT3)
Ewing sarcoma	t(11;22)(q24;q12) EWSR1-FLI1 t(21;22) EWSR1-ERG
Desmoplastic small round cell tumor	t(11;22)(p13;q12) EWSR1-WT1
Alveolar rhabdomyosarcoma	t(2:13)(q35;q14) PAX3-FOXO1A t(1;13) (p36;q14) PAX7-FOXO1A t(X;2)(q13;q35) PAX3-AFX

FOXO1A, Forkhead box 01A receptor, also denoted in some texts as FKHR.

STAGING

1. **How is STS staged?**
   - The components for staging are:
     - Grade: three-tier grading system is recommended in the most recent American Joint Committee on Cancer (AJCC) staging system.
     - Size
       - T1 <5 cm in greatest dimension
       - T2 is >5 cm in greatest dimension
     - Depth
       - Ta are tumors superficial to investing fascia.
       - Tb are tumors deep to investing fascia.
     - Nodal disease
       - N0 denotes no lymph node metastasis.
       - N1 denotes the presence of lymph node metastasis.
       - Nodal metastatic disease is observed in fewer than 10% of patients with STS.
       - Epithelioid sarcoma, synovial sarcoma, rhabdomyosarcoma, and angiosarcoma have a propensity to spread to lymph nodes.
     - Metastatic disease
       - M0 denotes no evidence of metastatic disease.
       - M1 denotes the presence of metastatic disease.

2010 Seventh Edition of the American Joint Committee on Cancer (AJCC) Staging System for Soft Tissue Sarcoma

Stage	T	Grade Using a Three-Grade System	N	M
IA	T1a, T1b	Grade 1	N0	M0
IB	T2a, T2b	Grade 1	N0	M0
IIA	T1a, T1b	Grades 2, 3	N0	M0
IIB	T2a, T2b	Grade 2	N0	M0
III	T2a, T2b	Grade 3	N0	M0
	Any	Any	N1	M0
IV	Any	Any	Any	M1

Source: From Edge S, Byrd DR, Compton CC, et al. eds. *AJCC Cancer Staging Handbook: From the AJCC Cancer Staging Manual.* 7th ed. New York, NY: Springer-Verlag; 2010. Reproduced with permission of Springer-Verlag.

2. What are important factors when staging GISTs?

- Location
  - Gastric GISTs have a better prognosis than non-gastric GISTs.
  - Rarely, GISTs can originate in the omentum, mesentery, or retroperitoneum, which have a poor prognosis similar to small bowel GISTs.
- Size of <5 cm is associated with a good prognosis, while >10 cm is associated with a higher rate of recurrence.
- Mitotic rate of <5 per 50 high powered fields (hpf) is associated with a good prognosis, while mitotic index of >5 per 50 hpf is associated with a higher rate of recurrence.
- Spread to lymph nodes or a distant site is associated with a worse prognosis.

3. What are the important factors for osteosarcoma staging?

- Grade of the tumor according to a four-tier system
- Tumor size and degree of invasion: T1 denotes tumor of <8 cm, T2 denotes tumor of >8 cm, and T3 denotes discontinuous tumor in primary bone site.
- Osteosarcoma can present with skip metastasis within the medullary canal.
- Lymph node involvement: N0 denotes no lymph node metastasis, N1 denotes lymph node metastasis.
  - Lymph node involvement is rare.
- Presence of distant metastatic disease and organ involved: M0 denotes no distant metastasis, M1a denotes lung metastasis, and M1b denotes other distant metastasis.
  - At diagnosis, 10% to 20% of patients with osteosarcoma will have metastatic disease.
  - Bone marrow involvement is rare.

2010 Seventh Edition of the American Joint Commission on Cancer (AJCC) Staging System for Bone Sarcomas

Stage	T	Grade	N	M
IA	T1	Low (Grades 1–2)	N0	M0
IB	T2			
IIA	T1	High (Grades 3–4)		
IIB	T2			
III	T3	Any		
IVA	Any	Any		M1a
IVB	Any	Any	N1	Any
	Any	Any	Any	M1b

Source: From Edge S, Byrd DR, Compton CC, et al. eds. *AJCC Cancer Staging Handbook: From the AJCC Cancer Staging Manual.* 7th ed. New York, NY: Springer-Verlag; 2010. Reproduced with permission of Springer-Verlag.

4. **Is Ewing sarcoma staged the same way as osteosarcoma?**
   - Staging for Ewing sarcoma is typically divided into two categories: localized and metastatic disease.
   - One third of patients present with metastatic disease.
   - Ewing sarcoma most commonly metastasizes to the lung, followed by the bone.
   - Ewing sarcomas may rarely involve lymph nodes, meninges, or the central nervous system (CNS).

SIGNS AND SYMPTOMS

1. **What are presenting symptoms of STSs?**
   - Painless, growing masses
   - Generally firmer than benign tumors (lipomas) and typically deeper than subcutaneous fat

2. **What are the most common primary anatomic sites for STSs?**
   - Thigh, buttock, and groin 46%
   - Torso 18%
   - Upper extremity 13%
   - Retroperitoneum 14%
   - Head and neck 9%

3. **What are common presenting symptoms of GISTs?**
   - Early satiety
   - Abdominal discomfort
   - Palpable mass
   - Gastrointestinal (GI) bleeding

4. **How do Ewing sarcomas present?**
   - In children, Ewing sarcomas and other primitive neuroectodermal tumors usually arise in the bone.
   - In adults, Ewing sarcomas may be more commonly found in soft tissue.
   - Local symptoms may include pain, local swelling, and functional impairment of the affected limb.
   - Systemic symptoms may include fever, fatigue, and weight loss, which correlate with a higher chance of developing metastatic disease.

5. **What are some presenting signs/symptoms of osteosarcoma?**
   - Painful, hardened mass

6. **What are common sites affected by osteogenic sarcomas?**
   - Osteosarcomas usually arise in the intramedullary metaphyses of long bones.
     - Most commonly the distal femur, proximal tibia (around the knee), or proximal humerus
     - Osteosarcoma in the axial skeleton is more common in adults than in teenagers
   - Ewing sarcomas usually arise in the diaphysis of long or flat bones.
     - Femur (20%); pelvis (20%); fibula, tibia, or humerus (10% each)
     - Proximal and pelvic involvement associated with worse prognosis

DIAGNOSIS

1. **What kind of biopsy is needed to diagnose sarcoma?**
   - Enough tissue is needed to perform immunohistochemistry (IHC) staining, cytogenetics, and molecular analysis in order to determine the sarcoma subtype.
   - Core needle biopsy (with adequate number of passes), incisional or excisional biopsy can be performed.
   - Biopsies should be performed by experienced personnel who are practiced in sarcoma biopsies.
   - Fine needle aspiration (FNA) is usually inadequate.

2. **What are the appropriate tests to do on the specimen once it is received?**
   - IHC for vimentin (mesenchymal cell marker) and cytokeratin (to exclude epithelial origin)
   - Further IHC characterization based on histologic appearance to further refine subtype (ie, actin as a smooth muscle cell marker for leiomyosarcoma)
   - Molecular diagnostic testing relevant to the histologic features to evaluate for the presence of specific translocations or genetic changes

3. **How is sarcoma graded?**
   - There are different grading systems depending on the pathologist and institution: two grades (low and high), three grades (low, intermediate, and high), or four grades (1–4).
   - Histologic grade is based on a variety of histologic features, including cellularity, pleomorphism, mitotic rate, and tumor necrosis.

- Grade is an important component in staging for every sarcoma and, therefore, also important in projecting overall survival.

4. **Are there unique pathologic features in different sarcoma subtypes?**
   - Osteosarcoma grading often correlates with the site of origin within the bone.
     - Intramedullary osteosarcomas are usually high grade.
     - Bone surface osteosarcomas are usually low grade (parosteal osteosarcoma), involving the bone cortex.
     - Periosteal osteosarcoma is an aggressive, high-grade cortical sarcoma best treated like classic osteosarcoma.
     - Osteosarcomas usually have malignant spindle cells, osteoblasts, and bone matrix (osteoid).
   - Chondrosarcomas are usually low-to-intermediate grade that resemble cartilage macroscopically and microscopically.
   - Ewing sarcomas are usually CD99 positive in a membranous staining pattern on IHC, but fluorescence in situ hybridization (FISH) and polymerase chain reaction (PCR) can be performed to detect the translocation.
   - Ewing sarcomas are always considered high grade.
   - Most GISTs have mutations in the *c-KIT* gene (80%), some with mutations in the *PDGFRA* gene (5%–10%), and the rest are considered wild type (10%–15%). Arise from interstitial cells of Cajal (pacemaker cells of GI tract).

5. **What are appropriate imaging modalities for the localized disease?**
   - CT or MRI may be used for tumor localization.
     - MRI is superior in imaging extremity and trunk sarcomas.
     - CT is generally preferred for abdominal and pulmonary tumors.
   - By x-ray, osteosarcomas present with lytic and blastic features in admixed bone. If osteosarcomas extend to the soft tissue, they can cause a periosteal reaction (Codman triangle) and ossification in a pattern perpendicular to the surface of the bone (sunburst pattern).
   - By x-ray, chondrosarcomas appear as a radiolucent area with bony destruction and discrete calcified areas, usually involving the medullary cavity. They may cause what appears to be a multinodular growth pattern with scalloped edges.
   - Ewing sarcoma usually affects the bone shaft in an infiltrative pattern called "onion skinning," which can be seen on CT but is harder to see on plain films.

6. **How does one evaluate for metastatic disease?**
   - Chest imaging should be done as sarcomas typically spread hematogenously and have a high propensity to metastasize to the lungs.
   - Bone scan should be performed in certain subtypes that have a predilection to metastasize to the bone, such as osteosarcoma, Ewing sarcoma, and angiosarcoma.
   - PET scans are not used routinely, as they are often, but not always, positive in high-grade sarcomas but may not be helpful in very low-grade sarcomas.
   - For GISTs, CT of the abdomen and pelvis is sufficient or a PET scan can be considered.

- It is not necessary to do a CT of the chest routinely since this sarcoma rarely metastasizes to the lungs without having widespread abdominal disease.

PROGNOSIS

1. **What is the median survival for metastatic sarcoma?**
   - Median survival is 12 to 18 months after diagnosis of metastatic disease.
   - However, 20% to 25% of patients live more than 2 years.

2. **What are independent predictors of prognosis in nonmetastatic STS?**
   - Age—older patients tend to fare more poorly.
   - Histologic subtype
     - MPNST and angiosarcoma generally have a poor prognosis.
   - Histologic grade—higher grade sarcomas have higher risk of metastasis
   - Tumor site
     - STSs of head and neck are associated with a poor prognosis.
   - Tumor size
     - Tumors <5 cm are associated with a 77% 5-year disease-free survival rate.
     - Tumors between 10 and 15 cm are associated with a 50% 5-year disease-free survival rate.
     - Tumors >20 cm are associated with a 17% 5-year disease-free survival rate.
   - Molecular markers are still being investigated in regard to their role in prognosis.
   - Large (>5 cm) and moderate to high-grade tumors have a poor prognosis with approximately 50% of patients developing metastatic disease.

3. **What determines prognosis in Ewing sarcoma?**
   - Diagnosis at younger age and tumors <8 cm are better in terms of prognosis.
   - Twenty percent of patients presenting with metastatic Ewing may be long-term survivors of the disease.
   - Lactate dehydrogenase (LDH) is a prognostic indicator in Ewing sarcoma.

4. **What determines prognosis in GIST?**
   - Size of tumor, site of origin, mitotic rate, and presence of tumor rupture.
   - Patients with GISTs that have high-risk features (>10 cm or mitotic rate >10 per 50 hpf) have more than a 50% risk of recurrence within 2 years.

TREATMENT

Treating Localized Disease

1. **When is surgery indicated in STS?**
   - Primary treatment for most STS is surgery.
   - Limb-sparing procedures can usually be performed. No difference in disease-free survival or overall survival when doing limb salvage with adjuvant radiation rather than amputation alone.

2. **In which circumstances is adjuvant chemotherapy warranted for STS?**
   - Adjuvant chemotherapy in adult STS is controversial.

- Data from a meta-analysis showed an improvement in overall survival with an anthracycline-based regimen used in the adjuvant setting for larger, high-grade STSs of extremity.
- In appropriate settings, it is reasonable to offer adjuvant chemotherapy to fit patients with high-risk tumors (high-grade, >5 cm) with the expectation of a small, but potentially meaningful improvement in overall survival.
  - Doxorubicin, ifosfamide typically used for most adult STSs.
  - Gemcitabine, docetaxel is sometimes used for uterine leiomyosarcoma.
- Adjuvant or neoadjuvant chemotherapy is used in pediatric-type rhabdomyosarcoma (embryonal or alveolar types), regardless of age. Agents typically include vincristine, dactinomycin, cyclophosphamide, and doxorubicin.

3. When should neoadjuvant treatment be used in STS?

- Neoadjuvant versus adjuvant therapy may be considered when the potential for limb-sparing surgery is in question and tumor shrinkage may improve resectability.
- Regarding radiation, neoadjuvant versus adjuvant radiation is associated with similar long-term outcomes. In some individual situations, preoperative versus postoperative radiation may be preferable.

4. What is recommended as adjuvant treatment in GIST tumors?

- If a tumor is determined to be at a high risk for recurrence, treatment with at least 3 years of adjuvant imatinib at 400 mg daily should be considered based on a study demonstrating improved progression-free survival (PFS) and overall survival with 3 years of imatinib therapy as compared to 1 year.

5. How do you treat localized osteosarcoma?

- Resection of high-grade osteosarcoma is curative in 20% of patients. The addition of neoadjuvant or adjuvant chemotherapy improves the cure rate to 60% to 80%.
- Treatment is dependent on grade.
  - If low grade, treated with surgery alone
  - If high grade, treated with chemotherapy and surgery
- Osteosarcoma is typically radiation resistant, so adjuvant radiation is not typically used. Radiation can be used for palliative purposes.

6. What are the advantages of neoadjuvant chemotherapy in osteosarcoma?

- Similar 5-year event-free survival with neoadjuvant versus adjuvant chemotherapy (60%–65%)
- Response to chemotherapy can be assessed at the time of operation, based on the amount of necrosis found (however, there is no evidence that changing chemotherapy regimens postoperatively can help improve overall survival if the disease is resistant to neoadjuvant chemotherapy).
- Starting chemotherapy preoperatively may allow for more careful surgical planning.

7. **What chemotherapy regimen should be used for osteosarcoma in the neoadjuvant and adjuvant setting?**
   - Patients with high-grade osteosarcoma are typically treated neoadjuvantly and adjuvantly with six cycles of doxorubicin and cisplatin. Cisplatin is often held after four cycles due to ototoxicity.
   - High-dose methotrexate is used in younger patients with very good kidney function.
   - Chemotherapy is typically given for at least two to three cycles prior to surgery.
   - Carboplatin is substituted for cisplatin in some patients, but a head-to-head comparison has not yet been done.

8. **How is chondrosarcoma treated?**
   - Resection is all that is typically needed.
   - Most chondrosarcomas are low-to-intermediate grade, and there are no known effective systemic agents; thus neoadjuvant and adjuvant therapies are not indicated.
   - Some variants, such as mesenchymal chondrosarcoma and dedifferentiated chondrosarcoma, are high grade with a high metastatic potential and are treated with adjuvant chemotherapy. Mesenchymal chondrosarcoma is treated like Ewing sarcoma. Dedifferentiated chondrosarcoma is treated like osteosarcoma.

9. **What is the ideal treatment for nonmetastatic Ewing sarcoma?**
   - Cure rate from local control measures alone is 15% as there is a high rate of distant disease recurrence.
   - Preoperative and adjuvant chemotherapy with vincristine, doxorubicin, and cyclophosphamide (VAC) alternating with ifosfamide and etoposide (IE) was shown to have a better progression-free and overall survival compared with VAC alone (category 1).
   - Five-drug regimen is continued for 12 to 14 cycles total, divided before and after resection.
   - Actinomycin-D should be substituted for doxorubicin after a cumulative dose of more than 450 mg/m^2 of doxorubicin has been given.
   - After surgical resection, radiation may be indicated.

10. **What are treatment options for locally advanced/unresectable Ewing sarcoma?**
    - Ewing sarcoma is radiosensitive, so primary radiation therapy can be used in addition to chemotherapy instead of surgery.
    - Local failure rates may be slightly higher with radiation versus complete resection of primary tumor, but long-term functional outcomes may be better with radiation, particularly for pelvic tumors.

11. **When is radiation indicated in the treatment of STS?**
    - Among bone sarcomas, radiation is used when warranted in the adjuvant setting or for local control of Ewing sarcoma.

- Adjuvant radiation to the site of the primary tumor is typically used for all STSs of the extremities or trunk that are larger than 5 cm (and frequently used for tumors over 2 cm), independent of the grade.
- However, radiation is not often used adjuvantly for abdominal or visceral STSs since the doses of radiation that are necessary to have an effect are not tolerated in the abdomen. In some cases, neoadjuvant therapy has been increasingly used and can better target the tumor instead of surrounding organs and therefore be associated with less toxicity.
- Adjuvant radiation therapy has been shown to be helpful in decreasing local rate of recurrence by one third to one half.

12. What kind of surveillance should be done after completion of definitive therapy?

- Surveillance frequency is based on tumor location, grade, and overall risk of recurrence.
- Serial tumor bed imaging with MRI for extremity STS is recommended every 6 months for the first 2 years.
- Chest imaging with chest x-ray and physical exam should be performed every 3 months in high-risk STS (>5 cm, high grade) and bone sarcoma (high-grade osteosarcoma, Ewing sarcoma). Surveillance can be performed less frequently for lower risk tumors (STS <5 cm, low grade and chondrosarcoma).
- After 2 years, follow-up evaluations are spaced to every 4 to 6 months for a minimum of 5 years.
- Follow-up evaluations are often continued beyond 5 years as late recurrences do occur.

Primary Treatment for Metastatic Sarcoma

1. What are initial options for treating newly diagnosed metastatic STS?

- Most trials show no survival benefit with combination versus single-agent chemotherapy in metastatic sarcoma, even though tumor response rates were higher with combination chemotherapy.
- Anthracyclines and alkylating agents (ifosfamide) yield response rates of 10% to 25% for each drug in the metastatic setting.
  - Doxorubicin and ifosfamide are additive, but not synergistic, so they can be used separately with no significant change in overall survival rate.
  - Studies have shown a higher tumor response rate (but not improved overall survival rate) with greater doses of doxorubicin and ifosfamide.
- Ifosfamide tends to have good activity against synovial sarcoma and myxoid/round cell liposarcoma but is less active against leiomyosarcoma.
- The combination of gemcitabine and docetaxel was shown to be superior in progression-free and overall survival to single-agent gemcitabine and is particularly active against leiomyosarcomas.
- Dacarbazine has some activity against STSs but only approximately 10% response rate.
  - Pazopanib is approved for nonadipocytic STS patients who have received prior chemotherapy based upon a phase 3 study demonstrating an improvement in PFS (4.6 vs. 1.6 months) compared to placebo.

- ○ Trabectedin is approved for patients with advanced or unresectable leiomyosarcoma or liposarcoma who have previously received an anthracycline given its improvement in PFS compared to dacarbazine.
- ○ Eribulin is approved for patients with advanced or unresectable liposarcoma who have previously received an anthracycline based upon a study that demonstrated an improvement in overall survival to 15.6 months versus 8.4 months in patients treated with dacarbazine. Olaratumab is approved in combination with doxorubicin for patients with advanced or unresectable STS and with a histologic subtype for which an anthracycline containing regimen is appropriate. This is based on a phase 2 study demonstrating an improvement in overall survival of 26.5 months in patients receiving doxorubicin with olaratumab versus 14.7 months in patients treated with doxorubicin alone.
- Paclitaxel is usually only effective in treatment of angiosarcoma and KS.
- No consensus as to the duration of therapy for metastatic disease. Some treat until progression or toxicity.

2. **What are initial options for treating metastatic osteosarcoma?**
- Treatment with doxorubicin-based regimen if not used previously.
- Ifosfamide with or without etoposide in the relapsed setting has shown response rates of 50% to 60%.
- If limited in number and without the presence of any other metastases, resection of lung metastases in osteosarcoma has the potential for cure.

3. **What is the recommended treatment for metastatic Ewing sarcoma?**
- The same chemotherapy regimens can be used for metastatic Ewing sarcoma as are used in the neoadjuvant/adjuvant setting, but there is no benefit to alternating VAC with IE in the metastatic setting, and they are often given sequentially instead.
- If standard agents have already been used, patients may respond to topoisomerase I inhibitors, either as single agents or in combination.
- Metastases to bone and soft tissues can be treated with 4,500 to 5,600 cGy of radiation as recommended by the Intergroup Ewing's Sarcoma Study (IESS).
- Pulmonary metastases can be treated with whole-lung irradiation of 1,200 to 1,500 cGy if complete resolution of pulmonary metastatic disease is possible with chemotherapy.
- Cyclophosphamide and topotecan have been associated with an overall response rate of up to 44% in patients with recurrent metastatic Ewing sarcoma, with 25% of patients maintaining response after 23 months.
- Irinotecan and temozolomide are also other options for recurrent metastatic Ewing sarcoma.

4. **How are advanced GISTs treated?**
- Cytotoxic chemotherapy and intraperitoneal chemotherapy have been attempted and studied, but are largely ineffective.
- Tyrosine kinase inhibitors (TKIs) against c-KIT or PDGFRA are the standard of care for GIST and are associated with good response rates.
  - ○ Imatinib is used first line with daily dose of 400 mg and achieves disease control in 80% of patients with a c-KIT mutation in exon 11.

- Can increase to 600 mg and to 800 mg if patient progresses on 400 mg dose. Usually c-KIT exon 9 mutations respond better to higher doses of imatinib.
- Side effects include nausea, vomiting, diarrhea, rash, mucositis, and diuretic-resistant peripheral edema.
- Those with PDGFRA mutation had lower response rate compared with exon 11 c-KIT mutation.
  - Sunitinib is used as second-line therapy for imatinib-refractory or imatinib-intolerant disease.
- Patients with exon 9 c-KIT mutation or wild-type GIST have the best response rates to sunitinib.
  - Regorafenib can be used as third-line therapy for patients who are refractory or intolerant to both imatinib and sunitinib.
- If limited number of disease sites, debulking surgery or local ablative strategies should be considered.
  - Patients should remain on TKI prior to and following surgery since they usually experience rapid recurrence once treatment is discontinued.
- If multiple sites of disease demonstrate progression, consider changing systemic therapy.
- Monitor patients on therapy with imaging every 3 to 6 months.

5. **When should radiation be considered in metastatic disease?**
   - Focal radiation should be considered for bone metastases that are painful or at risk for pathologic fracture.
   - Stereotactic body radiation therapy can be used for small, limited lung metastases to achieve disease control.

6. **How is local recurrence treated in most sarcomas?**
   - Re-resection is usually the preferred treatment with additional radiotherapy as possible.

SPECIAL CONSIDERATIONS

Kaposi Sarcoma

1. **What is Kaposi sarcoma (KS)?**
   - Indolent, soft-tissue vascular tumor involving skin, mucosa, and viscera
   - Associated with herpes virus (KSHV/HHV8) infection
   - Four different types of KS are indistinguishable by histology:
     - Classic KS
   - Primarily affects elderly men of Ashkenazi Jewish and/or Mediterranean descent
   - Peak incidence between the ages of 40 and 70 years
   - Usually affects distal extremities, particularly lower legs and feet

- Extracutaneous involvement is unusual but in approximately 10% of patients can involve the oral mucosa and GI tract.
- More indolent than the AIDS-KS and rarely accounts for mortality
  - Endemic KS—mostly seen in Africa
  - Iatrogenic sarcoma is usually seen in patients with immune disorders and those on immune suppression.
  - Epidemic or AIDS-related KS—most common neoplasm in patients with AIDS.

2. **What is the next step once KS is suspected?**
   - Screening for visceral involvement with stool guaiac and chest x-ray is recommended.
   - Additional evaluation with CT scanning is done only if indicated clinically.

3. **What is the prognosis of AIDS-related KS?**
   - There is no cure for AIDS-related KS.
   - Good-prognosis disease
     - Limited to skin, lymph nodes, or minimal oral involvement
     - CD4 count $\geq$200 cells/mm^3
     - No opportunistic infections or thrush
     - Good performance status (Karnofsky performance status [KPS] >70)
     - No B symptoms
   - Poor-prognosis disease
     - Tumor associated with edema/ulceration, extensive oral disease, GI or visceral disease
     - CD4 count is <200 cells/mm^3
     - History of opportunistic infections or thrush
     - Poor performance status (KPS <70)
     - Presence of other HIV-related illnesses

4. **What is the treatment for AIDS-related KS?**
   - Highly active antiretroviral therapy (HAART) is the only therapy recommended if disease is confined to the skin, oral cavity, and asymptomatic visceral disease.
   - If progressive disease, or if extensive cutaneous or symptomatic visceral disease, treatment with HAART + systemic therapy is indicated.
     - Liposomal doxorubicin or paclitaxel is usually used in the first- or second-line setting.
     - Vinorelbine, etoposide, or interferon (IFN) alpha are possible options for progressive disease.
     - Symptomatic localized disease can be treated with radiation and intralesional chemotherapy.

QUESTIONS

1. Which of the following is *not* a common side effect of imatinib?
   A. Periorbital edema
   B. Fatigue
   C. Liver function test abnormalities
   D. Neuropathy
   E. Muscle cramps

2. Which of following is a feature of a low-risk gastrointestinal stromal tumor (GIST)?
   A. Ileal location
   B. Mitotic index <5/50 high powered fields
   C. Size >10 cm
   D. Tumor rupture

3. All of the following treatments could be considered for a patient with metastatic liposarcoma *except:*
   A. Doxorubicin
   B. Ifosfamide
   C. Eribulin
   D. Pazopanib

4. A 55-year-old man presents with a firm, painless mass that has been enlarging on his left thigh. Biopsy reveals an undifferentiated pleomorphic sarcoma. Which of the following is the next step in management?
   A. Doxorubicin and ifosfamide
   B. Surgical resection
   C. MRI of the left lower extremity and CT chest
   D. Bone scan

5. A 22-year-old woman develops pain in her right posterior chest wall. CT chest demonstrates a 7.1 × 6.5 × 5.5 cm mass arising from the right eighth rib. No lung nodules are noted. CT-guided biopsy reveals high-grade osteosarcoma. Bone scan reveals uptake in the right eighth rib but no other sites of metastatic disease. What is the best treatment plan for this patient?
   A. Methotrexate, doxorubicin, and cisplatin followed by surgery
   B. Chemotherapy alone
   C. Surgery alone
   D. Radiation followed by surgery
   E. Best supportive care

ANSWERS

1. **D. Neuropathy.** All other answers are common side effects of imatinib.

2. **B. Mitotic index <5/50 high powered fields.** All others are features of high-risk GIST.

3. **D. Pazopanib.** Food and Drug Administration (FDA) approval for pazopanib is for nonadipocytic soft-tissue sarcoma (STS). All other agents are FDA-approved.

4. **C. MRI of the left lower extremity and CT chest.** Preoperative imaging to determine the extent of disease allows for accurate staging of sarcoma and formulating a treatment plan. A bone scan generally has no role in the staging of soft-tissue sarcoma (STS).

5. **A. Methotrexate, doxorubicin, and cisplatin followed by surgery.** The optimal treatment of localized osteosarcoma includes combination treatment with chemotherapy and surgical resection. Chemotherapy increases the chance of cure and should be added to surgery. Radiation has no role in the curative setting. Best supportive care is not appropriate for this potentially curable patient.

VIII

MELANOMA

Melanoma

31

Darren King and Christopher Lao

EPIDEMIOLOGY

1. **What are the various subtypes of melanoma? Describe the characteristics of each.**

   - *Superficial spreading:* most common subtype, appears as the classic irregular pigmented macule
   - *Nodular:* often appears as a rapidly growing, homogeneous darkly pigmented nodule (microscopically either spindled or epithelioid)
   - *Lentigo maligna:* develops in chronically solar damaged skin, typically of the head and neck in older patients
   - *Acral lentiginous:* less common in Whites, more common in people of Asian and African descent, not clearly related to sun exposure
   - *Desmoplastic:* rare, amelanotic, aggressive, and deeply invasive
   - *Mucosal:* arises from the mucosal surface of the nose, esophagus, oral cavity, genitourinary tract, anus, and rectum
   - *Uveal:* arises in the uvea of the eye, manifest as pain or change in visual acuity, often diagnosed without a biopsy. This is the most common primary intraocular malignancy in adults. Metastasis is hematogenous with liver as a common site.

ETIOLOGY AND RISK FACTORS

1. **Define the risk factors for melanoma.**

   - Light skin, intermittent sun exposure, history of blistering sunburn, exposure to ultraviolet (UV) A and B, UV radiation via tanning beds and with psoralen as a treatment for psoriasis, numerous common (>100) nevi, atypical nevi, large congenital nevi, prior history of melanoma
   - Dysplastic nevus syndrome is characterized by numerous atypical nevi and development of melanoma at an early age with lifetime risk of 100%

2. **What inherited genetic mutations/polymorphisms have been associated with increased risk of melanoma?**

   - Susceptibility in families with mutated tumor suppressor gene, *CDKN2A*, which encodes p16INK4A and p19ARF
   - CDK4 mutations
   - Melanocortin 1 receptor gene (*MCIR*)
   - BRCA2 mutation
   - BAP1 mutation (associated with uveal melanoma and mesothelioma)

3. What sporadic (somatic) gene mutations are seen in melanoma?

- BRAF is the most common somatic mutation seen in melanoma (50%–60% of cases), with higher incidence in superficial spreading subtype. The V600E mutation makes up approximately 80% of cases, while most of the remainder are V600K.
- NRAS is mutated and activated in 15% to 20% of melanomas. This protein occurs upstream of BRAF, and mutations in both NRAS and BRAF are extremely rare.
- c-KIT mutations are seen in up to 10% of cases of melanoma, primarily in those occurring in areas not exposed to sun (acral, mucosal) or in lentigo maligna.
- GNAQ/GNA11 and BAP mutations are seen in uveal melanomas.

STAGING

1. Define the staging for melanoma.

Primary Tumor Stage, Cutaneous Melanoma

Tx	Primary tumor cannot be assessed
T0	No evidence of primary tumor
Tis	Melanoma in situ
T1	<1 mm in thickness
	T1a without ulceration
	T1b with ulceration
T2	1.01–2 mm in thickness
	T2a without ulceration
	T2b with ulceration
T3	2.01–4 mm in thickness
	T3a without ulceration
	T3b with ulceration
T4	>4 mm in thickness
	T4a without ulceration
	T4b with ulceration

Nodal Disease Staging

Nx	Patients in whom the regional nodes cannot be assessed (eg, previously removed for another reason)
N0	No regional metastases detected
N1	One lymph node*
N2	Two or three lymph nodes#
N3	Four or more metastatic lymph nodes, or matted lymph nodes, or in-transit metastasis/satellite(s) with metastatic lymph node

*N1a, micrometastasis in the lymph node; N1b, macrometastasis in the lymph node.

#N2a, micrometastasis in the two or three lymph nodes; N2b, macrometastasis in at least one of the two to three lymph nodes; N2c, in-transit metastasis or satellite metastasis without a lymph node involvement.

Staging of Metastasis

M0	No detectable evidence of distant metastases
M1a	Metastases to skin, subcutaneous, or distant lymph node, normal serum LDH
M1b	Lung metastases, normal LDH
M1c	Nonpulmonary visceral metastases with a normal LDH, or any distant metastases and an elevated LDH

LDH, lactate dehydrogenase.

Melanoma Seventh Tumor, Node, and Metastasis (TNM) Stage Group

Stage 0	Tis	N0	M0
Stage IA	T1a	N0	M0
Stage IB	T1b	N0	M0
	T2a	N0	M0
Stage IIA	T2b	N0	M0
	T3a	N0	M0
Stage IIB	T3b	N0	M0
	T4a	N0	M0
Stage IIC	T4b	N0	M0
Stage III	Any T	N1, N2, or N3	M0
Stage IV	Any T	Any N	M1

SIGNS AND SYMPTOMS

1. **What are the characteristic features of a primary melanoma lesion?**
   - Asymmetry of the lesion
   - Irregularity of borders
   - Variegate color
   - Diameter >6 mm
   - Enlargement or evolution over time
   - This is the "ABCDE" mnemonic (Asymmetry, Borders, Color, Diameter, Evolution)

DIAGNOSIS

1. **What is the recommended diagnostic test for a suspicious pigmented lesion?**
   - Excisional biopsy with a 1 to 2 mm rim of normal-appearing skin. A punch biopsy is also a consideration. A wide excision for diagnostic purposes should not be performed as this might affect future management.

2. **What genetic mutations should be tested in patients with stage III or IV disease?**

   - BRAF V600E and K mutation (except in uveal melanomas, which do not harbor BRAF mutations)
   - KIT (~10%–15% of acral lentiginous and mucosal melanomas). KIT targeted therapy can be considered if KIT mutation is identified.

PROGNOSTIC FACTORS

1. **What are the various prognostic variables in melanoma?**

   - Primary lesion:
     - Breslow depth (tumor thickness): this is the most important prognostic factor
     - Lymph node involvement
     - Mitotic rate
     - Ulceration
   - Lactate dehydrogenase (LDH): any distant metastasis with an elevated LDH or visceral metastasis is staged as M1c while lung metastasis with a normal LDH is staged as M1b
   - Additional poor prognostic variables: poor performance status, older age, male gender, tumor location in the head and neck area

TREATMENT OF PRIMARY/LOCALIZED MELANOMA

1. **What is the surgical management of a primary melanoma?**

   - Wide local excision
   - For melanomas <1 mm in depth: 1 cm margin
   - For melanomas >1 mm but <2 mm: 1 to 2 cm margin
   - For melanomas >2 mm: 2 cm margin

2. **When should sentinel lymph node mapping be considered?**

   - In patients with clinically negative nodes and primary melanoma >1 mm thick or <0.75 mm thick but associated with ulceration, >1 mitosis/mm^2, positive deep margins or lymphovascular invasion. There is an improvement in progression-free survival (PFS) with sentinel lymph node mapping, but no improvement in overall survival (OS).
   - If there is evidence of lymph node involvement on the sentinel lymph node biopsy, a completion lymph node dissection is the standard of care.

3. **What are the indications for adjuvant therapy?**

   - For many years, the only Food and Drug Administration (FDA)-approved adjuvant therapy was high-dose interferon alpha (IFNa) 2b. For patients at high risk of relapse (stage IIB/IIC/III) who have no serious coexisting illness and have an estimated life expectancy of 10 years or more, postoperative treatment with high-dose IFNa may be considered.
   - IFNa is associated with an improved relapse-free survival (relative risk reduction of 17%–26%). An OS advantage was demonstrated at 5 years, but no clear

benefit after 10 years. Given the significant side effects from IFN use, observation alone is also considered acceptable.

- In 2015 the FDA approved the use of ipilimumab (see the following) as adjuvant treatment in stage III disease.

TREATMENT OF METASTATIC DISEASE

1. **What are the treatment options for metastatic melanoma?**
   - Categories of treatment for metastatic melanoma include chemotherapy, molecularly targeted therapy, surgical resection, and radiation.

2. **What is the role of chemotherapy in treatment of metastatic melanoma?**
   - Chemotherapy has traditionally proven ineffective in improving overall survival in metastatic melanoma.
   - The only chemotherapeutic agent that is FDA approved for the treatment of metastatic melanoma is dacarbazine, an alkylator. Objective response rate (ORR) in clinical trials is in the 10% to 20% range, although responses are not durable and long-term response is only seen in 1% to 2% of patients
   - Temozolomide is an oral alkylating agent that crosses the blood–brain barrier and has been used off-label and in clinical trials in metastatic melanoma.
   - Other single agents, as well as combination chemotherapy with paclitaxel/carboplatin, have been investigated, all with very modest activity.
   - With the advent of molecularly targeted therapy and immunotherapy, chemotherapy is now considered a second- or third-line approach to treatment of metastatic melanoma.
   - In patients with recurrent, metastatic, or in-transit melanoma confined to a single limb, chemotherapy (typically melphalan) may be administered via isolated limb perfusion.

3. **What is the role of molecularly targeted therapy in metastatic melanoma?**
   - The FDA has approved two BRAF inhibitors (vemurafenib and dabrafenib) and one MEK inhibitor (trametinib) in treatment of unresectable stage III or metastatic disease based on mutational status.
   - Vemurafenib has been approved by the FDA for use in unresectable or metastatic melanoma harboring a BRAF V600E mutation. This oral agent has shown a PFS and OS advantage compared to dacarbazine. Potential side effects include development of cutaneous squamous cell carcinoma or keratoacanthoma, arthralgias, rash, nausea, and hand–foot syndrome. EKG should be monitored for QT prolongation while on therapy.
   - Dabrafenib has also been FDA approved for use in unresectable or metastatic melanoma with a BRAF V600E mutation, also based on comparison to dacarbazine. Potential side effects include arthralgias, fever, uveitis/iritis, squamous cell carcinoma (lower incidence than with vemurafenib), and cardiomyopathy.
   - Trametinib is an oral MEK inhibitor, which acts downstream of BRAF in the MAPK pathway. It has been approved by the FDA as monotherapy for unresectable or metastatic melanoma with a BRAF V600E or V600K mutation. As a single agent, side effects include rash, diarrhea, cardiac toxicity, and ocular toxicity.

- Dabrafenib and trametinib are also used in combination, with improvement in PFS compared to dabrafenib alone. Rates of squamous cell carcinoma are lower with combination therapy, compared to dabrafenib alone. The most common side effect seen with combination dabrafenib/trametinib is fever (70% of patients), which may cause dose interruptions and can be managed with corticosteroids.
- Patients with c-KIT mutations have been treated off-label with tyrosine kinase inhibitors such as imatinib.

4. What is the role of immunotherapy in treatment of metastatic melanoma?

- Approved immunotherapy for metastatic melanoma includes IL-2 and the checkpoint inhibitors ipilimumab (anti-CTLA-4 monoclonal antibody), nivolumab (monoclonal PD-1 antibody), pembrolizumab (monoclonal PD-1 antibody), and the combination of ipilimumab and nivolumab.
- A relative contraindication to use of immunotherapy is the presence of preexisting autoimmune conditions, as these may be exacerbated by therapy. Immunotherapy with checkpoint inhibitors in general can cause unpredictable and potentially severe autoimmune inflammatory states to multiple organ systems.
- Due to the (beneficial) recruitment of antitumor T cells to the sites of metastatic disease by the checkpoint inhibitors, increased inflammation can occur at tumor sites. This may lead to CT scans showing transient increases in size of lesions—this is referred to as "pseudoprogression," and in the absence of new lesions or clinical worsening, should not be taken as a sign of treatment failure, but rather monitored with subsequent scans. Given the rapid growth in use of checkpoint-inhibitor-based therapy, RECIST criteria for radiographic progression have now been replaced by immune-related response criteria (irRC) for patients receiving treatment with these drugs.
- An additional form of approved immunotherapy for melanoma is oncolytic virus therapy. In 2015, the FDA approved talimogene laherparepvec (T-VEC) as treatment for unresectable cutaneous, subcutaneous, or nodal melanoma. This drug is a genetically modified herpes simplex virus, which targets cancer cells and replicates while producing the growth factor GM-CSF. Cells eventually lyse, releasing GM-CSF and virus- and tumor-derived antigens, thus eliciting a local immune response.

5. What is the role of IL-2 in treatment of metastatic melanoma?

- For many years, IL-2 was the only approved immunotherapy for metastatic melanoma. It is a T-cell activator.
- Although ORR is only 16%, many of these responders achieve a durable complete response (CR).
- Treatment is given inpatient due to the need for close monitoring for hypotension, acute renal failure, fever, nausea/vomiting/diarrhea, and respiratory failure. Many of these serious side effects are due to capillary-leak syndrome and resolve after discontinuation.
- Due to these toxicities, use of IL-2 is limited to younger, otherwise healthy patients.

6. **What is the role of ipilimumab in treatment of metastatic disease?**
   - Ipilimumab is a monoclonal antibody directed against CTLA-4. Blocking this target causes sustained T-cell activation, leading to antitumor immune activity.
   - This was the first agent shown to improve OS in metastatic melanoma.
   - In a phase 3 clinical trial, ipilimumab (with or without gp100 peptide vaccine) compared to gp100 vaccine was associated with a median OS of 10.1 versus 6.4 months. Four-year OS rate is close to 20%. Ipilimumab in combination with dacarbazine was associated with a median OS of 11.2 months compared with 9.1 months for dacarbazine alone.
   - Side effects include fatigue, rash, itching, and, especially, immune-related toxicities: enterocolitis, hypophysitis, uveitis, dermatitis, and transaminitis. Prolonged use of high-dose steroids with interruption of treatment is required if significant immune-related toxicities develop.
   - Ipilimumab has now also been approved as adjuvant treatment for stage III melanoma.

7. **What are the roles of nivolumab and pembrolizumab in treatment of metastatic disease?**
   - Nivolumab and pembrolizumab are FDA-approved monoclonal antibodies that target PD-1, a coinhibitory receptor found on T cells. By blocking PD-1 from its ligand, PD-L1, nivolumab and pembrolizumab augment the antitumor immune response. In one trial comparing pembrolizumab to ipilimumab, pembrolizumab showed an ORR of 33% compared to 12% with ipilimumab alone.
   - Nivolumab was granted FDA approval based on a randomized control trial comparing it to investigator's choice of chemotherapy, which showed an ORR of 31.7% versus 10.6%.
   - Toxicity profiles of nivolumab and pembrolizumab also show autoimmune/inflammatory side effects, although the rate appears to be lower than with single agent ipilimumab.

8. **What is the role of combination immunotherapy in metastatic melanoma?**
   - Combination treatment with ipilimumab and nivolumab has been very promising, gaining FDA approval in 2015 for patients with metastatic disease without a BRAF mutation, and with expansion in 2016 to include patients regardless of mutational status.
   - In a phase 1 clinical trial, the combination of ipilimumab and nivolumab at maximal dosing showed an objective response in 53% of patients.
   - In a subsequent trial, patients receiving ipilimumab plus nivolumab showed an ORR of 50% compared to 40% for single agent nivolumab and 14% for single agent ipilimumab.
   - Rate of autoimmune/inflammatory phenomena is higher with combination therapy than in single-agent immunotherapy.

9. **How should molecularly targeted and immunotherapy be sequenced in eligible patients with metastatic disease?**
   - BRAF inhibitors have been shown to provide rapid, though not very durable, responses. Immunotherapy, conversely, can take longer to produce an objective response, but this response may be much more durable.
   - As a result, one approach to sequencing therapy is to use BRAF inhibitors as frontline therapy in patients with rapidly progressive/symptomatic disease to achieve faster control, while patients with more indolent disease may be started on checkpoint-inhibitor therapy as frontline treatment.

10. **What is the role of radiation therapy in metastatic melanoma?**
   - Metastatic melanoma is relatively radioresistant, but radiation therapy can be tried in the palliative setting and in the case of cord compression.
   - In the case of brain metastases, durable control is not usual with whole-brain radiation therapy (WBRT). However, some patients who undergo stereotactic radiosurgery for oligometastatic disease may have long-term benefit.

11. **What is the role of surgical resection in metastatic melanoma?**
   - Surgical resection of symptomatic metastases can provide fast and effective palliation.
   - Resection of isolated visceral metastases can provide long-term survival improvement in a subset of patients.
   - Surgical resection is the standard of care for patients with stage III disease with in-transit metastases.

QUESTIONS

1. A 60-year-old male with melanoma with lung metastasis has begun frontline treatment with nivolumab. The patient's disease is BRAF wild type. He has been tolerating therapy without signs or symptoms of toxicity. He is feeling well. He undergoes his first set of follow-up CT scans for restaging. These show interval growth in several lung nodules compared to pretreatment CT—one nodule has grown from 2 to 3 cm, and another from 1 to 2 cm. Multiple other pulmonary nodules are stable in size. What should be the next step in treatment?
   A. Continue nivolumab
   B. Change from nivolumab to pembrolizumab
   C. Add ipilimumab to nivolumab
   D. Discontinue nivolumab and start standard chemotherapy with dacarbazine

2. A 55-year-old male undergoes complete resection of a 5 mm superficial spreading melanoma of the left thigh. Due to palpable inguinal lymph nodes, he undergoes a therapeutic left inguinal lymph node dissection. This reveals macrometastatic nodal disease, and he is staged as stage IIIC. Mutational testing is negative for BRAF and c-KIT mutations. Staging PET/CT shows no additional sites of disease. The patient's oncologist informs him that his risk of relapse is high, and the patient asks what can be done to reduce this risk. Which of the

following statements is the most accurate regarding adjuvant treatment options in stage III melanoma?

A. Adjuvant use of either interferon or ipilimumab has shown improvement in overall survival (OS) but not relapse-free survival (RFS) in stage III melanoma

B. Adjuvant use of either interferon or ipilimumab has shown improvement in RFS but not OS in stage III melanoma

C. Adjuvant use of ipilimumab has shown improvement in OS in stage III melanoma while interferon has not

D. Adjuvant use of interferon has shown improvement in OS in stage III melanoma while ipilimumab has not

3. A 60-year-old female is undergoing combination treatment with ipilimumab/nivolumab for metastatic melanoma with lung and liver involvement. She presents to the clinic for her fourth dose of treatment complaining of fatigue. Her blood pressure is noted to be low, at 80/45, and she is tachycardic to the 120s. She is afebrile, and appears fatigued but comfortable. Basic labs show a normal basic metabolic panel (BMP), liver function tests (LFTs), and thyroid-stimulating hormone (TSH). Complete blood count (CBC) is unremarkable. The patient is started on intravenous fluids (IVFs) while in clinic. What should be the next step in management?

A. Initiate broad-spectrum antibiotics

B. Perform echocardiogram

C. Perform adrenocorticotropic hormone (ACTH) stimulation test

D. Proceed with treatment as planned following IVF administration

4. A 50-year-old male has been receiving ipilimumab/nivolumab as treatment for metastatic melanoma. After three doses of treatment, he develops profuse watery diarrhea with abdominal cramping and anorexia. CT abdomen/pelvis is consistent with colitis. He is admitted to the hospital and started on high-dose steroids for immune-related colitis. After 1 week on steroids, his stool volume has not significantly decreased, and he continues to have abdominal discomfort. Testing for *Clostridium difficile* is negative. In anticipation of the next therapeutic step in management, what diagnostic test should be performed?

A. Repeat CT abdomen/pelvis

B. Colonoscopy

C. Testing for hepatitis B

D. Purified protein derivative (PPD) testing for tuberculosis (TB)

5. A 35-year-old female with multiple sclerosis is diagnosed with melanoma metastatic to the lungs. She is found to carry a BRAF V600E mutation. Clinically she is well-appearing. What would be the most appropriate first line of therapy to use?

A. Dabrafenib/trametinib

B. Trametinib monotherapy

C. Ipilimumab/nivolumab

D. Nivolumab monotherapy

E. Dacarbazine

6. **A 75-year-old male is diagnosed with melanoma of the rectal mucosa following workup for hematochezia. Which of the following genes is most likely to be mutated in this tumor?**

A. *BRAF*

B. *NRAS*

C. *c-KIT*

D. *CDKN2A*

ANSWERS

1. **A. Continue nivolumab.** The finding of initial tumor growth at some sites of disease early in a treatment course with a checkpoint inhibitor may be a sign of pseudoprogression, rather than true disease progression. Because of this unique effect of immunotherapy, a new set of response criteria have been developed, the immune-related response criteria (irRC) to substitute for RECIST. Nivolumab should be continued as the patient is clinically doing well and is tolerating treatment. There is no evidence for efficacy in changing from one PD-1 inhibitor to another, or for adding ipilimumab once nivolumab has already been started. Standard chemotherapy with dacarbazine has shown inferior results compared to checkpoint-inhibitor therapy.

2. **B. Adjuvant use of either interferon or ipilimumab has shown improvement in RFS but not OS in stage III melanoma.** No therapy has yet been shown to improve OS as adjuvant treatment in stage III melanoma. Both interferon (in 1995) and ipilimumab (in 2015) received Food and Drug Administration (FDA) approval for use as adjuvant therapy based on improvement in RFS, not OS. There is an ongoing clinical trial comparing interferon and ipilimumab in the adjuvant setting with OS as a primary end point (phase 3 Eastern Cooperative Oncology Group [ECOG] 1609).

3. **C. Perform adrenocorticotropic hormone (ACTH) stimulation test.** A common side effect of the ipilimumab/nivolumab combination is autoimmune phenomena, which can lead to endocrinopathies. Incidence seems to increase after the third or fourth doses of treatment. This includes hypophysitis, leading to a secondary adrenal insufficiency. Because symptoms may be nonspecific, there should be a low threshold for testing the pituitary axis with serum cortisol, ACTH stimulation, or consideration of brain MRI. Cardiac and infectious toxicities are not commonly associated with checkpoint-inhibitor therapy. In the presence of hypophysitis, treatment must be held and steroids initiated.

4. **D. Purified protein derivative (PPD) testing for tuberculosis (TB).** In patients on checkpoint-inhibitor therapy with immune-mediated colitis that is not improving with steroids, the next step in therapeutic management is initiation of infliximab. Infliximab is a monoclonal antibody targeting TNF-α. Due to risk for reactivation, patients should undergo testing for TB prior to receiving infliximab.

5. **A. Dabrafenib/trametinib.** Although checkpoint inhibitors are approved as monotherapy (nivolumab) and in combination (ipilimumab/nivolumab) in patients regardless of BRAF mutation status, the patient is at high risk for exacerbation of her multiple sclerosis due to immune activation with these drugs. Molecularly targeted therapy would thus likely have a safer toxicity profile, with the combination of dabrafenib/trametinib more efficacious than trametinib alone. Efficacy of dacarbazine in the frontline setting is low.

6. **C. c-KIT.** Melanomas arising from mucosal surfaces not exposed to the sun are most likely to harbor a c-KIT mutation.

IX

CENTRAL NERVOUS SYSTEM MALIGNANCIES

Central Nervous System Tumors

Erin F. Cobain, Aaron Mammoser, and Larry Junck

Central Nervous System Tumors (General)

ETIOLOGY AND RISK FACTORS

1. **What is the etiology of central nervous system (CNS) tumors?**
   - The majority are sporadic
   - A small proportion is associated with genetic syndromes, radiation, or immunosuppression

2. **What are the common genetic syndromes associated with primary brain tumors?**
   - Neurofibromatosis type I: neurofibromas (especially important on spinal nerve roots), optic nerve glioma (a type of pilocytic astrocytoma), other pilocytic astrocytoma, diffuse glioma (grades II–IV), malignant peripheral nerve sheath tumor
   - Neurofibromatosis type II: bilateral vestibular schwannoma (acoustic neuroma), meningioma, ependymoma of cervical spinal cord
   - Tuberous sclerosis: subependymal giant cell astrocytoma, hamartomas
   - Turcot syndrome: Lynch syndrome with glioma (especially glioblastoma), or familial adenomatous polyposis with medulloblastoma or pineoblastoma
   - Li–Fraumeni syndrome: high-grade glioma, medulloblastomas, and primitive neuroectodermal tumor
   - Cowden syndrome: dysplastic gangliocytoma of the cerebellum

SIGNS AND SYMPTOMS

1. **What are the common presenting features of CNS tumors?**
   - Headache
   - Seizures
   - Focal neurologic symptoms (focal weakness, gait disturbance, visual symptoms, language deficit)
   - Cognitive deficits and behavior changes

CLASSIFICATION AND DIAGNOSIS

1. **For diffuse gliomas, grades II–III, what are the three molecular classes?**
   - Most favorable: codeletion in chromosomes 1p and 19q (nearly always have isocitrate dehydrogenase [IDH] mutation as well). The majority of oligodendrogliomas fall into this class, as do some oligoastrocytomas (mixed histopathology).

- Intermediate: IDH mutation but no codeletion. Histopathologically, oligodendrogliomas, oligoastrocytomas, and pure astrocytomas may all fall into this class.
- Most unfavorable: No IDH mutation or codeletion. These are usually astrocytomas, but occasionally oligoastrocytomas.
- In addition to molecular class being highly prognostic, regardless of treatment, codeletion is highly predictive and IDH mutation moderately predictive of response to PCV chemotherapy (procarbazine, CCNU, vincristine) and probably temozolomide chemotherapy.

2. **What are the most important molecular predictors for glioblastoma?**
   - Methylation of the methylguanine methyltransferase (MGMT) promoter (present in about one third, both predictive of temozolomide benefit but also prognostically favorable regardless of treatment)
   - IDH mutation (favorable, present in ~5%–8%, generally in young adults)

3. **What are the most important clinical factors in determining prognosis for primary CNS tumors?**
   - Age (in adults, young age is favorable)
   - Performance status (PS)

4. **What is the best imaging modality for primary CNS tumors?**
   - MRI brain. Gadolinium enhancement is a hallmark of high-grade tumors.

5. **What primary CNS tumor types may require additional diagnostic evaluation beyond MRI brain?**
   - Medulloblastoma, CNS germ cell tumors, ependymoma require MRI of total spine. These types and primary CNS lymphoma require cerebrospinal fluid (CSF) examination.

Diffuse Gliomas

1. **What is the most common primary malignant brain tumor?**
   - Glioblastoma (grade IV astrocytoma)

2. **How is secondary glioblastoma defined, and what is its molecular signature?**
   - Glioblastoma arising in a tumor previously diagnosed as grade II or III glioma
   - Usually has IDH mutation

3. **What is the standard treatment for newly diagnosed glioblastoma?**
   - For most adults up to age 65 to 70, maximum safe surgical removal, followed by conformal radiation to 60 Gy over 6 weeks with concomitant daily temozolomide, followed by six to 12 cycles of temozolomide (5 days of every 28 days).
   - For most adults over age 65 to 70, maximum safe surgical removal, followed by conformal radiation to 40 Gy over 3 weeks with concomitant daily temozolomide, followed by six cycles of temozolomide.

- For the elderly, especially if very old or with poor functional status, other options after surgery include conformal radiation to 40 Gy over 3 weeks without chemotherapy or (especially if tumor has MGMT promoter methylation) cyclic temozolomide monotherapy.
- For those with severe disability at any age, 3 weeks of radiation to 40 Gy without temozolomide. Another option is supportive care.
- The addition of bevacizumab to chemoradiation with temozolomide provides no overall survival benefit.
- Patients may exhibit pseudoprogression on imaging, most commonly within 3 months after completion of treatment. It is difficult to distinguish from tumor progression. However, it is reasonable to continue temozolomide with or without corticosteroid therapy and repeat imaging in 1 to 2 months before switching therapy.

4. What are the most common treatments for recurrent glioblastoma?

- Resection, if the tumor is not in an eloquent area, especially if functional status is good and if time since previous resection approaches or exceeds 1 year.
- Bevacizumab has a substantial chance of clinical and MRI improvement but uncertain survival benefit.
- Lomustine (CCNU) monotherapy may provide modest delay in progression and extension of survival, but with low probability of clinical or MRI improvement.
- Adding bevacizumab to lomustine delays tumor progression but does not extend survival compared to lomustine alone. Generally, this combination is not recommended.

5. What is the standard treatment for newly diagnosed anaplastic glioma (grade III)

- Maximal surgical resection followed by radiation (consider hypofractionated radiation in age >65–70 or Karnofsky performance status [KPS] <70)
- For oligodendroglial tumors (including oligoastrocytomas) with codeletion in 1p/19q, two large studies have shown that PCV chemotherapy after radiation provides substantial benefit.
- For oligodendroglial tumors with IDH mutation but no codeletion, PCV chemotherapy after radiation has been shown to be moderately beneficial.
- For oligodendroglial tumors without IDH mutation or codeletion, PCV chemotherapy provides no benefit.
- For anaplastic astrocytomas, no conclusive studies have been done to assess the benefit of PCV chemotherapy.
- For anaplastic gliomas lacking codeletions, cyclic temozolomide after radiation has been shown to be of benefit. The benefit of temozolomide concomitant with radiation for these tumors is under assessment.
- For anaplastic gliomas with codeletions, temozolomide is known to have fairly high activity. Comparison of temozolomide with PCV as initial treatment, together with radiation, is under assessment.

6. **What agent is approved for treatment of recurrent anaplastic astrocytoma?**
   - Temozolomide

7. **What is the standard treatment for newly diagnosed diffuse glioma (grade II astrocytoma, oligoastrocytoma, oligodendroglioma)?**
   - For most patients, optimal surgical resection
   - If a patient is asymptomatic other than well-controlled seizures, and tumor is small or moderate in size and lacks enhancement, it may be reasonable to delay surgery (ie, watch-and-wait approach)
   - Radiation may be employed following surgery; however, trials have not demonstrated a survival benefit for radiation early after surgery versus radiation delayed to time of progression
   - Chemotherapy with procarbazine/CCNU/vincristine (PCV) following radiation improves overall survival in patients with low-grade gliomas (LGGs) when compared to radiation treatment alone.
   - Small studies report the use of cyclic temozolomide monotherapy after resection, mainly in patients with codeleted tumors having no neurologic symptoms other than well-controlled seizures, with some indications of benefit.

8. **What are high-risk features in LGGs?**
   - Pignatti criteria (≥3 criteria of 5 associated with high risk):
     - Age older than 40
     - Astrocytoma histology
     - Maximum dimension >6 cm
     - Tumor crossing midline
     - Preoperative neurologic deficit

9. **What are the most common types of very low-grade (grade I) glioma?**
   - Pilocytic astrocytoma
   - Ganglioglioma
   - Subependymal giant cell astrocytoma (seen almost exclusively in patients with tuberous sclerosis)
   - These tumors are most commonly seen in children and young adults

10. **What are the most common locations for pilocytic astrocytoma and what are the characteristics on imaging?**
    - Cerebellum (40%), supratentorial regions (35%)
    - On MRI, often cystic with an enhancing mural nodule

11. **What is the standard treatment for grade I astrocytomas?**
    - Surgical resection is usually curative

Medulloblastoma

EPIDEMIOLOGY

1. **In what age group do medulloblastomas typically occur?**
   - Children, but they also occur in adults, especially young adults.

DIAGNOSIS

1. **What is the most common location for this tumor?**
   - Posterior fossa: cerebellar vermis (especially in young children) or hemispheres (older children and adults)
   - Some cases present with acute hydrocephalus, with symptoms of headache, vomiting, somnolence, and gait disturbance.

2. **What are the signs and symptoms at presentation?**
   - Cerebellar dysfunction: gain instability, diplopia, dysarthria. Also, hydrocephalus including nausea/vomiting, headache, somnolence, gait disturbance.

3. **What are the four molecular subtypes of medulloblastoma?**
   - WNT: best prognosis
   - Sonic hedgehog (SHH): intermediate prognosis
   - Group 3: characterized by overexpression of MYC, worst prognosis
   - Group 4: intermediate prognosis

TREATMENT

1. **How is medulloblastoma typically treated?**
   - Surgical removal of as much of the mass lesion as possible
   - Radiation therapy to the craniospinal axis with a boost to the site of primary tumor
   - Platinum-containing chemotherapy regimen: cisplatin, cyclophosphamide, lomustine vincristine

2. **What staging characteristics identify medulloblastoma tumors to be at high risk for recurrence?**
   - Postoperative residual >1.5 cm
   - Dissemination within nervous system demonstrated by MRI or CSF analysis

Primary Central Nervous System Lymphoma (Non-AIDS)

EPIDEMIOLOGY

1. **What is the typical age at diagnosis?**
   - In immunocompetent patients, older adults, with median age 60 years
   - In HIV patients, median 30 years

DIAGNOSIS

1. **What is primary central nervous system lymphoma (PCNSL)?**
   - PCNSL is an aggressive, uncommon variant of extranodal non-Hodgkin lymphoma (NHL) involving brain, leptomeninges, eyes, or spinal cord without evidence of systemic disease.
   - Pathology is generally diffuse large B-cell lymphoma (DLBCL).
   - About 20% have leptomeningeal dissemination and 15% have ocular disease at presentation; thus, lumbar puncture (if safe) and slit-lamp examination are important.

2. **What is the best neuroimaging modality in PCNSL?**
   - MRI with and without gadolinium.

3. **What is the MR imaging characteristic of PCNSL?**
   - Solitary or multiple homogeneously enhancing lesions, usually with minimal vasogenic edema (less than expected with similarly sized metastatic lesion or glioma)
   - Supported by relative darkness on T2 images and evidence for restricted diffusion
   - Disappearance (partial or complete) on MRI after initiation of steroid therapy strongly suggests PCNSL.

4. **What are the typical locations of PCNSL?**
   - Periventricular white matter, subcortical/cortical locations, leptomeninges, and vitreous
   - About 50% are single and 50% are multiple at diagnosis

5. **What is the diagnostic procedure of choice for PCNSL?**
   - When imaging findings suggest PCNSL, cytologic and flow cytometry examination of the CSF can sometimes establish the diagnosis.
   - In most case, stereotactic biopsy is needed for diagnosis.
   - Resection is not generally recommended when PCNSL is suspected.

STAGING

1. **What is the staging workup of PCNSL?**
   - Once diagnosis of PCNSL is confirmed, the International PCNSL Collaborative Group recommends:
   - CNS staging with:
     - Total spine MRI preferably before lumbar puncture to avoid contrast artifact
     - CSF exam (if lumbar puncture is safe; if not safe at initial evaluation, consider doing later when partial response has been achieved)
     - Ophthalmology evaluation including slit-lamp exam.
   - Systemic staging with:
     - CT of the chest, abdomen, and pelvis, or body PET
     - HIV test

- ○ Lactate dehydrogenase (LDH) (of prognostic value)
- ○ Testicular exam in males
- ○ Possible bone marrow biopsy

SIGNS AND SYMPTOMS

1. What are the clinical presentations of PCNSL?
- Mental status changes (most common presentation)
- Focal neurologic symptoms
- Seizure (uncommon)
- Headache (uncommon)
- Visual symptoms such as "floaters" due to vitreous involvement

PROGNOSTIC FACTORS

1. What are the prognostic factors of PCNSL?
- From the International Extranodal Lymphoma Study Group, the following are negative prognostic predictors:
  - ○ Age older than 60
  - ○ Eastern Cooperative Oncology Group (ECOG) PS >1
  - ○ Elevated serum LDH
  - ○ Elevated CSF protein
  - ○ Involvement of deep brain regions
  - ○ Immunocompromised state also confers a worse prognosis

TREATMENT

1. What is the role of steroids in PCNSL?
- When PCNSL is suspected, steroid therapy should be avoided prior to diagnosis (if safe to do so) to avoid:
  - ○ "Vanishing tumor" syndrome with regression of tumor mass
  - ○ Interference with histopathologic diagnosis
- Once diagnosis is established, steroid therapy is generally appropriate.

2. What is the current standard therapy of PCNSL?
- Selection of primary therapy depends on the general health and age
  - ○ For healthy patients with KPS >40, a high-dose methotrexate-based regimen is recommended. Evidence supports inclusion of rituximab and cytarabine.
  - ○ For patients with KPS <40, whole-brain radiation therapy (WBRT) may be considered

3. What are commonly used chemotherapy regimens in PCNSL?
- High-dose methotrexate with rituximab, procarbazine, and vincristine, followed by low-dose WBRT, then cytarabine consolidation
- High-dose methotrexate with rituximab and temozolomide, followed by consolidation with etoposide and cytarabine

4. **Why is high-dose methotrexate used in PCNSL?**
   - High level of single-drug activity
   - Moderate passage across blood–brain barrier
   - CSF penetrance

5. **What is the role of intrathecal chemotherapy in PCNSL?**
   - Intrathecal chemotherapy (usually with methotrexate or cytarabine) has not been studied prospectively. However, two large retrospective studies demonstrated no benefit of adding intrathecal therapy to high-dose methotrexate.
   - Intrathecal chemotherapy adds complexity and risk of complications.
   - Intrathecal methotrexate contributes to cognitive decline.
   - Prophylactic intrathecal chemotherapy has no evidence for clinical benefit.

6. **What is the response and survival rate following high-dose methotrexate in PCNSL?**
   - Complete response: 60% to 66% with the better multidrug methotrexate-based regimens
   - Overall median survival: 25 to 50 months

7. **What is the treatment of recurrent PCNSL following systemic therapy?**
   - If recurrence occurs later than 1 year, retreating with the same or different high-dose methotrexate-based regimen is an option.
   - If recurrence occurs earlier than 1 year, WBRT with or without systemic therapy is recommended.
   - Promising results have been observed with high-dose cytarabine and autologous stem cell transplant for early recurrence. Studies are ongoing to evaluate this approach.
   - Best supportive care is also an option, particularly for those with poor performance status.

Meningioma

EPIDEMIOLOGY

1. **What is meningioma?**
   - Extra-axial CNS tumors arising from the arachnoid cap cells in the meninges

2. **What is the incidence of meningioma?**
   - Incidence of 1.8 per 100,000 in males and 3.4 per 100,000 in females
   - Common in middle to late adult life

DIAGNOSIS

1. **What is the best imaging modality for diagnosis of meningioma?**
   - MRI with gadolinium

2. What are the MR imaging characteristics of meningioma?
   - Dome-shaped mass with broad dural attachment
   - Smooth well-defined contours
   - Isointense with gray matter
   - Homogeneous enhancement
   - Enhancing dural tail

GRADING, PROGNOSTIC FACTORS

1. What factors impact rate of recurrence in meningioma?
   - Tumor grade
   - Extent of resection

2. What are the molecular subtypes of meningioma and what are their anticipated clinical courses?
   - Mutation of NF2 (on chromosome 22) is the most common acquired driver mutation
   - Tumors with NF2 mutations and/or chromosome 22 losses are more likely to be atypical and to follow a more aggressive course

3. What is the grading system of meningioma?

Grade	Incidence (%)
I—benign	92
II—atypical	6
III—anaplastic	2

4. What is the risk of recurrence after gross total resection based on grade of meningioma?

Grade	Risk of Recurrence (%)
I	1–16
II	20–41
III	56–63

TREATMENT

1. What are the treatment options for meningioma?
   - Observation: if small (ie, <3 cm) and asymptomatic (or symptomatic with well-controlled seizure)
   - Surgery: if accessible and if treatment is needed (large, growing, or symptomatic)
   - Radiation: if treatment is needed and not a surgical candidate

2. **What are the indications for radiation in meningioma following resection?**
   - All grade III meningioma (even after gross total resection)
   - Incompletely resected grade II
   - Completely resected grade II (radiation optional)
   - Large (ie,>3 cm) unresectable grade I or large residual after resection of grade I
   - Symptomatic unresectable grade I (including symptoms other than seizures)

3. **Which type of radiation modality is used in meningioma?**
   - Fractionated conformal radiotherapy
   - Stereotactic radiosurgery (SRS) (generally only if maximum dimension is <3 cm)

4. **What systemic therapies are used in meningioma?**
   - Sunitinib, octreotide, and bevacizumab are all in use
   - No high-quality evidence supporting any of these

Brain Metastasis

EPIDEMIOLOGY

1. **How common is brain metastasis compared to primary brain tumors?**
   - Incidence of metastatic brain tumors is two to four times that of primary brain tumors.

2. **What proportion of patients with cancer develop brain metastases?**
   - About 10% of cancer patients develop symptomatic brain metastases.

3. **What are the most common cancers of origins of brain metastasis?**
   - Lung cancer
   - Breast cancer
   - Melanoma

SIGNS AND SYMPTOMS

1. **What are the common presenting symptoms of brain metastases?**
   - Headache (40%–50%)
   - Focal neurologic impairment (40%)
   - Mental status change (30%)
   - Seizure (15%–25%)

2. **What part of the brain is affected more by metastases?**
   - Cerebral hemisphere: 80%
   - Cerebellum: 15%
   - Brainstem: 5%

TREATMENT

1. **When multiple metastatic lesions are present, what is the role of resection?**
   - To obtain biopsy sample when diagnosis cannot be obtained systemically
   - To relieve mass effect, uncommonly one large metastasis is resected in a patient who otherwise has a reasonable prognosis.

2. **What is the role of radiotherapy for metastases?**
   - To decrease local recurrence (WBRT or SRS)
   - To decrease recurrence at new sites in the brain (WBRT only)
   - To decrease likelihood of neurologic disability and death

3. **What is the best modality of treatment for limited (1–3) metastatic lesions?**
   - For single metastasis, surgical resection if safe, followed by SRS if tumor bed <30 mm
   - For single unresectable metastasis or for two to three metastases, if all are <30 mm in size, SRS alone
   - Compared to treatment with SRS, WBRT is associated with identical survival, worse quality of life, worse cognitive function, but lower rate of recurrence elsewhere in brain
   - For most patients with one to three metastases <3 cm in size, SRS is preferred over WBRT

4. **In what situation is WBRT recommended?**
   - Any unresectable tumor >3 cm, or tumor bed >3 cm after resection
   - Four or more metastases

QUESTIONS

1. A 56-year-old man presents to the neurology clinic due to concerns of intermittent right arm numbness. Imaging reveals the presence of a large left parietal mass. He undergoes surgery and has a subtotal resection of the tumor. Final pathology returns as anaplastic astrocytoma, isocitrate dehydrogenase (IDH) mutated. Which of the following statements is true regarding this patient's prognosis?
   A. IDH mutated tumors have an inferior prognosis
   B. IDH mutated tumors have a superior prognosis
   C. Prognosis is not impacted by IDH mutation status in anaplastic astrocytoma

2. A 63-year-old man presented to his primary care physician due to increasing difficulty with word finding. MRI brain was ordered and the patient was found to have a ring-enhancing mass in the right frontal lobe. He underwent subtotal resection of the tumor and recovered well following the surgery. Pathology demonstrated glioblastoma with methylguanine methyltransferase (MGMT) promoter methylation.

Following surgery, the patient is advised to begin adjuvant radiation concurrent with temozolomide followed by six cycles of postradiation temozolomide. Which of the following statements about this patient's recommended treatment strategy is true?

A. MGMT promoter hypermethylation predicts benefit from temozolomide therapy
B. MGMT promoter hypermethylation portends a worse prognosis
C. Consideration should be given to the addition of bevacizumab to planned treatment with temozolomide plus radiation
D. The addition of temozolomide to radiation following surgery does not improve overall survival

3. A 53-year-old woman was diagnosed with a left parietal lobe glioblastoma approximately 3 months ago. She underwent maximum surgical resection and postoperative imaging did reveal minimal residual tumor. She subsequently underwent radiation therapy concurrent with temozolomide. She now returns to the clinic to begin postradiation temozolomide; however, MRI imaging has revealed increased contrast enhancement in the area of the residual tumor. The patient feels well and has not developed any new symptoms since initiating therapy. What should you advise the patient?

A. Stop temozolomide and initiate bevacizumab for treatment of recurrent disease
B. Biopsy the area of concern to confirm disease recurrence
C. Continue with adjuvant postradiation temozolomide as previously planned
D. Continue with adjuvant postradiation temozolomide as previously planned, but add bevacizumab

4. A 59-year-old man presents to his primary care physician with his wife, who is concerned that the patient has "not been acting like himself" recently. She believes his behavior has been more impulsive. MRI of the brain reveals a solitary enhancing lesion approximately 3 cm in size with minimal vasogenic edema. The scan is read as suspicious for primary central nervous system (CNS) lymphoma. Cerebrospinal fluid (CSF) exam confirms a diagnosis of large B-cell lymphoma. There is no evidence of disease outside of the CNS on staging imaging. The most appropriate initial therapy for this patient is as follows:

A. Radiation therapy concurrent with temozolomide
B. High-dose methotrexate-based chemotherapy
C. Whole-brain radiation therapy (WBRT)
D. Rituximab, cyclophosphamide, doxorubicin, vincristine, and prednisone (R-CHOP)

5. A 42-year-old woman with a history of stage II ER-negative, HER2/neu-positive breast cancer diagnosed 5 years previously is brought to the emergency room after a seizure witnessed by her family members. MRI reveals the presence of a right temporal lobe mass with surrounding vasogenic edema, concerning for a neoplastic process. CT

of chest/abdomen/pelvis to complete her staging shows several liver metastases. Biopsy of a liver lesion confirms the diagnosis of recurrent HER2/neu-positive breast cancer. In addition to urgent administration of steroids, what is the most appropriate initial treatment for her solitary brain metastasis?

A. Surgical resection
B. Whole-brain radiation therapy (WBRT)
C. Lapatinib
D. Intrathecal chemotherapy

ANSWERS

1. **B. IDH mutated tumors have a superior prognosis.** IDH mutated anaplastic astrocytomas have superior outcomes compared to those without mutations. Additional molecular markers that have been associated with improved prognosis include methylation of the methylguanine methyltransferase (MGMT) promoter as well as codeletion of 1p/19q.

2. **A. MGMT promoter hypermethylation predicts benefit from temozolomide therapy.** MGMT promoter hypermethylation in patients with glioblastoma predicts benefit from temozolomide therapy. MGMT promoter hypermethylation also portends a better prognosis regardless of treatment received. The addition of bevacizumab to standard chemoradiotherapy following optimal surgical debulking of glioblastoma has not been shown to improve overall survival and, therefore, is not recommended in this setting. Finally, temozolomide plus radiation therapy has been demonstrated to be superior to radiation therapy alone following maximum surgical debulking in glioblastoma.

3. **C. Continue with adjuvant postradiation temozolomide as previously planned.** The scenario described in this question may represent pseudo-progression, which is a common imaging finding in patients who have just received radiation plus temozolomide for treatment of glioblastoma.

4. **B. High-dose methotrexate-based chemotherapy.** High-dose methotrexate-based chemotherapy is the recommended treatment for primary CNS lymphoma. Evidence supports combination therapy. While R-CHOP is most commonly used for the treatment of systemic diffuse large B-cell lymphoma (DLBCL), it does not penetrate the CNS well and is not recommended as treatment for lymphoma arising in the CNS. Radiation plus temozolomide is the appropriate treatment for glioblastoma following maximum surgical debulking. WBRT may be used to treat recurrent primary CNS lymphoma; however, it is not recommended initially due to shorter survival and risk of neurocognitive injury.

5. **A. Surgical resection.** In the case of solitary brain metastasis, surgical resection of the lesion is the preferred approach. Resection followed by WBRT has been demonstrated to result in superior survival over WBRT alone. If the postoperative tumor bed is <3 cm, resection would typically be followed by stereotactic radiosurgery (SRS). SRS as the initial approach could also be appropriate. While lapatinib may have some penetration into the central nervous system (CNS), use of systemic therapy alone is not appropriate in this scenario.

Cervical, Vulvar, and Vaginal Cancers

Kari E. Hacker and Karen McLean

ETIOLOGY AND RISK FACTORS

1. **What are risk factors for cervical cancer?**
   - Human papillomavirus (HPV) is associated with 99% of cases. The most common HPV viral types associated with cervical cancer are 16 and 18, and the two viral types most frequently associated with genital warts are 6 and 11.
   - Highest rates are among Latin American, African American, and Native American women. More common in lower socioeconomic and education classes that have lower rates of Pap screening.
   - Smoking, male partners with multiple sex partners, HIV, immunosuppression, and oral contraceptive use increase the risk.

2. **What are risk factors for vulvar or vaginal cancer?**
   - The majority (80%) of vulvar lesions are associated with HPV 16.
   - Other risk factors include chronic inflammation, prior history of cervical cancer, immunodeficiency, and tobacco use.
   - Bimodal distribution of vulvar cancer: disease is HPV-associated in young women, while it is associated with lichen sclerosis in older women.
   - Diethylstilbestrol (DES) exposure in utero increases the risk of vaginal clear cell carcinoma 50-fold.

STAGING

1. **How is cervical cancer staged using International Federation of Gynecology and Obstetrics (FIGO) staging?**

Stage	Description
IA	Confined to the cervix, microscopic disease
IB	Confined to the cervix, macroscopic disease
IIA	Invasion beyond cervix, but not to pelvic wall or lower third of vaginal wall
IIB	Invasion beyond cervix, with parametrial involvement
III	Extension to pelvic wall, lower third of vagina, or causing hydronephrosis
IVA	Extension to adjacent organs (bowel or bladder)
IVB	Distant metastasis

2. **What information is used to assign a FIGO stage for cervical cancer?**
   - FIGO (international standard) cervical cancer staging is based on clinical exam rather than surgical staging due to a disproportionate prevalence in developing countries and nonoperative management for advanced-stage disease. There is also a less commonly used American Joint Committee on Cancer (AJCC) surgical staging system.

3. **How is vulvar cancer staged (FIGO staging)?**

Stage	Description
0	Carcinoma in situ
IA	Tumor confined to vulva or perineum, stromal invasion <1 mm, inguinal/groin nodes negative
IB	Tumor confined to vulva or perineum, stromal invasion >1 mm, inguinal/groin nodes negative
II	Tumor extends to adjacent perineal structures (anus, lower one third of urethra or vagina), inguinal/groin nodes negative
III	Tumor may or may not extend to adjacent perineal structures (anus, lower one third of urethra or vagina), inguinal/groin nodes positive
IVA	Tumor invades upper two thirds of urethra or vagina, bladder or rectal mucosa, or fixed to pelvic bone, or fixed or ulcerated inguinofemoral lymph nodes
IVB	Distant metastatic disease (including pelvic lymph nodes)

SIGNS AND SYMPTOMS

1. **What are the most common presentations of cervical cancer?**
   - Vaginal bleeding or discharge, including postcoital bleeding
   - Hematuria or rectal bleeding
   - Lumbosacral or leg pain and edema with locally advanced disease

2. **What are the common signs and symptoms of vulvar malignancies?**
   - Pruritus (45%), mass (45%), pain, ulceration, and bleeding

DIAGNOSTIC WORKUP

1. **What is the workup for suspected cervical cancer?**
   - Initial workup focuses on obtaining diagnostic tissue biopsy and includes bimanual pelvic and rectal exam, Pap test, colposcopy and biopsy, and cervical conization.
   - Workup for metastatic disease can include chest x-ray (CXR), CT scan, MRI, or fluorodeoxyglucose (FDG)-PET. Imaging is optional for stage IB1 and smaller tumors.
   - Cystoscopy and sigmoidoscopy are indicated for suspected bladder or rectal involvement, respectively.

2. What is the most common histologic type of cervical cancer?

- Eighty percent are squamous cell carcinomas.
- Twenty percent are adenocarcinoma or adenosquamous, originating in the squamous–columnar junction or transformation zone of the cervix.

3. How is vulvar cancer diagnosed?

- Tissue biopsy including surrounding skin, dermis, and underlying connective tissue.

4. What are the common histologies of vulvar malignancies?

- Ninety percent are squamous cell carcinomas.
- Melanoma is the second most common vulvar malignancy.
- Adenocarcinomas represent less than 10% of primary vulvar malignancies.
- Paget disease is a rare intraepithelial lesion accounting for 1% to 5% of lesions and can be associated with underlying adenocarcinoma of another primary site (15%–35%).

5. What histologies are associated with vaginal cancers?

- Eighty percent to 90% have squamous cell histology.
- Clear cell carcinoma is associated with in utero DES exposure.
- Adenocarcinomas, melanomas, and sarcomas can also be present.

PROGNOSTIC FACTORS

1. What factors influence prognosis of cervical cancer?

- Poor prognostic factors include para-aortic and/or pelvic lymph node involvement, larger primary tumor size, younger age, advanced stage, and uterine invasion.

TREATMENT

1. How is cervical cancer treated?

Stage	Treatment
Preinvasive dysplasia	Local therapy by one of the following methods: electrocautery, cryotherapy, laser, or surgical excision by LEEP or cervical conization
I, IIA	Surgery: radical hysterectomy,* parametrectomy, upper vaginectomy, and lymphadenectomy
IIB, III, IVA	Radiation (external beam plus brachytherapy) with concurrent radiosensitizing chemotherapy (usually cisplatin)
IVB	Palliative systemic chemotherapy ± tumor-directed radiation therapy

*Stage IA1 disease with microinvasion (<3 mm) can be managed with cervical conization for fertility preservation or simple hysterectomy alone if future fertility is not desired. Select cases of IA2 and IB1 disease can be managed with radical trachelectomy (removal of the cervix) for fertility preservation.

LEEP, loop electrosurgical excision procedure.

2. **How is vulvar cancer treated?**

Stage	Treatment
Preinvasive dysplasia	Local therapy by one of the following methods: wide local excision, carbon dioxide laser photoablation, or topical therapy*
IA	Surgery: radical hemivulvectomy, no lymphadenectomy
IB	Surgery: radical hemivulvectomy + lymphadenectomy
II, III, IVA	Either: a. Neoadjuvant radiation with 5-FU and/or cisplatin chemosensitization followed by surgical resection if persistent disease or: b. Radical surgical resection
IVB	Palliative systemic chemotherapy ± tumor-directed radiation therapy

*5-FU and imiquimod can be used off-label for treatment of high-grade vulvar dysplasia.
5-FU, 5-fluorouracil.

3. **What is the role of palliative chemotherapy in advanced cervical cancer?**
   - Recommended first-line treatment for metastatic or recurrent cervical cancer is cisplatin, paclitaxel, and bevacizumab.
   - Platinum doublets modestly improve response rates over single-agent therapy.
   - Active agents include cisplatin, ifosfamide, and paclitaxel.
   - Most agents have only brief responses.

4. **How is vulvar cancer staged and treated?**
   - Surgical staging.
   - See earlier table for stage-based treatment.

5. **What treatment modalities are used to treat vaginal cancers?**
   - Radiation (external beam radiotherapy and/or brachytherapy). Consider chemosensitization with 5-fluorouracil (5-FU) or cisplatin based on experience with other lower genital tract malignancies.
   - Surgery is used in select stage I cases.
   - No clear role for systemic chemotherapy alone in up-front treatment.

SPECIAL CONSIDERATIONS
1. **Prevention: What agents are available to decrease cervical cancer risk?**
   - There are three Food and Drug Administration (FDA)-approved HPV vaccines: a quadrivalent vaccine Gardasil (against HPV strains 6, 11, 16, 18), a bivalent vaccine Cervarix (against HPV strains 16 and 18), and a nonavalent vaccine Gardasil 9 (against HPV strains 6, 11, 16, 18, 31, 33, 45, 52, 58).

- HPV vaccination is recommended for females aged 9 to 26 and males aged 9 to 21. High-risk males may receive the vaccine up to age 26.

2. Screening: What are the current American Society for Colposcopy and Cervical Pathology/American Society for Clinical Pathology (ASCCP/ASCP) screening guidelines for cervical cancer?

Age	Screening Method	Interval
<21	No screening	
21–29	Cytology alone	3 yrs
30–65	Cytology and HPV cotesting (preferred)	5 yrs
	Cytology alone (acceptable)	3 yrs
>65	No screening*	
After hysterectomy	No screening*	
HPV-vaccinated	Follow age-specific recommendations	

*Screening should be continued in these groups if there is a history of moderate dysplasia (CIN2) or more severe cervical pathology diagnosis.

Although the Food and Drug Administration has approved an HPV-alone screening test, the ASCCP has not yet recommended this approach for cervical cancer screening.

QUESTIONS

1. It is recommended that a human papillomavirus (HPV) vaccine series be administered to which of the following patient populations:
   A. Only males 9 to 21 years old
   B. Only females 9 to 26 years old
   C. All sexually active women
   D. Males 9 to 21 years old and females 9 to 26 years old
   E. It is not recommended as routine vaccination for any patients

2. A 32-year-old woman presents with stage IVB squamous cell carcinoma of the cervix. Preferred first-line treatment is:
   A. Chemotherapy with cisplatin, paclitaxel, and bevacizumab
   B. Surgery with radical hysterectomy (uterus, cervix, parametrium, and upper vagina)
   C. Pelvic radiation with chemosensitization
   D. Surgery with simple hysterectomy (uterus and cervix only)

3. A 65-year-old woman presents with a left-sided vulvar lesion that extends to within 5 mm of the midline and biopsy reveals squamous cell carcinoma of the vulva with a depth of invasion of 1.5 mm. Recommended treatment is:
   A. Radiation therapy to the vulva
   B. Systemic chemotherapy with cisplatin and paclitaxel
   C. Surgery with radical vulvectomy
   D. Surgery with radical vulvectomy with inguinal lymphadenectomy

4. The majority of cervical cancer worldwide is believed to be secondary to infection with which strains of the human papillomavirus (HPV)?
   A. HPV 6 and 11
   B. HPV 16 and 18
   C. HPV 34 and 36
   D. HPV 56 and 62

5. Patients exposed to diethylstilbestrol (DES) in utero are 50 times more likely to develop which of the following lower genital tract malignancies?
   A. Squamous cell carcinoma of the cervix
   B. Clear cell adenocarcinoma of the vagina
   C. Paget disease of the vulva
   D. Squamous cell carcinoma of the vagina

6. Vulvar dysplasia may be treated with:
   A. Surgical resection
   B. Laser ablation
   C. Topical treatment with imiquimod
   D. All of the above

ANSWERS

1. **D. Males 9 to 21 years old and females 9 to 26 years old.** The Centers for Disease Control and Prevention recommends that an HPV vaccine series (consisting of three shots) be administered to males aged 9 to 21 and females aged 9 to 26 years. The preferred age for vaccination is 11 or 12 years old. Males who are at high risk for HPV infection (homosexual, immunosuppressed) should receive a vaccination series up to age 26 if they have not been previously vaccinated.

2. **A. Chemotherapy with cisplatin, paclitaxel, and bevacizumab.** Systemic chemotherapy with cisplatin, paclitaxel, and bevacizumab has been shown to result in improved overall survival, progression-free survival, and overall response rate when compared to cisplatin and paclitaxel alone in patients with metastatic or recurrent cervical cancer. Patients with micro-invasive cervical squamous cell cancer (stage IA1) are recommended to undergo a simple hysterectomy.

3. **D. Surgery with radical vulvectomy with inguinal lymphadenectomy.** Patients with squamous cell carcinoma of the vulva confined to the vulva/perineum should undergo surgical resection with radical vulvectomy. Inguinal lymphadenectomy by either sentinel lymph node dissection or full lymphadenectomy is recommended if the depth of invasion of the primary lesion is greater than 1 mm. If the tumor extends to adjacent structures such as the urethra or anus, primary radiation therapy with chemosensitization can be considered rather than resection. Systemic chemotherapy is reserved for patients with recurrent or metastatic disease.

4. **B. HPV 16 and 18.** While HPV 6 and 11 are responsible for the majority of genital and anal warts, HPV 16 and 18 are believed to be associated with ~70% of cases of cervical cancer. In addition to cervical cancer, HPV infection is believed to be responsible for 90% of anal cancers; 71% of vulvar, vaginal, or penile cancers; and 72% of oropharyngeal cancers.

5. **B. Clear cell adenocarcinoma of the vagina.** In utero exposure to DES increases a patient's risk for clear cell adenocarcinoma of the vagina but not any other lower genital tract malignancies. Most of these cancers are diagnosed in patients in their late teens through their 20s.

6. **D. All of the above.** All of these treatments are valid options for patients with preinvasive vulvar lesions. Topical treatments are currently not Food and Drug Administration (FDA)-approved but a systematic review showed that clinical response rates are as high as 50%.

Ovarian Cancer

Lan G. Coffman and Ronald J. Buckanovich

ETIOLOGY AND RISK FACTORS

1. **What are the risk factors?**
   - Older age
   - Personal or family history of breast or ovarian cancer
   - Early menarche and late menopause
   - Nulliparity, infertility, or age over 35 at first birth

2. **What factors are protective?**
   - Salpingo-oophorectomy
   - Multiparity
   - Use of oral contraceptives for 5 years
   - Lactation

3. **Do hereditary factors play a role in ovarian cancer?**
   - Up to 15% to 20% of ovarian cancer has been associated with germline mutations, mainly in genes related to DNA repair including *BRCA1* and *BRCA2*
   - Genetic evaluation is recommended for all women with a personal history of ovarian cancer
   - Hereditary breast and ovarian cancer syndrome
     - *BRCA1* and *BRCA2* are tumor suppressor genes that are involved in DNA repair
     - Founder mutations in *BRCA1* and *BRCA2* are found in 2.5% of Ashkenazi Jewish women
     - Inherited in an autosomal dominant fashion
     - Risk-reducing bilateral salpingo-oophorectomy is recommended by 35 to 40 years of age or upon completion of childbearing
     - *BRCA1*
       - Located on chromosome 17q
       - Mutation confers lifetime risk of ovarian cancer of 16% to 44%
     - *BRCA2*
       - Located on chromosome 13q
       - Mutation confers lifetime risk of ovarian cancer of 20%

- Hereditary nonpolyposis colorectal cancer (HNPCC or Lynch syndrome)
  - Caused by a mutation in one of the DNA mismatch repair genes (*MSH2*, *MLH1*, and *PMS2*)
  - Increased risk for colon cancer, breast cancer (lobular), endometrial cancer, and ovarian cancer (generally endometrioid histology)
  - Mutation confers lifetime risk of ovarian cancer of about 5%

MOLECULAR MECHANISM AND CELL OF ORIGIN

- Ovarian cancer is associated with high rates of mutations in DNA repair pathways.
- Controversy exists regarding the true cell of origin. However, recent evidence suggests that many tumors start in the fallopian tube epithelium.
- Primary peritoneal, fallopian tube, and high-grade serous ovarian epithelial cancers are considered to be similar diseases, perhaps sharing the same cell of origin, and are clinically treated as the same entity.
- Serous tubal intraepithelial lesions found within the fallopian tube are a possible precursor lesion giving rise to primary peritoneal, fallopian tube, and ovarian epithelial cancer.

SCREENING

1. **Who should be screened for ovarian cancer?**
   - Screening is not recommended for the general population although there are ongoing trials to address this question.
   - Screening may be considered for high-risk populations.
     - Women with positive family history (increases risk by two- to threefold)
     - Women with known BRCA or HNPCC (Lynch syndrome) mutations

2. **How is ovarian cancer screening accomplished?**
   - Regular CA-125 measurement and transvaginal ultrasounds using an algorithm such as the ROCA (risk of ovarian cancer algorithm)

3. **How can ovarian cancer be prevented?**
   - Prophylactic salpingo-oophorectomy is the most effective means of preventing ovarian cancer reducing the risk by 80%.

PATHOLOGY

- "Epithelial" ovarian cancer (EOC) comprises 90% of ovarian tumors.
  - The most common is papillary serous (70%), followed by endometrioid, clear cell, mucinous, transitional cell, or carcinosarcoma (malignant mixed Müllerian tumor).
  - Clear cell is the most aggressive subtype (always grade 3).
- The remaining subtypes include:
  - Metastatic from breast, colorectal, or gastric primary (Krukenberg tumor)

o Sex cord–stromal tumors:
  ▪ Granulosa cell tumors
  ▪ Inhibin A and B levels are tumor markers
  ▪ Sertoli–Leydig
  ▪ Testosterone is a tumor marker
o Germ-cell tumors:
  ▪ Monitor beta-human chorionic gonadotropin (beta-HCG), alpha-fetopro-tein, and lactate dehydrogenase (LDH) levels
  ▪ Treated similarly to germ-cell tumors of the testes in men

SIGNS AND SYMPTOMS

1. What are the signs and symptoms of ovarian cancer?

- Symptoms include abdominal/pelvic pain, bloating, increased abdominal girth, early satiety, urinary urgency or frequency.
- Signs on physical exam include adnexal mass, ascites, umbilical lymph node (Sister Mary Joseph nodule), and pleural effusion.
- Adnexal masses:
  o In premenopausal women, approximately 5% of adnexal masses are ovarian cancer.
  o In postmenopausal women, approximately 30% of adnexal masses are ovarian cancer.
- Paraneoplastic syndromes:
  o Trousseau syndrome (thrombosis)
  o Cerebellar degeneration (anti-Yo antibodies in cerebrospinal fluid [CSF])
  o Dermatomyositis (rash and elevated creatinine kinase)
  o Leser–Trelat syndrome (seborrheic keratoses)
  o Palmar fasciitis

DIAGNOSIS

1. What tests should be ordered?

- History and physical, routine lab work, and CA-125
- Alpha-fetoprotein and beta-HCG in patients under 30 years old to rule out germ-cell tumor
- Ultrasound or CT scan of abdomen and pelvis
- Chest imaging

2. What type of surgery is indicated?

- Laparotomy, total abdominal hysterectomy, bilateral salpingo-oophorectomy with comprehensive staging are indicated for all patients.
- Unilateral salpingo-oophorectomy is indicated for stage I if fertility is desired.
- Referral to experienced gynecologic oncologist is critical.

- Patients who had an ovarian cancer removed but did not have adequate staging should be referred to a gynecologic oncologist for consideration of completion staging operation.

3. **Which patients should have a debulking operation?**
   - Cytoreductive surgery is indicated for all stages of disease, including stage IV disease if possible.
   - Goal of cytoreductive surgery is to reduce disease down to <1 cm, which implies "optimally debulked."
   - Smaller amount of residual disease is associated with longer survival.

PROGNOSTIC FACTORS

1. **Aside from stage, what are favorable prognostic factors?**
   - Age less than 65
   - Good performance status
   - Nonclear cell histology
   - *BRCA* mutation

STAGING

1. **How are the tumor, node, and metastasis (TNM) and International Federation of Gynecology and Obstetrics (FIGO) stages for ovary, fallopian tube, and primary peritoneal cancer defined?**

TNM	FIGO Stage	
T1	I	Tumor limited to ovaries or fallopian tubes (one or both)
T1a	IA	Tumor limited to one ovary (capsule intact) or fallopian tube; no tumor on ovarian or fallopian tube surface. No malignant cells in ascites or peritoneal washings
T1b	IB	Tumor limited to both ovaries (capsules intact) or fallopian tubes. No tumor on ovarian or fallopian tube surface. No malignant cells in ascites or peritoneal washings
T1c	IC	Tumor limited to one or both ovaries or fallopian tubes with any of the following: surgical spill (T1c1), capsule ruptured, tumor on ovarian or fallopian tube surface (T1c2), malignant cells in ascites or peritoneal washings (T1c3)
T2	II	Tumor involves one or both ovaries or fallopian tubes with pelvic extension or primary peritoneal cancer
T2a	IIA	Extension to and/or implants on uterus and/or tube(s) and/or ovaries

(continued)

(continued)

TNM	FIGO Stage	
T2b	IIB	Extension to and/or implants on other pelvic intraperitoneal tissues
T3	III	Tumor involves one or both ovaries or fallopian tubes or primary peritoneal cancer with cytologically or histologically confirmed spread to the peritoneum outside the pelvis and/or metastasis to the retroperitoneal lymph nodes
T3 N1	IIIA1	Positive retroperitoneal lymph nodes only
T3a2-N0/N1	IIIA2	Microscopic extrapelvic peritoneal involvement ± positive retroperitoneal lymph nodes
T3b-N0/N1	IIIB	Macroscopic peritoneal metastasis beyond pelvis ≤2 cm in greatest dimension ± positive retroperitoneal lymph nodes
T3c-N0/N1	IIIC	Peritoneal metastasis beyond pelvis >2 cm in greatest dimension and/or regional lymph node metastasis ± positive retroperitoneal lymph nodes
Any T, any N, M1	IV	Distant metastasis excluding peritoneal metastasis
	IVA	Pleural effusion with positive cytology
	IVB	Parenchymal metastases and metastases to extra-abdominal organs (including inguinal lymph nodes and lymph nodes outside of the abdominal cavity)

2. What is the most common stage at the time of diagnosis?

- Seventy percent are diagnosed at stage III or IV.

TREATMENT

First-Line Therapy

1. What is the treatment of patients with early-stage EOC?

- For early-stage disease (stage I), the 5-year survival rate is 93%.
- Surgery alone is the treatment for patients with stage IA or IB with low-grade (grade 1) tumors. No chemotherapy is indicated.
- For high-risk early stage (stage IA or B grade 2–3, or stage IC), surgery and three to six cycles of intravenous (IV) carboplatin with taxane are indicated.

2. What is the standard first-line treatment for patients with advanced EOC?

- In general, surgical debulking followed by treatment with six cycles of platinum and taxane combination is the standard of care.
- Intraperitoneal (IP) chemotherapy is recommended for stage III patients who are optimally debulked (<1 cm of residual disease) and fit. IP chemotherapy conveys a survival advantage of about 16 months compared to standard IV therapy. IP chemotherapy can be considered in stage II disease.

- Dose-dense paclitaxel and carboplatin has a demonstrated survival benefit over standard IV chemotherapy in women with suboptimal, non-clear-cell histology.
- Chemotherapy regimens include:
  - IV paclitaxel day 1, IP cisplatin day 2 with IP paclitaxel day 8 every 3 weeks × six cycles
  - IV paclitaxel and IV carboplatin every 3 weeks × six cycles
  - IV docetaxel and IV carboplatin every 3 weeks × six cycles
  - Dose-dense paclitaxel on days 1, 8, and 15; and IV carboplatin every 3 weeks × six cycles
- Bevacizumab, a monoclonal antivascular endothelial growth factor antibody, in the adjuvant setting has been shown to increase progression-free survival, and may improve survival in a subset of patients with poor-prognosis disease, but is not currently approved for adjuvant therapy in the United States.

3. Is there any role for neoadjuvant chemotherapy?
- Yes, for patients who are not surgical candidates or those who are not surgical candidates at the time of diagnosis
- Patients who receive neoadjuvant therapy still benefit from interval debulking.

4. Is there any role for maintenance chemotherapy after complete response?
- Maintenance paclitaxel has been shown to increase progression-free survival, but has not shown a benefit in overall survival.

5. What are treatment options for elderly patients with poor performance status?
- Low-dose weekly chemotherapy with single agent carboplatin or in combination with paclitaxel

6. How should patients who had complete response to their primary therapy be monitored?
- Patients with early-stage disease who had fertility-preserving surgery should be monitored by ultrasound and should consider completion surgery after childbearing is finished.
- Patients with stage I to IV disease should be monitored with regular office visits, including pelvic exams and CA-125 measurement if initially elevated. CT imaging should only be pursued if there is a clinical indication (rising CA-125, concerning exam, or new symptoms).
- Frequency is every 2 to 4 months for the first 2 years, then 3 to 6 months for 3 years, and then annually after 5 years.
- All women with a diagnosis of ovarian cancer should be referred for genetic counseling per National Comprehensive Cancer Network (NCCN) guidelines.

7. What are borderline ovarian tumors and how are they treated?
- Tumors with malignant cytological features but low malignant potential and noninvasive
- Treated surgically with no role for chemotherapy (even in stage III disease)

8. **How are nonepithelial ovarian cancers treated?**
   - Sex cord–stromal tumors:
     - Surgery followed by bleomycin, etoposide, and cisplatin for stages IB to IV
     - Surgery followed by radiation for limited-stage disease
   - Germ-cell tumors:
     - Surgical resection, followed by chemotherapy (3–4 cycles of bleomycin, etoposide, and cisplatin) for the following subtypes:
       - Dysgerminoma (stages II–IV)
       - Embryonal or endodermal sinus tumor (any stage)
       - Immature teratoma (stage I: grades 2–3, and stages II–IV)
     - After surgery, observation alone is sufficient for stage I dysgerminoma and low-grade stage I immature teratoma.

Refractory and Resistant Disease

1. **How are the terms refractory and recurrent defined?**
   - Platinum refractory disease is defined as progression or persistent disease while receiving primary platinum-based therapy.
   - Platinum resistant disease is defined as achievement of a complete remission with relapse in <6 months after completion of primary platinum-based therapy.
   - Platinum-sensitive disease is defined as the achievement of a complete clinical remission with relapse more than 6 months after primary platinum-based therapy.

2. **How is platinum refractory or platinum-resistant disease treated?**
   - Single-agent palliative chemotherapy with non-platinum-based agent such as gemcitabine, liposomal doxorubicin, topotecan, oral etoposide, or weekly taxane therapy. All have equal efficacy and choice is based on best side-effect profile for the patient.
   - Bevacizumab as a single agent or in combination with chemotherapy (cyclophosphamide or weekly paclitaxel)
   - Olaparib, a poly ADP ribose polymerase (PARP) inhibitor, has recently been approved for treatment of ovarian cancer in women with *BRCA* mutations who have had three previous lines of therapy.
     - PARP inhibitors work through inducing "synthetic lethality" by inhibiting DNA repair mechanisms in cells that already have impaired DNA damage repair due to *BRCA* mutations
     - Olaparib has demonstrated progression-free survival benefit without overall survival benefit to date
   - Best supportive care

3. **How is recurrent platinum-sensitive disease treated?**
   - Consider secondary cytoreductive surgery if:
     - Recurrence >1 year after completion of therapy
     - Isolated site of recurrence
     - No ascites on imaging

- First recurrence treated with platinum-based therapy, generally carboplatin and paclitaxel. Can consider carboplatin with liposomal doxorubicin, docetaxel, or gemcitabine if significant neuropathy.
- Second recurrence treated with platinum-based chemotherapy with carboplatin or cisplatin, either as single agent or in combination with another agent as mentioned earlier.
- Bevacizumab as a single agent or in combination with chemotherapy.

QUESTIONS

1. A 63-year-old woman presents with abdominal pain and bloating. Abdominal ultrasound demonstrates a complex adnexal mass and ascites. She undergoes a total abdominal hysterectomy, bilateral salpingo-oophorectomy, lymphadenectomy, and omental biopsies, which demonstrate bilateral ovarian tumors with lymph node involvement, omental caking, and ascites. Tumor was debulked to less than 1 cm of residual disease. Pathology demonstrates high-grade serous adenocarcinoma. She has recovered well from surgery and has no significant comorbidities. What is the next best step in treatment?
   A. Observation
   B. Adjuvant hormonal therapy with an aromatase inhibitor for 5 years
   C. Intravenous carboplatin and paclitaxel every 3 weeks for six cycles
   D. Intravenous paclitaxel on day 1, intraperitoneal cisplatin on day 2, and intraperitoneal paclitaxel on day 8 of a 21-day cycle for six cycles
   E. Intravenous carboplatin and docetaxel every 3 weeks for six cycles

2. A 24-year-old woman is diagnosed with a right ovary yolk sac tumor with ovary capsule rupture. Post operative alpha-fetoprotein is 500. CT imaging of the chest, abdomen, and pelvis are without evidence of disease. What is the best next step in treatment?
   A. Completion staging with a total abdominal hysterectomy, bilateral salpingectomy, left oophorectomy, and lymphadenectomy
   B. Intravenous carboplatin and paclitaxel every 3 weeks for six cycles
   C. Intravenous cisplatin and etoposide every 3 weeks with weekly bleomycin for three or four cycles
   D. Observation
   E. Intravenous paclitaxel on day 1, intraperitoneal cisplatin on day 2 and intraperitoneal paclitaxel on day 8 of a 21-day cycle for six cycles

3. A 42-year-old woman presents with a pelvic mass. Surgical staging demonstrates a 5 cm ovarian mass with capsular rupture and multiple peritoneal implants without evidence of invasion. She is optimally debulked with less than 1 cm of residual disease. Pathology demonstrates an epithelial serous ovarian tumor of low malignant potential. The patient recovers well from surgery and presents to discuss adjuvant treatment options. Which of the following is the best next step?
   A. Adjuvant intravenous carboplatin and paclitaxel for three to six cycles
   B. Intravenous paclitaxel on day 1, intraperitoneal cisplatin on day 2, and intraperitoneal paclitaxel on day 8 of a 21-day cycle for six cycles

C. Observation
D. Intravenous carboplatin and paclitaxel with Avastin every 3 weeks for six cycles followed by 6 months of Avastin maintenance therapy
E. Initiate Olaparib at 400 mg daily

4. A 65-year-old woman with a history of high grade serous adenocarcinoma of the fallopian tube treated with surgical debulking and adjuvant carboplatin/paclitaxel therapy for six cycles, completed 18 months ago, presents with pelvic pain. CT imaging demonstrates a localized pelvic mass but no other evidence of disease. CA-125 is 1,060. She otherwise feels well without significant comorbidities or functional limitations. What is the best next step in treatment to maximize overall survival?
   A. Surgical debulking followed by intravenous carboplatin and paclitaxel every 3 weeks for six cycles
   B. Intravenous Doxil every 4 weeks for six cycles
   C. Aromatase inhibitor therapy
   D. Intravenous carboplatin and paclitaxel every 3 weeks for six cycles
   E. Recommend hospice referral

5. A 52-year-old woman with recurrent high-grade serous ovarian cancer presents with abdominal pain and bloating with a rising CA-125 2 months after completion of six cycles of intravenous carboplatin and paclitaxel. CT scan confirms recurrent disease. She has a good performance status and wants to pursue additional therapy. What is an appropriate next step in therapy?
   A. Intravenous Doxil every 4 weeks
   B. Restart intravenous carboplatin and paclitaxel every 3 weeks
   C. Restart intravenous carboplatin and paclitaxel every 3 weeks with the addition of Avastin
   D. Secondary surgical debulking
   E. Intravenous carboplatin and docetaxel every 3 weeks

6. A 49-year-old woman presents for follow-up. She was diagnosed at age 43 with high-grade serous adenocarcinoma of the ovary and has had multiple recurrences. She is currently undergoing treatment with her third line of chemotherapy. She denies a family history of breast or ovarian cancer. Which of the following is correct?
   A. BRCA1/2 testing is not indicated as it will not affect the management of her disease
   B. National Comprehensive Cancer Network (NCCN) guidelines recommend genetic testing given her personal history of ovarian cancer
   C. *BRCA1/2* mutations are negative prognostic factors in ovarian cancer
   D. Germline heterozygous *BRCA2* mutations convey a higher risk for developing ovarian cancer at a younger age compared to *BRCA1* mutations

ANSWERS

1. **D. Intravenous paclitaxel on day 1, intraperitoneal cisplatin on day 2, and intraperitoneal paclitaxel on day 8 of a 21-day cycle for six cycles.** In women with stage III "optimally debulked" (<1 cm of residual disease) high-grade epithelial ovarian cancer who are otherwise fit, intraperitoneal chemotherapy is recommended based on overall survival benefit of 16 months demonstrated in GOG172 compared to standard platinum-based intravenous therapy (1).

2. **C. Intravenous cisplatin and etoposide every 3 weeks with weekly bleomycin for three or four cycles.** Germ-cell tumors of the ovary are treated similarly to germ-cell tumors of the testes. In yolk sac tumors, which are a poor risk germ-cell tumor, adjuvant chemotherapy with bleomycin, cisplatin, and etoposide is indicated for even early-stage, resected disease.

3. **C. Observation.** Ovarian epithelial tumors of low malignant potential, also known as borderline tumors, are noninvasive tumors and treatment is with surgical resection. Chemotherapy is not indicated even with advanced-stage disease.

4. **A. Surgical debulking followed by intravenous carboplatin and paclitaxel every 3 weeks for six cycles.** In patients with a disease-free interval of >6 months and localized disease, secondary cytoreductive surgery where complete cytoreduction is achieved conveys a survival benefit (2). Patients most likely to benefit from secondary debulking have recurrence >1 year from completion of chemotherapy, localized disease, and no ascites. Further, ovarian cancer that has recurred >6 months following completion of last platinum therapy is considered platinum-sensitive and these patients should receive platinum-based chemotherapy after cytoreductive surgery.

5. **A. Intravenous Doxil every 4 weeks.** Ovarian cancer that recurs within 6 months of previous platinum therapy is considered platinum-resistant. Therefore further platinum-based chemotherapy is not warranted. Doxil is an active therapeutic option in women with platinum-resistant ovarian cancer.

6. **B. National Comprehensive Cancer Network (NCCN) guidelines recommend genetic testing given her personal history of ovarian cancer.** NCCN recommend genetic testing for all women diagnosed with ovarian cancer, regardless of family history. Olaparib, a poly ADP ribose polymerase (PARP) inhibitor, has recently been approved by the Food and Drug Administration (FDA) for the treatment of recurrent ovarian cancer in women with germline *BRCA1/2* mutations. Therefore mutational status may affect this patient's treatment options. *BRCA1/2* mutations are associated with a better prognosis and are predictive of response to platinum therapy. *BRCA1* mutations convey a higher risk of earlier onset ovarian cancer compared to *BRCA2* mutations.

REFERENCES

1. Armstrong DK, Bundy B, Wenzel L, et al. Intraperitoneal cisplatin and paclitaxel in ovarian cancer. *N Engl J Med*. 2006;354(1):34–43.
2. Bristow RE, Zahurak ML, Diaz-Montes TP, et al. Impact of surgeon and hospital ovarian cancer surgical case volume on in-hospital mortality and related short-term outcomes. *Gynecol Oncol*. 2009;115(3):334–338.

35

Endometrial Cancer

Lan G. Coffman and Ronald J. Buckanovich

EPIDEMIOLOGY

- Mortality—2 × higher in African Americans than in Whites.
  - Likely due to increased incidence of aggressive subtypes and issues of access to health care

ETIOLOGY AND RISK FACTORS

1. **What are the most common risk factors for developing endometrial cancer?**
   - Age
   - Hypertension
   - Diabetes
   - Endogenous estrogen excess:
     - Obesity
     - Polycystic ovary disease and chronic anovulation
     - Estrogen-secreting tumors of the ovary (such as granulosa cell tumors)
     - Liver disease
   - Exogenous unopposed estrogen sources:
     - Hormone replacement therapy (HRT)
     - Selective estrogen receptor modulators (SERMs), for example, tamoxifen
   - Site-specific activity stimulates uterine lining.
   - Endogenous prolonged estrogen exposure:
     - Early menarche
     - Late menopause
     - Nulliparity
     - Irregular menses and infertility
   - Genetic syndromes:
     - Hereditary nonpolyposis colorectal cancer (HNPCC), aka Lynch syndrome
       - Lynch syndrome is found at a similar rate in endometrial cancer as colon cancer (~5%).
       - Women with Lynch syndrome have a 40% to 60% lifetime risk of developing endometrial cancer.

■ Screening for genetic mutations associated with Lynch syndrome (such as mismatch repair proteins, ie, MLH1, MSH2, MSH6, PMS2, and microsatellite instability) should be considered in all patients with endometrial cancer, especially in those under 50 or with a significant family history of colon, endometrial, or ovarian cancer.

2. **What are protective factors against developing endometrial cancer?**
   ● Oral contraceptives
     ○ Fifty percent decrease in relative risk if used for 12 months
     ○ Protective effect persists for at least 15 years after cessation of use
   ● Postmenopausal progestin therapy
     ○ Progestin suppresses endometrial proliferation.
   ● Physical activity

3. **When do you worry about endometrial hyperplasia?**
   ● Endometrial hyperplasia is generally considered to be a precursor to endometrial cancer.
   ● Simple endometrial hyperplasia can typically be treated with progestins.
   ● There is a risk of concurrent adenocarcinoma, which was missed at the time of biopsy—mnemonic to remember is **"penny, nickel, dime, quarter"** for 1%, 5%, 10%, and 25% based on simple/complex hyperplasia ± atypia (see the following table).
   ● Unless fertility preservation is desired, patients with complex atypical hyperplasia (CAH) should have a hysterectomy with considerations for staging.

Type of Hyperplasia	Appearance	Risk of Progression (%)	Mnemonic
Simple	Dilated glands with some outpouching, abundant endometrial stroma	1	"Penny"
Complex	Crowded glands, little endometrial stroma, complex gland pattern, and outpouching formations	5	"Nickel"
Simple with atypia	Presence of cytologic atypia (hyperchromatic, enlarged epithelial cells with an increased N:C ratio)	10	"Dime"
Complex with atypia (CAH)		25	"Quarter"

SCREENING AND PREVENTION

● Routine screening is not indicated in asymptomatic women.

- Women with HNPCC can undergo yearly transvaginal ultrasound (TVUS) or endometrial biopsy after age 35 or consider risk-reducing surgery with total abdominal hysterectomy (TAH) and bilateral salpingo-oophorectomy (BSO) after completion of childbearing.
- Women taking tamoxifen should have routine annual gynecologic exams.
- Endometrial biopsy is indicated for any patients with postmenopausal bleeding or spotting.

SIGNS AND SYMPTOMS

1. **What are the most common signs and symptoms of endometrial cancer?**
   - Abnormal vaginal bleeding—seen in 90%
     - Premenopausal women with menorrhagia should undergo endometrial biopsy.
     - All postmenopausal women with vaginal bleeding should be evaluated.
   - Abnormal glandular tissue on Pap smear in asymptomatic women
   - Palpable tumor or fullness palpated on bimanual exam
   - Signs of advanced disease—pain, ascites, bloating, early satiety

STAGING

1. **What are important steps in the pretreatment evaluation?**
   - Physical exam with pelvic exam
   - Tumor markers
     - CA-125 clinically useful for predicting extrauterine spread
   - Radiographic studies
     - Pelvic/abdominal imaging unnecessary if surgical staging planned
     - If necessary, MRI is most sensitive
     - Chest radiograph is standard part of initial assessment
   - Assessment for hereditary cancer syndromes, such as Lynch syndrome

2. **What is the typical approach to surgical staging for endometrial cancer?**
   - Total extrafascial hysterectomy with BSO with pelvic and para-aortic lymph node dissection
     - Biopsy of areas suspicious for metastases
     - Cytoreduction often done when metastases are evident
     - Omentectomy done in event of papillary serous or clear cell histology
   - May be done via abdominal, vaginal, laparoscopic, or robot-assisted approaches

3. **How is endometrial cancer staged?**
   - Endometrial cancer is staged according to the joint 2010 International Federation of Gynecology and Obstetrics (FIGO)/tumor, node, and metastasis (TNM) classification system:

TNM Categories	FIGO Stages	Definition
Primary Tumor (T) (Surgical–Pathologic Findings)		
Tx		Primary tumor cannot be assessed
T0		No evidence of primary tumor
Tis		Carcinoma in situ
T1	I	Tumor confined to corpus uteri
T1a	IA	Tumor limited to endometrium or invades less than one half of the myometrium
T1b	IB	Tumor invades one half or more of the myometrium
T2	II	Tumor invades stromal connective tissue of the cervix, but does not extend beyond uterus
T3a	IIIA	Tumor involves serosa and/or adnexa (direct extension or metastasis)
T3b	IIIB	Vaginal involvement (direct extension or metastasis) or parametrial involvement
T any, N1	IIIC	Metastasis to pelvic and/or para-aortic lymph nodes
T4	IVA	Tumor invades bladder mucosa and/or bowel mucosa (bullous edema is not sufficient to classify a tumor as T4)
T any, N any, M1	IVB	Distant metastasis (includes metastasis to inguinal lymph nodes and intraperitoneal disease)

PATHOLOGY

1. **What are the most common types of endometrial cancer?**
   - Two major classes of endometrial cancer exist:
     - Type I (endometrioid tumors)—80% of cases, estrogen related
     - Type II (papillary serous, clear cell, or carcinosarcoma tumors)—20% of cases, unrelated to estrogen stimulation, but carry much higher risk of metastatic disease
   - Carcinosarcoma of the uterus is a poorly differentiated carcinoma with areas of sarcomatoid differentiation and is treated as a carcinoma rather than a sarcoma

DIAGNOSTIC CRITERIA

1. **How is endometrial cancer diagnosed?**
   - Endometrial biopsy—in-office procedure as initial diagnostic test

- Hysteroscopy with dilation and curettage less common as initial step
  - Performed if initial biopsy negative for malignancy, but high suspicion of cancer still exists (eg, hyperplasia with atypia, persistent bleeding)
- Transvaginal ultrasonography—helpful to distinguish bleeding due to atrophy versus anatomic lesion in postmenopausal women
  - Endometrial thickness <4 to 5 mm has low risk.

PROGNOSTIC FACTORS

1. **What are the major prognostic factors in endometrial cancer?**
   - Stage of disease
   - Grade of tumor (higher is worse)
   - Depth of myometrial invasion (deeper is worse)
   - Tumor extension behind the uterine fundus
   - Histologic type (serous, clear cell, and carcinosarcoma have worse prognosis)
   - Larger tumors of at least 2 cm have worse prognosis
   - Older age
   - Lymphovascular space involvement (LVSI)
   - Lower uterine segment (cervical) involvement
   - Tumor hormone receptor status—(estrogen receptor/progesterone receptor) (ER/PR) positivity associated with longer progression-free survival (PFS)

TREATMENT

1. **Primary treatment is surgical.**
   - TAH/BSO ± lymph node resection
   - Surgery completes staging of disease in addition to therapeutic resection of the cancer.
   - Primary radiation therapy (RT) can be used for patients who are poor surgical candidates.

2. **How do we decide who needs adjuvant treatment?**
   - Stage I disease (confined to the uterus):
     - Consider adjuvant RT in patients with high-risk disease due to two or more of the following:
       - Grade 3 disease
       - more than 50% myometrial invasion
       - LVSI
       - Age >60
   - Stage II disease (tumor involves cervix)
     - Adjuvant RT
   - Stage III disease (tumor extends beyond the uterus)
     - Adjuvant chemotherapy +/− RT

- Serous, clear cell, or carcinosarcoma histology is considered high risk, even in stage I disease. Therefore adjuvant chemotherapy and radiation therapy is warranted regardless of stage (though there is debate on the best approach in stage IA disease).

3. **What type of RT is used?**
   - External beam pelvic RT (45–50 Gy)
   - Vaginal brachytherapy

   Note: Adjuvant RT improves local control, but is not proven to improve survival.

4. **What type of adjuvant chemotherapy is used?**
   - Commonly used combination regimens include:
     - Intravenous paclitaxel + carboplatin for six cycles
     - Intravenous paclitaxel + ifosfamide for six cycles can be considered for carcinosarcoma histology
   - Important considerations:
     - Chemotherapy has shown survival advantage over whole abdominal irradiation.
     - Paclitaxel-containing regimens may improve response, particularly in serous histology.
   - Single-agent therapy options include platinum, doxorubicin, docetaxel, and topotecan.

5. **What is the role of chemoradiation?**
   - Adjuvant RT reduces risk of local recurrence for women with high-risk disease and is often used along with chemotherapy when adjuvant chemotherapy is warranted (see the previous discussion).
   - The ideal sequencing of chemotherapy and RT is unclear.
     - RT can be given before or after completion of chemotherapy
     - RT can be approached in a "sandwich" fashion with three cycles of chemotherapy followed by RT, followed by three additional cycles of chemotherapy.
     - Concurrent chemoradiation can also be considered.
     - Ongoing clinical trials are investigating exact timing of chemotherapy + RT.

6. **How do you treat locally recurrent disease?**
   - Local recurrence occurs in 7% to 11% of patients.
   - **Surgical resection** may improve PFS for patients with local recurrence after initial surgery.
     - Pelvic exenteration considered for isolated central pelvic recurrence
     - Contraindications include extension to the pelvic sidewall and/or retroperitoneal involvement.
     - Must be able to tolerate surgery; pelvic exenteration has high morbidity.
   - **RT** is more commonly offered to patients with local recurrence.
     - Combination of external beam RT and brachytherapy

○ Local control can be achieved in 40% to 75% of patients.

○ Survival rate is highest in patients with isolated vaginal recurrence.

7. **How do you treat distant recurrent or metastatic disease? What is the role of hormonal therapy in this setting?**

- Hormonal therapy is preferred first over chemotherapy in recurrent or metastatic disease with low symptom burden, indolent pace of disease, and low grade due to improved toxicity profile.

- Produces response in 15% to 30% of patients, average length of response is 1 year.

- Treatment options include:

  ○ Megestrol

  ○ Medroxyprogesterone

  ○ Tamoxifen

  ○ Aromatase inhibitors

- In patients with negative ER/PR status or high-grade histology (grade 3, serous, clear cell, or carcinosarcoma) or rapid progression, chemotherapy is offered.

  ○ Best regimen for salvage chemotherapy has not been established.

  ○ If chemonaïve consider a platinum-doublet therapy such as carboplatin + paclitaxel.

  ○ Single agent liposomal doxorubicin, gemcitabine, and topotecan have modest activity.

SPECIAL CONSIDERATIONS

1. **What are the recommendations for posttreatment surveillance?**

- Physical examination including pelvic exam every 3 to 6 months for 2 years, then every 6 months or annually

- Vaginal cytology does not have proven benefit and is not recommended by the National Comprehensive Cancer Network (NCCN) or Society of Gynecologic Oncology (SGO)

- Measurement of serum CA-125 is optional at each visit

- CT/MRI only as clinically indicated

QUESTIONS

1. A 71-year-old otherwise healthy female presents with postmenopausal bleeding. Endometrial biopsy demonstrates adenocarcinoma. Surgical staging including total abdominal hysterectomy, bilateral salpingo-oophorectomy, and lymphadenectomy was performed. Pathology demonstrates a 2.3 cm grade 1 endometrioid adenocarcinoma invading 1.2 cm into a 2 cm myometrium with positive lymphovascular invasion. Disease was confined to the uterus without cervical involvement. What is the next step in treatment?
A. Observation
B. Adjuvant radiation therapy
C. Adjuvant platinum-based chemotherapy followed by radiation therapy
D. Adjuvant concurrent chemoradiation

2. A 56-year-old woman recently diagnosed with endometrial cancer presents to discuss recommended genetic screening. She was adopted and does not know any of her family history. She has not had a colonoscopy. Which of the following is true?
   A. No further testing is recommended
   B. Recommend age-appropriate colon cancer screening and immuno-histochemical staining of tumor tissue for MLH1, MSH2, MSH6, and PMS2. Refer for genetic counseling if protein stains are retained
   C. Recommend age-appropriate colon cancer screening and immuno-histochemical staining of tumor tissue for MLH1, MSH2, MSH6, and PMS2. Refer for genetic counseling if protein stains are absent
   D. Recommend germline BRCA 1/2 testing

3. A 68-year-old female presents with biopsy-proven recurrent grade 1 endometrioid endometrial adenocarcinoma metastatic to the lung and pelvis. Tumor tissue stains positive for estrogen receptor (ER). She is asymptomatic from her current disease. She has residual peripheral neuropathy from her previous adjuvant carboplatin and paclitaxel chemotherapy completed 1 year ago. What is the most appropriate next step in management?
   A. Hormonal therapy with an aromatase inhibitor
   B. Doublet chemotherapy with a platinum and taxane
   C. Surgical resection of dominant lung nodule
   D. Doublet chemotherapy with a platinum and anthracycline

4. A 59-year-old woman undergoes a total abdominal hysterectomy with bilateral salingo-oophorectomy and lymphadenectomy for endome-trial cancer. Pathology is consistent with a high-grade papillary serous adenocarcinoma invading 1.5 cm into a 2 cm myometrium with posi-tive lymphovascular invasion. Disease is confined to the uterus without cervical involvement. What is the best next step in treatment?
   A. Observation
   B. Adjuvant radiation therapy
   C. Adjuvant carboplatinum and paclitaxel sequenced with radiation therapy
   D. Adjuvant hormonal therapy with an aromatase inhibitor

5. A 72-year-old woman with a history of stage la endometrial cancer who underwent total abdominal hysterectomy and bilateral salpingo-oophorectomy 1 year ago presents with vaginal bleeding. Physical exam demonstrates a nodule on the vaginal cuff. Biopsy demonstrates recurrent grade 1 endometrioid endometrial cancer. Physical exami-nation suggests disease may be adherent to the pelvic sidewall. CT chest/abdomen/pelvis and pelvic MRI demonstrate a 3 cm mass at the top of the vagina without further evidence of disease. The patient is otherwise fit and wishes to pursue therapy. What is the next best step in treatment?
   A. Pelvic exenteration
   B. Local radiation therapy

C. Observation
D. Carboplatin and paclitaxel chemotherapy

6. A 58-year-old woman is diagnosed with a 1 cm grade 1 endometrioid endometrial cancer after undergoing a total abdominal hysterectomy and bilateral salpingo-oophorectomy for presumed benign indications. Disease invaded 0.2 cm into a 2 cm myometrium without lymphovascular invasion. What is the next best step in treatment?
   A. Observation
   B. Completion staging with pelvic and aortic lymphadenectomy
   C. Adjuvant chemotherapy with carboplatin and paclitaxel
   D. Adjuvant radiation therapy

ANSWERS

1. **B. Adjuvant radiation therapy.** This patient has stage Ib disease with three risk factors including positive lymphovascular invasion, depth of invasion, and age and therefore warrants local radiation therapy, given the increased risk for local recurrence.

2. **C. Recommend age-appropriate colon cancer screening and immunohistochemical staining of tumor tissue for MLH1, MSH2, MSH6, and PMS2. Refer for genetic counseling if protein stains are absent.** Hereditary nonpolyposis colorectal cancer (HNPCC) or Lynch syndrome is found in ~5% of women with endometrial cancer. It is a syndrome characterized by loss of DNA mismatch repair proteins including MLH1, MSH2, MSH6, and PMS2. Immunohistochemistry of tumor tissue looking for loss of these mismatch repair proteins is an accepted initial screening method to identify women who should be referred for germline genetic testing.

3. **A. Hormonal therapy with an aromatase inhibitor.** Hormonal therapy (ie, aromatase inhibitors, megestrol, or tamoxifen) is a well-tolerated treatment in women with low-grade metastatic endometrial cancer, especially with ER positivity. Hormonal therapy is most appropriate in women without large symptom burden or rapidly growing disease as it is most effective in controlling and/or slowing disease growth.

4. **C. Adjuvant carboplatinum and paclitaxel sequenced with radiation therapy.** This patient has a stage Ib high-grade papillary serous endometrial cancer. Given the increased rates of distant recurrence with high-grade papillary serous histology, adjuvant chemotherapy in addition to local radiation therapy is recommended.

5. **B. Local radiation therapy.** Radiation therapy is appropriate for locally recurrent disease. Surgical resection is sometimes an option, but in the case of pelvic sidewall adhesion it is generally not considered.

6. **A. Observation.** Observation is appropriate in this case (stage Ia, grade 1, no lymphovascular space involvement [LVSI], and tumor <2 cm), given the low risk for disease recurrence. Further lymph node assessment is not needed for this early-stage tumor, given the very low risk of nodal involvement.

XI

CANCER OF UNKNOWN PRIMARY

Cancer of Unknown Primary | 36

Benjamin Y. Scheier and Laurence H. Baker

EPIDEMIOLOGY

1. **How is cancer of unknown primary (CUP) typically classified?**
   - Adenocarcinoma (70%), squamous cell carcinoma (~5%), neuroendocrine carcinoma (~1%), poorly differentiated carcinoma (20%–25%)

2. **What are the five most common primary sites in CUP eventually diagnosed during life or at autopsy?**
   - Lung (23.7%), pancreas (21.1%), ovary (6.4%), kidney (5.5%), and colorectal (5.3%)

DIAGNOSIS

1. **What is important in the workup of a patient with CUP?**
   - History and physical: performance status, nutritional status, comorbidities, pain/symptoms
   - Histologic tissue evaluation with immunohistochemistry
   - CT of the chest, abdomen, and pelvis
   - Symptom-driven assessment: endoscopy, digital rectal exam, breast exam/mammography, pelvic exam, laryngoscopic exam
   - Breast MRI in women with axillary adenopathy and a normal mammogram
   - PET/CT may be helpful (can detect primary tumor in approximately 30% of patients)
   - Tumor markers (see the following)
   - Emphasis should be on identifying treatable/curable subset of patients and tumor types

2. **What tumor markers may be useful in diagnosis?**
   - Beta-human chorionic gonadotropin (beta-HCG) and alpha-fetoprotein (AFP), especially in poorly/undifferentiated carcinomas, which may suggest germ-cell tumor primary site.
   - Prostate-specific antigen (PSA) is specific for prostate cancer: consider in men with adenocarcinoma and bone-only metastases.
   - CEA, CA19-9, CA-125, and CA15-3 are nonspecific.

3. **Should you obtain molecular profiling/tumor of origin testing?**
   - There are no prospective data supporting its clinical use. It may have diagnostic utility. The Food and Drug Administration (FDA) approved the Pathwork Tissue of Origin test in 2008.

4. **Following are some commonly used immunoperoxidase stains that are useful in the diagnosis of CUP:**
   - Cytokeratin 7 and 20 (CK 7, CK 20), thyroid transcription factor-1 (TTF-1), PSA, ER/PR, leukocyte common antigen, S100 protein, HMB 45, neuron-specific enolase, chromogranin, vimentin, and desmin
     - Which of these should stain positive in neuroendocrine tumors?
       - Cytokeratin
       - Neuron-specific enolase
     - Which of these should stain positive in sarcomas?
       - Vimentin and desmin
     - Which of these are helpful in identifying a melanoma?
       - S100 protein
       - HMB 45 (see Figure 36.1)

5. **Cytokeratin staining is positive in which tumor type(s)?**
   - Carcinoma
   - Neuroendocrine

6. **TTF-1 is commonly positive in which cancer type?**
   - Lung adenocarcinoma

7. **CK 20 is commonly positive in which cancer type?**
   - Colon

8. **CK 7 positive and cytokeratin 20 negative is common in which malignancy?**
   - Lung

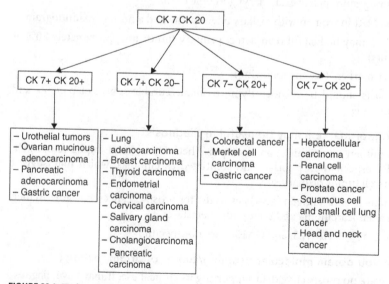

FIGURE 36.1 ■ Approach to immunohistochemical markers in cancer of unknown primary.
Source: From Ref. (1). Varadhachary GR, Abbruzzese JL, Lenzi R. Diagnostic strategies for unknown primary. *Cancer.* 2004;100:1776–1785.

9. **What additional markers should be considered after a preliminary workup with CK 7 and CK 20?**

Cancer	Marker
Urothelial carcinoma	Uroplakin III, thrombomodulin, high molecular weight cytokeratin
Breast carcinoma	Gross cystic disease fluid protein, ER, PR
Lung (mainly adenocarcinoma)	Thyroid transcription factor-1 (TTF-1), surfactant A and B
Medullary thyroid cancer	TTF-1, calcitonin
Merkel cell carcinoma	CD117
Hepatocellular carcinoma	Hep par-1
Prostate cancer	PSA, prostate acid phosphatase (PAP)
Cholangiocarcinoma	CK 19
Mesothelioma	Calretinin

Source: From Ref. (1). Varadhachary GR, Abbruzzese JL, Lenzi R. Diagnostic strategies for unknown primary. *Cancer.* 2004;100:1776–1785.

PROGNOSIS

1. **What are poor prognostic features in CUP?**
   - Male gender
   - Adenocarcinoma histology
   - Poorly differentiated neuroendocrine histology
   - Multiple involved organ sites
   - Supraclavicular lymphadenopathy
   - Hepatic or adrenal involvement

TREATMENT

1. **Is chemotherapy helpful?**
   - Chemotherapy increases overall survival by 3 to 6 months compared to best supportive care. There is less than a 30% response rate.

2. **How are adenocarcinomas of unknown primary usually treated?**
   - Combination chemotherapy, usually containing a platinum; that is:
     - Paclitaxel, carboplatin, ($\pm$) etoposide
     - Docetaxel and carboplatin
     - Gemcitabine and cisplatin
     - Gemcitabine and docetaxel

3. **How are women with adenocarcinoma of unknown primary with peritoneal carcinomatosis treated?**
   - As ovarian primary: consider surgical cytoreduction in the appropriate candidate, followed by platinum-based combination chemotherapy.

4. **How are women with adenocarcinoma of unknown primary and axillary lymph node metastasis treated?**
   - As stage II or III breast cancer (occult breast primary found in 55%–75%)

5. **How are squamous cell CUPs with high cervical nodes evaluated and treated?**
   - As head and neck primaries
     - Check p16 staining (human papillomavirus [HPV]) for level I to IV nodes; if positive, most likely indicates oropharyngeal primary.
   - Panendoscopy should be performed with biopsies of the following:
     - Pyriform sinus, nasopharynx
     - Base of tongue, and tonsils (bilateral simple tonsillectomies)

6. **How are squamous cell CUPs with inguinal lymph nodes treated?**
   - As genital or anorectal primary
   - Consider inguinal lymph node dissection, followed by inguinal radiotherapy +/− chemotherapy

7. **How are high-grade neuroendocrine CUPs treated?**
   - Treat as small cell lung cancer (ie, platinum combined with etoposide)

8. **How do you treat CUP with the extragonadal germ-cell syndrome?**
   - Consider in middle-aged men, midline adenopathy, elevated AFP/beta-HCG
   - Treat as poor risk germ-cell tumor: responsive to platinum, response often durable

9. **How do you treat CUP with isolated bone metastases?**
   - In a man, check PSA and evaluate for prostate primary. If a woman, consider breast primary
   - If solitary metastasis, consider radiotherapy followed by observation

10. **How do you treat CUP with isolated brain metastasis/metastases?**
    - Single site: resect +/− adjuvant radiotherapy
    - Multiple lesions: whole-brain radiotherapy

QUESTIONS

1. A 58-year-old woman has multiple liver lesions identified on CT scan of the chest, abdomen, and pelvis obtained during a routine workup for abdominal pain. There was no evidence of a primary tumor. A core biopsy of one of the liver lesions is performed, revealing a moderately differentiated adenocarcinoma with the following immunohistochemistry profile: CK 7 negative, CK 20 positive, CD X2 positive.
   Which of the following is the most likely primary site?
   A. Lung
   B. Colorectal
   C. Ovarian
   D. Gastric

2. A 49-year-old woman presents with a palpable and painless 3 cm left axillary mass. CT scan of the chest, abdomen, and pelvis is obtained, which reveals several enlarged axillary lymph nodes but no primary site identified. Bilateral mammograms show no abnormalities in the breasts. A core biopsy is obtained, which reveals adenocarcinoma. What would you recommend next?
   A. Bilateral mastectomy and bilateral axillary lymph node dissection
   B. Gemcitabine and docetaxel
   C. MRI of the breasts
   D. Left axillary lymph node dissection

3. A 61-year-old woman presents with a painless lump in her right groin that has been growing slowly over the past 3 months. She is otherwise asymptomatic. A basic physical exam and laboratory assessment is unremarkable, aside from the palpable fixed mass, measuring about 4 cm, in the left inguinal region. Biopsy is performed showing poorly differentiated squamous cell carcinoma. CT of the chest, abdomen, and pelvis shows no primary tumor.
   What would you recommend next?
   A. Gynecologic exam with colposcopy and anoscopy
   B. PET/CT
   C. Radiotherapy
   D. Chemotherapy

4. A 71-year-old man, previously healthy, presents with a growing 2.5 cm left-sided chest mass over the past 6 months. A biopsy demonstrates adenocarcinoma, and a PET/CT scan shows no avid lesions aside from the chest wall mass. He has no comorbidities and has an Eastern Cooperative Oncology Group (ECOG) performance status of zero.
   What would you recommend next?
   A. Observation
   B. Surgery followed by radiation
   C. Chemotherapy
   D. Radiation therapy alone

ANSWERS

1. **B. Colorectal.** Immunohistochemical stains can often guide diagnosis of a primary site. Cytokeratin stains are a helpful first triage point. CK 7 negative/CK 20 positive tumors are often colorectal, Merkel cell, or gastric primaries. CD X2 is very specific for colorectal tumors.

2. **C. MRI of the breasts.** Women with isolated adenocarcinoma with axillary lymph node metastases require a thorough workup for a breast primary site. An MRI is useful in women with a normal mammogram and breast ultrasound. If no further sites are identified, following a stage II breast adenocarcinoma treatment paradigm should be considered.

3. **A. Gynecologic exam with colposcopy and anoscopy.** Squamous cell carcinoma isolated to inguinal lymph nodes represents a potentially curable subset of cancer of unknown primary (CUP). Attention to identifying a primary site via thorough gynecologic and anorectal examinations is indicated.

4. **B. Surgery followed by radiation.** Isolated metastases should be treated aggressively for cure in the appropriate candidates. Observation is not appropriate in treatment candidates. Resection followed by radiotherapy, with or without chemotherapy should be considered, in accordance with National Comprehensive Cancer Network (NCCN) guidelines.

REFERENCE

1. Varadhachary GR, Abbruzzese JL, Lenzi R. Diagnostic strategies for unknown primary. *Cancer*. 2004;100:1776–1785.

37

Genetics and Tumor Biology

Carlos J. Gallego, Jessica N. Everett, Shawna Kraft, and
Elena M. Stoffel

INTRODUCTION

- Inherited cancer syndromes comprise approximately 5% to 10% of all cancers.
- Majority of cancer syndromes are inherited in autosomal dominant manner.
- Genes affected may be proto-oncogenes, tumor suppressor genes, or mismatch repair genes.
- Patients aware of genetic predisposition may start screening for certain cancers at a younger age.
- Genes, clinical features, and surveillance of inherited cancer syndromes are detailed in Table 37.1.

HEREDITARY BREAST CANCER SYNDROMES

1. **What are the most common hereditary syndromes associated with breast cancer?**
   - Hereditary breast and ovarian cancer syndrome (*BRCA1*, *BRCA2* genes)
   - PTEN hamartoma tumor or Cowden syndrome (*PTEN*)
   - Li–Fraumeni syndrome (*TP53*)

2. **In which populations are BRCA founder mutations highly prevalent?**
   - Ashkenazi Jewish and Polish

3. **What is the penetrance of breast and ovarian cancer in women with pathogenic BRCA variants?**
   - *BRCA1*: 55% to 70% breast cancer and 40% ovarian cancer by age 70 years
   - *BRCA2*: 45% to 70% breast cancer and 15% ovarian cancer by age 70 years

4. **What is the impact of bilateral prophylactic mastectomy in cancer risk reduction in women with pathogenic BRCA variants?**
   - 90% for breast cancer

5. **What is the impact of bilateral salpingo-oophorectomy in cancer risk reduction in women with pathogenic BRCA variants?**
   - 80% for ovarian cancer
   - 50% for breast cancer

(*text continues on page 407*)

TABLE 37.1 ■ Clinical Manifestations and Screening Recommendations for Inherited Cancer Syndromes

Cancer Syndrome	Gene Involved	Incidence	Clinical Manifestations	Screening Recommendations for Carriers
Hereditary Breast Cancer Syndromes				
Hereditary breast-ovarian cancer (HBOC) syndrome	BCRA1 and BRCA2	1 in 500–1,000 (1 in 40 people of Ashkenazi Jewish descent)	• Early-onset breast and ovarian cancers • Lifetime risk of breast cancer of 50%–85%, risk of ovarian cancer 15%–40% • Increased risk of pancreatic, stomach, fallopian tube, and primary peritoneal cancers (two- to fourfold increase in relative risk)	• Annual mammogram and breast MRI beginning at age 25 or individualized based on family history • Self-breast exams • Clinical breast exam every 6–12 months starting at age 25 • Transvaginal ultrasound and CA-125 twice yearly starting at age 35 or 5–10 yrs earlier than age of first diagnosis of ovarian cancer in family • Consider prophylactic mastectomy or chemoprevention with tamoxifen • Recommend bilateral salpingo-oophorectomy (BSO) at age 35–40 and once childbearing is over

(continued)

TABLE 37.1 ■ Clinical Manifestations and Screening Recommendations for Inherited Cancer Syndromes (*continued*)

Cancer Syndrome	Gene Involved	Incidence	Clinical Manifestations	Screening Recommendations for Carriers
PTEN hamartoma tumor syndrome (Cowden syndrome)	*PTEN*	1 in 200,000	• Mucocutaneous lesions • GI polyps • Macrocephaly • Thyroid abnormalities • Trichilemmoma and papillomatous papule formation • Palmar keratosis • Macular speckling of glans • Increased risk of breast, thyroid, endometrial, and kidney cancers	• Clinical breast exam starting at 20–25 yrs • Annual mammogram and breast MRI starting at 30–35 yrs • Consider risk-reducing mastectomy • Annual thyroid ultrasound
Li-Fraumeni syndrome	*TP53*	Rare; exact incidence unknown	• Increased risk of many malignancies at a young age, including: sarcoma, breast cancer, brain tumor, leukemia, lung cancer, adrenocortical carcinoma • Risk of cancer is 90% by 60 yrs old	• Annual physical exam, CBC, chemistries • Mammogram and breast MRI starting at 20–25 yrs • Colonoscopy starting at 25 yrs, continue every 2–5 yrs • Consider surveillance with whole body/brain MRI

(continued)

TABLE 37.1 ■ Clinical Manifestations and Screening Recommendations for Inherited Cancer Syndromes (continued)

Cancer Syndrome	Gene Involved	Incidence	Clinical Manifestations	Screening Recommendations for Carriers
Hereditary Colon Cancer Syndromes				
Lynch syndrome (hereditary nonpolyposis colorectal cancer [HNPCC])	MLH1, MSH2, MSH6, PMS2, TACSTD1/ EPCAM	1 in 400	• Increased risk of colorectal cancer, as well as ovarian, endometrial, pancreas, small intestine cancers, and sebaceous skin cancer	• Annual colonoscopy starting at 20–25 yrs or 10 yrs earlier than earliest age of diagnosis in family, whichever is earlier • Consider endometrial surveillance (transvaginal ultrasound and endometrial biopsy) starting age 30–35 yrs or prophylactic TAH-BSO after childbearing • Periodic upper endoscopy • Annual skin surveillance

(continued)

TABLE 37.1 ■ Clinical Manifestations and Screening Recommendations for Inherited Cancer Syndromes (continued)

Cancer Syndrome	Gene Involved	Incidence	Clinical Manifestations	Screening Recommendations for Carriers
Familial adenomatous polyposis (FAP)	APC	1 in 5,000–10,000	• Thousands of adenomas throughout GI tract, polyposis usually develops in second or third decade of life • Risk of colon cancer is 90% by age 45 • Additional risk of extracolonic cancers, including ampullary, thyroid, CNS tumors, hepatoblastoma • Osteomas of the mandible • Epidermoid cysts • Desmoid tumors • Congenital hypertrophy of retinal pigment epithelium	• At-risk children should undergo genetic testing by age 10–12 yrs • Colonoscopy yearly for mutation carriers beginning age 10–12 yrs • EGD with side-viewing scope every 1–3 yrs once colonic polyps develop • Colectomy strongly recommended once polyps become too numerous for surveillance or if large adenomas, villous histology, high-grade dysplasia • After colectomy surveillance of ileal pouch/rectum every 6 months—3 yrs depending on polyp burden
MYH-associated polyposis	MUTYH		• Similar to FAP, but recessive inheritance	• Same as FAP

(continued)

TABLE 37.1 ▪ Clinical Manifestations and Screening Recommendations for Inherited Cancer Syndromes (continued)

Cancer Syndrome	Gene Involved	Incidence	Clinical Manifestations	Screening Recommendations for Carriers
Peutz–Jeghers syndrome	LKB1/STK11	1 in 200,000	• Hamartomatous GI polyp formation (78% in upper jejunum) • Main complication is intussusception • Mucocutaneous hyperpigmentations • Increased risk of breast, colon, stomach, small intestine, pancreatic, lung cancers • Increased risk of GU cancers, including adenoma malignum (cervix), sex cord tumors, Sertoli cell tumors	• EGD and colonoscopy at age 15 yrs, consider double balloon enteroscopy for removal of small bowel polyps • Small bowel imaging (video capsule endoscopy or MR enterography) every 1–3 yrs beginning age 8 yrs • Annual testicular exams from birth to age 12 • Annual pelvic exam, transvaginal ultrasound beginning age 25 yrs • Annual breast MRIs beginning age 25 yrs • Pancreas cancer screening (MRCP alternating with endoscopic ultrasound, annually beginning age 30 yrs)

(continued)

TABLE 37.1 ■ Clinical Manifestations and Screening Recommendations for Inherited Cancer Syndromes (continued)

Cancer Syndrome	Gene Involved	Incidence	Clinical Manifestations	Screening Recommendations for Carriers
Juvenile polyposis syndrome (JPS)	SMAD4 and BMPR1A	1 in 100,000	• Hamartomatous juvenile polyps throughout GI tract • Increased risk of GI and pancreas malignancies • Can be associated with congenital anomalies (cardiac) or hereditary hemorrhagic telangiectasia (HHT) (SMAD4 mutations only)	• Colonoscopy every 1–2 yrs starting at age 15 yrs • Upper GI surveillance (EGD) every 1–2 yrs
Multiple Endocrine Neoplasias				
Multiple endocrine neoplasia, type 1 (MEN1)	MEN1	1–2 in 100,000	• "3 Ps:" • Parathyroid adenomas • Pancreatic endocrine tumors • Pituitary tumors	• Yearly PTH, calcium, and 25-OH vitamin D starting at age 10 yrs • Yearly gastrin, chromogranin A, pancreatic polypeptide, glucagon, VIP, proinsulin, insulin, C-peptide, prolactin, IGF-1 starting at age 10 yrs • MRI of pancreas and adrenal gland yearly beginning at age 10 yrs, brain MRI every 3–5 yrs beginning at age 10 yrs • CT or MRI of chest (thymic neuroendocrine tumor screening) every 2–5 yrs beginning at age 10 yrs

(continued)

TABLE 37.1 ■ Clinical Manifestations and Screening Recommendations for Inherited Cancer Syndromes (continued)

Cancer Syndrome	Gene Involved	Incidence	Clinical Manifestations	Screening Recommendations for Carriers
Multiple endocrine neoplasia, type 2 (MEN2)	RET	Unknown	• Medullary thyroid cancer (MTC) • Pheochromocytoma • Hyperparathyroidism (HPT)	• Prophylactic thyroidectomy, timing based on type of RET mutation (early childhood)
Other Inherited Cancer Syndromes				
Hereditary diffuse gastric cancer syndrome	Type 1 E-cadherin (CDH1)		• 70% lifetime risk of gastric cancer • 40% lifetime risk of lobular breast cancer	• Endoscopy has poor sensitivity since lesions are submucosal • Recommend prophylactic gastrectomy after age 20 • Consider early breast imaging in women
Familial atypical multiple mole melanoma syndrome (FAMMM)	CDKN2A, CDK4	Unknown	• Multiple malignant melanomas and atypical nevi, often diagnosed at a young age • Risk for pancreatic cancer up to 17%	• Baseline skin exam at 10 yrs, then every 6–12 months • Education about sun avoidance • Consider surveillance for pancreatic cancer (MRCP alternating with endoscopic ultrasound yearly)

(continued)

TABLE 37.1 ■ Clinical Manifestations and Screening Recommendations for Inherited Cancer Syndromes (continued)

Cancer Syndrome	Gene Involved	Incidence	Clinical Manifestations	Screening Recommendations for Carriers
von Hippel–Lindau disease (VHL)	VHL	1 in 36,000	• CNS hemangioblastomas • Retinal hemangiomas • Clear-cell renal cell carcinoma • Pheochromocytoma • Renal, pancreatic, or epididymal cysts	• Retinal exam (annually) • Plasma metanephrines and normetanephrines (annually) • MRI abdomen and pelvis (annual) • MRI brain/spine (every other year)
Hereditary paraganglioma and pheochromocytoma	SDHA, SDHAF2, SDHB, SDHC, SDHD	Unknown	• Pancreatic neuroendocrine tumors • Head and neck paraganglioma • Adrenal and extra-adrenal pheochromocytoma • Malignant pheochromocytoma • Renal cell cancer • GI stromal tumor	• Plasma metanephrines and normetanephrines (annual) • MRI head/neck, abdomen every 2 yrs

CBC, complete blood count; CNS, central nervous system; EGD, esophagogastroduodenoscopy; GI, gastrointestinal; GU, genitourinary; MRCP, magnetic resonance cholangiopancreatography; PTH, parathyroid hormone; TAH, total abdominal hysterectomy.

6. **Patients with BRCA variants are also at an increased risk of developing what type of tumors?**
   - *BRCA1/2*: primary fallopian tube and primary peritoneal cancer
   - *BRCA2*: pancreatic, prostate, and male breast cancer

7. **What are the cardinal clinical features of Cowden syndrome?**
   - Mucocutaneous lesions, gastrointestinal polyps, macrocephaly, thyroid abnormalities, trichilemmoma and papillomatous papule formation, palmar keratosis, macular speckling of glans (Bannayan–Riley–Ruvalcaba syndrome)

8. **Patients with Cowden syndrome are at an increased risk of what type of tumors?**
   - Breast, thyroid, and endometrial cancers

9. **Patients with Li–Fraumeni syndrome are at an increased risk of what type of tumors?**
   - Sarcomas, breast cancer, brain tumors, leukemia, lung cancer, adrenocortical carcinomas (ACC).
   - All patients with ACC should be tested for *TP53* mutations (80% will have *TP53* variants in pediatric population with ACC).

HEREDITARY COLON CANCER SYNDROMES

1. **What are the most common hereditary syndromes associated with colon cancer?**
   - Lynch syndrome (*MLH1, MSH2, MSH6, PMS2, TACSTD1/EPCAM* genes).
   - Familial adenomatous polyposis (*APC*).
   - Peutz–Jeghers (*STK11*).
   - Juvenile polyposis (*SMAD4, BMPR1A*).

2. **Patients with Lynch syndrome are at an increased risk of what type of tumors?**
   - Colorectal, ovarian, endometrial, pancreas, small intestine, skin cancer.
   - All patients with sebaceous carcinoma should be evaluated for Lynch syndrome.

3. **What are the cardinal clinical features of familial adenomatous polyposis (FAP)?**
   - Hundreds to thousands of adenomas throughout the gastrointestinal (GI) tract, osteomas of the mandible, epidermoid cysts, desmoid tumors, congenital hypertrophy of retinal pigment epithelium. Sometimes FAP is associated with central nervous system (CNS) tumors (Turcot syndrome) or extracolonic tumors (Gardner syndrome).

4. **Patients with FAP are at an increased risk of what type of tumors?**
   - Colorectal cancer (average age 39 years old at diagnosis), ampullary, thyroid, CNS tumors, and hepatoblastoma.

5. **What is attenuated FAP?**
   - A milder form of FAP with fewer polyps and later age of colon cancer diagnosis.

6. **What is the inheritance pattern on MUTYH-associated polyposis? What is its clinical presentation?**
   - Autosomal recessive
   - Clinical presentation is very similar to FAP with multiple adenomas in the GI tract

7. **What are the cardinal features of Peutz–Jeghers syndrome?**
   - Hamartomatous polyps in the GI tract (78% in jejunum, increased risk of intussusception), mucocutaneous pigmentation.

8. **What are the cardinal clinical features of juvenile polyposis syndrome?**
   - Increased risk of colonic and pancreatic cancer. Congenital anomalies (clubbing, macrocephaly, gut malrotation).

MULTIPLE ENDOCRINE NEOPLASIA

1. **How are multiple endocrine neoplasias (MENs) classified?**
   - MEN1 (gene also *MEN1*), MEN2 (*RET* gene).
   - MEN2 is classified into MEN2a and MEN2b.

2. **Which tumors are characteristic of multiple endocrine neoplasia type 1 (MEN1)?**
   - Remember the "3 Ps": parathyroid adenomas (common presentation with hyperparathyroidism), pancreatic endocrine tumors, and pituitary tumors.

3. **Which tumors are characteristic of multiple endocrine neoplasia type 2 (MEN2)?**
   - Medullary thyroid cancer, pheochromocytoma, mucosal neuromas (more common in MEN2b).

4. **What are the clinical differences between MEN2a and MEN2b?**
   - MEN2b has younger age of tumor onset, hyperparathyroidism is less likely, marfanoid habitus and mucosal neuromas are more likely.

5. **Why is early diagnosis of MEN2 important?**
   - Medullary thyroid cancer is life-threatening.
   - Children with pathogenic variants of *RET* gene might be considered for prophylactic thyroidectomy.

OTHER HEREDITARY CANCER SYNDROMES

1. **Which are other common hereditary syndromes?**
   - Hereditary diffuse gastric cancer (HDGC) syndrome (*CDH1*).
   - Familial atypical multiple melanoma syndrome (*CDKN2A, CDK4*).
   - Von Hippel–Lindau (*VHL*).
   - Hereditary paraganglioma and pheochromocytoma (*SDHB, SDHC, SDHD*).

2. **Patients with HDGC are at an increased risk of what type of tumors?**
   - Gastric cancer (70% lifetime penetrance), lobular breast cancer (40% lifetime penetrance).
   - Prophylactic gastrectomy is recommended after age 20 years.

3. **What are the cardinal clinical features of familial atypical multiple mole melanoma syndrome?**
   - Multiple malignant melanomas and atypical nevi, increased risk of pancreatic cancer.

4. **What are the cardinal clinical features of von Hippel–Lindau (VHL)?**
   - CNS hemangioblastomas, retinal hemangiomas, clear-cell renal cell carcinoma, pheochromocytoma, pancreatic neuroendocrine tumors, cysts (renal, pancreatic, epididymal).

5. **What are the cardinal clinical features of hereditary paraganglioma and pheochromocytoma?**
   - Head and neck paraganglioma, adrenal and extra-adrenal pheochromocytoma, malignant pheochromocytoma.
   - Genetic evaluation is indicated for any isolated paraganglioma or pheochromocytoma (25% are hereditary, differential diagnosis includes VHL and MEN2).

TUMOR BIOLOGY AND TARGETED CANCER THERAPIES

1. **What are the most important Food and Drug Administration (FDA) approved targeted cancer therapies that have been demonstrated to benefit patients, particularly in populations with specific genomic drivers of malignancy?**

   See Table 37.2.

TABLE 37.2 ■ Targeted Cancer Therapies

Gene	Malignancy	Alteration	Cancer Therapy
Receptor Tyrosine Kinases			
ALK	Lung, neuroblastoma, anaplastic large cell lymphoma	Mutation or amplification	Crizotinib, alectinib, ceritinib
CDK4/6	Breast	Amplification	Palbociclib
EGFR	Lung, glioblastoma	Mutation or amplification	Erlotinib, gefitinib, osimertinib (T90M mutation)
ERBB2	Breast	Amplification	Lapatinib
c-MET	Lung, gastric	Amplification	Crizotinib
c-KIT	GIST	Mutation	Imatinib, sunitinib
PDGFRA	GIST, glioblastoma	Mutation	Sunitinib, sorafenib, imatinib

(continued)

TABLE 37.2 ■ Targeted Cancer Therapies (*continued*)

Gene	Malignancy	Alteration	Cancer Therapy
PDGFRB	CMML	Translocation	Sunitinib, sorafenib, imatinib
ROS1	Lung	Translocation	Crizotinib
VEGF	RCC, HCC, others	Amplification	Sunitinib, sorafenib, pazopanib, axitinib, cabozantinib
FLT3	AML	Internal tandem duplication	FLT3 inhibitors (eg, sorafenib)
Nonreceptor Tyrosine Kinases			
ABL	CML	Translocation (BCR-ABL)	Imatinib, dasatinib, nilotinib, bosutinib, ponatinib
JAK2	CML, myeloproliferative neoplasms	Mutation (V617F), translocation	Ruxolitinib
Serine–Threonine–Lipid Kinases			
BRAF	Melanoma, colon, thyroid	Mutation (V600E)	Vemurafenib, dabrafenib
MTOR	Renal cell	Increased activation	Temsirolimus, everolimus
PI3K	Lymphoma	Mutation	Idelalisib

2. **What are the most important FDA-approved monoclonal antibody-based therapies to know?**

See Table 37.3.

TABLE 37.3 ■ Monoclonal Antibody Therapies

Target	Malignancy	Monoclonal Antibody
CD20	B-cell non-Hodgkin lymphoma	Rituximab, tositumomab (labeled with I-131), Ibritumomab (labeled with Y-90), ofatumumab
CD52	B-cell CLL	Alemtuzumab
CTLA-4	Malignant melanoma	Ipilimumab
CD30	Refractory/relapsed Hodgkin lymphoma, anaplastic large cell lymphoma	Brentuximab
CD38		Daratumumab
	Multiple myeloma	

(*continued*)

TABLE 37.3 ■ Monoclonal Antibody Therapies (*continued*)

Target	Malignancy	Monoclonal Antibody
HER2	Breast	Trastuzumab
EGFR	Metastatic CRC	Panitumumab
	Head and neck cancer	Cetuximab
PD-1	Metastatic melanoma, RCC, lung, lymphoma, urothelial	Nivolumab, pembrolizumab, atezolizumab
SLAMF7	Multiple myeloma	Elotuzumab
VEGF	Multiple	Bevacizumab

CLL, chronic lymphocytic leukemia; CRC, colorectal cancer; RCC, renal cell carcinoma.

3. What are other important targeted therapies to know?

See Table 37.4.

TABLE 37.4 ■ Miscellaneous Therapies

Drug	Malignancy	Mechanism of Action
Tamoxifen	Breast	Selective estrogen receptor modulators (SERMs)
Fulvestrant	Breast	Destroys estrogen receptor
Anastrozole	Breast	Aromatase inhibitors
Exemestane		
Letrozole		
Leuprolide	Prostate	GnRH agonists
Goserelin		GnRH antagonist
Triptorelin		Antiandrogens
Degarelix		17 alpha-hydroxylase inhibitor
Bicalutamide		Androgen receptor antagonist
Flutamide		Androgen receptor antagonist
Nilutamide		Inhibitor of CYP17A1
Abiraterone		Androgen receptor antagonist
Enzalutamide		
Vorinostat	CTCL	HDAC inhibitor
Bortezomib	Multiple myeloma	Proteasome inhibitor
Ixazomib	Multiple myeloma	Proteasome inhibitor

CTCL, cutaneous T-cell lymphoma; HDAC, histone deacetylase.

QUESTIONS

1. A 52-year-old man is diagnosed with a localized colorectal cancer after his first colonoscopy. After surgical resection, the tumor tissue is sent for immunohistochemistry staining and is found to be deficient in MLH1 expression.
   What is the most likely etiology of this cancer?
   A. Malignant transformation of adenomatous polyp
   B. Germline mutation in mismatch repair gene
   C. Methylation of *MLH1* promoter
   D. Malignant transformation of hamartomatous polyp

2. A 35-year-old woman with a strong family history of breast cancer is referred to the cancer genetics clinic and is found to have a germline mutation in the *BRCA2* gene.
   Compared to patients with germline *BRCA1* mutations, this patient is at a *decreased* risk of developing what type of tumor?
   A. Thyroid cancer
   B. Pancreatic cancer
   C. Colorectal cancer
   D. Ovarian cancer

3. A 54-year-old man is evaluated because of anorexia, vague abdominal discomfort, and 30 lb weight loss during the past 3 months. His father and his brother died of stomach cancer. Upper endoscopy shows diffuse gastric mucosal abnormalities and no discrete mass. Random biopsies confirm HER2-negative adenocarcinoma with signet-ring cells. Germline testing of his blood reveals a *CDH1* mutation. The patient's 24-year-old son is subsequently tested and carries the same mutation.
   Which of the following should you recommend for this patient's son?
   A. History and physical examination every 6 months
   B. Surveillance endoscopy every year
   C. Diet low in nitrites, nitrates, spicy and smoked foods, and alcohol
   D. Total gastrectomy

4. A 26-year-old man presents to your clinic with paroxysmal hypertension and headaches. His father died at age 40 from an intracranial bleed during a hypertensive crisis. Bloodwork shows catecholamine hypersecretion and MRI shows an adrenal mass.
   Which of the following conditions is *not* in the differential diagnosis of this condition?
   A. Multiple endocrine neoplasia type 1
   B. Multiple endocrine neoplasia type 2
   C. Von Hippel–Lindau disease
   D. Hereditary paraganglioma–pheochromocytoma syndrome

5. A 66-year-old female patient with advanced renal cell carcinoma is being considered for immunotherapy after failing pazopanib and axitinib. Her tumor's PD-L1 expression is <1%.
   Which is the best option for therapy at this time?
   A. Everolimus
   B. Nivolumab
   C. Pembrolizumab
   D. Atezolizumab

ANSWERS

1. **C. Methylation of *MLH1* promoter.** Colorectal cancer that demonstrates microsatellite instability (MSI) is caused by either germline mismatch repair gene mutations (~15%), or "sporadic" somatic tumor *MLH1* promoter methylation (~85%). Malignant transformation of adenomatous polyps is seen in familial adenomatous polyposis, and hamartomatous polyps are seen in Peutz–Jeghers.

2. **D. Ovarian cancer.** When compared to patients with germline *BRCA1* variants, patients with *BRCA2* variants have a lower risk of developing ovarian cancer (40% vs. 15% penetrance at 70 years in *BRCA1* and *BRCA2*, respectively). Patients with *BRCA2* variants are at an increased risk of pancreatic, prostate, and male breast cancer when compared to the general population and patients with germline *BRCA1* variants. Thyroid and colorectal cancer are not associated with inherited breast and ovarian cancer syndromes.

3. **D. Total gastrectomy.** Hereditary diffuse gastric cancer (HDGC) is a relatively rare disorder, with a mutated *CDH1* gene as the only known cause. Carriers of a germline mutation in *CDH1* have a lifetime risk of >80% of developing diffuse gastric cancer. As periodic gastric surveillance is of limited value in detecting early stages of HDGC, prophylactic gastrectomy is advised for this patient group. Clinical surveillance and lifestyle modifications are not stand-alone recommendations for patients with *CDH1* germline mutations.

4. **A. Multiple endocrine neoplasia type 1.** This patient likely has a pheochromocytoma. Multiple endocrine neoplasia 2, Von Hippel–Lindau, and hereditary paraganglioma–pheochromocytoma syndrome are in the differential diagnosis of isolated pheochromocytoma. Patients with multiple endocrine neoplasia type 1 are at an increased risk of parathyroid adenomas, pancreatic endocrine tumors, and pituitary tumors, but not pheochromocytoma.

5. **B. Nivolumab.** Nivolumab demonstrated improved overall survival for renal cell carcinoma compared to everolimus irrespective of PD-L1 status. Pembrolizumab and atezolizumab are not Food and Drug Administration (FDA) approved for renal cell carcinoma although theoretically they may work.

SUPPORTIVE AND PALLIATIVE CARE

Oncologic Emergencies and Supportive Care

Angel Qin, Francis P. Worden, and Maria Silveira

Oncologic Emergencies

TUMOR LYSIS SYNDROME

1. **What is tumor lysis syndrome?**
   - Metabolic derangements due to tumor breakdown and release of intracellular potassium, phosphate, and nucleic acids into the systemic circulation

2. **What are the risk factors for tumor lysis syndrome?**
   - Highly proliferative tumors (eg, acute lymphoblastic leukemia, Burkitt lymphoma/leukemia; solid tumors include small cell lung cancer, breast cancer, and testicular cancer)
   - High tumor burden
   - High sensitivity to cytotoxic chemotherapy
   - Preexisting hyperuricemia, renal insufficiency, and hypovolemia

3. **What are the laboratory features associated with tumor lysis syndrome?**
   - *High*: potassium, phosphate, and uric acid
   - *Low*: calcium

4. **In addition to electrolyte abnormalities, what are the signs, symptoms, and manifestations of tumor lysis syndrome?**
   - Nausea, vomiting, diarrhea, lethargy
   - Muscle cramps, paresthesias, tetany
   - Acute renal failure (defined as serum creatinine $>1.5 \times$ the institutional upper limit of normal)
   - Confusion, hallucinations, seizures, syncope
   - Cardiac arrhythmias, heart failure
   - Sudden death

5. **What is the treatment for tumor lysis syndrome?**
   - Aggressive intravenous (IV) fluid hydration (with diuresis as needed to maintain adequate output)
   - Urinary alkalinization with sodium bicarbonate is controversial
   - Electrolyte repletion/removal; renal replacement therapy as indicated

- Hypouricemic agents
  - Allopurinol
    - Xanthine analog, which competitively inhibits xanthine oxidase
    - Decreases formation of new uric acid, does not reduce preexisting level
    - Needs to be renally dosed
    - Reduces degradation of other purines (6-mercaptopurine and azathioprine)
    - Adjust doses of medications also metabolized by the P450 system
  - Rasburicase
    - Recombinant urate oxidase, which catalyzes uric acid to allantoin
    - Decreases serum concentration of uric acid
    - Cannot be used in pregnant women or in G6PD deficiency (causes severe hemolysis and methemoglobinemia)

HYPERCALCEMIA OF MALIGNANCY

1. **What are the mechanisms by which hypercalcemia of malignancy occur?**
   - Osteolytic metastases with local cytokine release (including osteoclast activating factors)
     - Approximately 20% of cases
     - Usually seen in breast cancer and multiple myeloma
   - Parathyroid-hormone-related protein (PTHrP) secretion
     - Approximately 80% of cases
     - Usually seen in squamous cell carcinomas; renal, bladder, breast and ovarian cancer; leukemia; and lymphoma
   - Other causes (rare)
     - Calcitriol production: primarily lymphomas
     - Ectopic PTH production
     - Drugs: administration of estrogen or antiestrogens (ie, tamoxifen)

2. **What are the signs and symptoms of hypercalcemia?**
   - "Stones (renal), bones (pain), groans (abdominal), psychiatric overtones"
     - Neurologic: anxiety, depression, confusion, psychosis, somnolence, coma, and hyporeflexia
     - Cardiac: QT interval shortening, widened T waves, bradycardia, prolonged PR intervals, and arrhythmia
     - GI: nausea, vomiting, constipation, peptic ulcers, and pancreatitis
     - Renal: polyuria/polydipsia, acute/chronic renal insufficiency, distal renal tubular acidosis (RTA), nephrolithiasis, and nephrogenic diabetes insipidus
     - Musculoskeletal: bone pain, weakness, and fatigue

3. **What is the treatment for hypercalcemia?**
   - First line

○ Aggressive hydration ± diuresis
○ Bisphosphonates
  ▪ Pamidronate 30 mg IV if mild, 60 to 90 mg IV if severe
  ▪ Zoledronic acid 4 mg (8 mg reserved only for refractory/relapsed hypercalcemia)
  ▪ Denosumab 120 mg SQ (human monoclonal antibody against receptor activator of nuclear factor kappa-B ligand [RANKL])
● Second line
  ○ Calcitonin (can give with bisphosphonates; 4–8 IU/kg/day IM or SQ q6–12 hr; short-acting and risk of tachyphylaxis with repeated dosing)
  ○ Gallium, plicamycin/mithramycin, and corticosteroids

LEUKOSTASIS

1. **What is leukostasis?**
   ● Symptomatic hyperleukocytosis (typically white blood cell [WBC] counts >100,000)
   ● Most commonly seen with acute myeloid leukemia (AML) or chronic myelogenous leukemia (CML) in blast crisis

2. **What are the signs and symptoms of leukostasis?**
   ● Pulmonary: dyspnea, hypoxia, ± diffuse alveolar infiltrates
   ● Neurologic: headache, visual changes, confusion, somnolence, and coma
   ● Less common: EKG signs of myocardial ischemia or right ventricular overload, renal insufficiency, priapism, acute limb ischemia, and bowel infarction

3. **What is the treatment for leukostasis?**
   ● Aggressive intravenous fluid (IVF) hydration
   ● Leukapheresis
   ● Additional cytoreductive measures:
     ○ Induction chemotherapy (preferred)
     ○ Hydroxyurea (cannot be given to women who are pregnant or breastfeeding)
   ● Avoid blood transfusions if possible due to increased whole blood viscosity
   ● Monitor for/manage tumor lysis and disseminated intravascular coagulation (DIC)

FEBRILE NEUTROPENIA

1. **What is febrile neutropenia?**
   ● Fever: as per the Infectious Diseases Society of America (IDSA) guidelines, defined as a single temperature higher than 38.3°C (101.3°F) or sustained temperature higher than 38°C (100.4°F) for more than 1 hour
   ● Neutropenia: absolute neutrophil count (ANC) <500/uL or ANC <1,000/uL with predicted decline to <500/uL in 48 hours

2. **What are the signs and symptoms of febrile neutropenia?**
   ● Signs and symptoms may be minimal or absent

3. What should the evaluation of febrile neutropenia include?

- Thorough physical exam with particular attention to skin, sinuses, mouth/oropharynx, lungs, abdomen, perirectal area (avoid digital rectal exam), and indwelling catheters
- Laboratory studies including complete blood count (CBC) with differential, comprehensive metabolic panel, blood cultures × two sets (peripheral and from indwelling catheter or port if applicable), urinalysis and culture, site-specific cultures if applicable (stool, skin lesions, etc.)
- Ideally, cultures should be obtained prior to initiating antibiotics
- Radiologic studies, including routine chest x-ray; additional imaging for localizing symptoms as warranted

4. What are the associated pathogens found in febrile neutropenia?

- Infectious source identified in approximately 30% of patients
- Bacterial pathogens *most* common
  - ○ Gram-negative bacilli (particularly *Pseudomonas aeruginosa*)
  - ○ Initial increasing trend toward gram-positive organisms (*Staphylococcus* and *Streptococcus*) since the 1980s has started to swing toward gram-negative organisms given the rise of multidrug resistance
- Fungal and viral pathogens are also common; invasive fungal infections are especially prevalent in high-risk neutropenia
- Empiric treatment must provide broad coverage against gram-negatives including *Pseudomonas*; gram-positive and anaerobic coverage dependent on risk factors and presenting signs/symptoms

5. What is the treatment for febrile neutropenia?

- For select patients with anticipated brief neutropenia (<7 days) and few to no comorbidities or symptoms, outpatient therapy (ciprofloxacin and augmentin) with close monitoring may be acceptable. This is not commonly done.
- High-risk patients require inpatient hospitalization with IV antibiotics
- For uncomplicated infections, monotherapy with broad-spectrum beta-lactams with good pseudomonal coverage is as effective as combination therapy
  - ○ Cefepime, piperacillin–tazobactam, imipenem, meropenem, and ceftazidime based on institutional susceptibilities
- Combination therapy should be used in setting of severe sepsis/septic shock or high prevalence of multidrug-resistant (MDR) gram-negative rods
  - ○ Typically use a beta-lactam plus an aminoglycoside or fluoroquinolone
- Role of vancomycin:
  - ○ Should *not* be used initially unless one or more of the following apply:
    - Clinically suspected catheter-related infection
    - Gram-positive bacteria identified on blood culture, susceptibilities pending
    - Known colonization with methicillin-resistant *Staphylococcus aureus* (MRSA)

- Severe mucositis or soft-tissue infection
- Severe sepsis or septic shock
- Role of antifungal therapy:
  - Should be initiated for persistent fever after 4 to 7 days of broad-spectrum therapy
- Duration of antibiotics:
  - Documented infection: treat for standard duration indicated for specific infection and/or until neutropenia resolves, whichever is longer
  - Undocumented infection: treat until fever disappears and ANC of greater than 500 for at least 24 hours

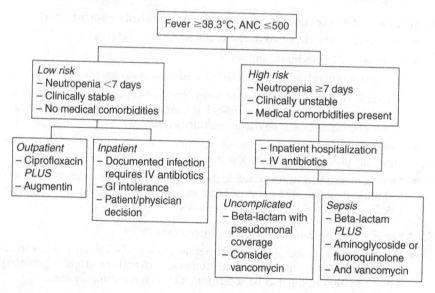

SPINAL CORD COMPRESSION

1. **What are the clinical signs and symptoms of cord compression?**
   - Back or radicular pain (pain is the most common and generally first complaint)
   - Muscle weakness
   - Change in bowel or bladder function (retention or incontinence)
   - Sensory loss or autonomic dysfunction
   - Ataxia
   - Neurologic examination should include percussion of spinal column, evaluation for motor and sensory weakness, and rectal exam to assess sphincter tone

2. **What are the preferred imaging modalities to diagnose cord compression?**
   - MRI with gadolinium contrast is the preferred testing modality
   - CT with myelogram is an acceptable alternative when MRI is not available or contraindicated

3. **What is the treatment for cord compression?**
   - Single most important prognostic factor for regaining ambulation is pretreatment neurologic status; therefore, need to avoid delays in initiating therapy
   - Steroids should be initiated immediately: loading dose 10 mg IV dexamethasone followed by 4 mg IV dexamethasone every 6 hours. Consider higher dose steroids if the patient is presenting with paraplegia or paraparesis
   - Emergent evaluations by Neurosurgery (for decompression) and Radiation Oncology. Consider minimally invasive procedures (eg, kyphoplasty or vertebroplasty) for patients who are not candidates for open surgery
   - Rigid brace if spine is unstable

SUPERIOR VENA CAVA SYNDROME

1. **What is superior vena cava (SVC) syndrome?**
   - Any condition that leads to obstruction and impedance of blood flow through the SVC
   - Usually external compression from primary or metastatic disease
   - May also be due to thrombosis
   - Development of venous collaterals leads to associated clinical manifestations
   - SVC syndrome is a clinical diagnosis and may develop acutely or gradually

2. **What are the symptoms of SVC syndrome?**
   - Dyspnea (most common symptom), orthopnea, cough
   - Facial swelling or head fullness
   - Arm swelling
   - Chest pain
   - Dysphagia, hoarseness
   - Headaches, confusion, coma (if cerebral edema present)
   - Positional worsening of symptoms (bending over, supine position)

3. **What are the signs associated with SVC syndrome?**
   - Superficial venous distension of the neck or chest wall
   - Facial and periorbital edema, plethora
   - Upper extremity edema
   - Lethargy, mental status changes

4. **What imaging studies are useful in SVC syndrome?**
   - Chest radiograph may show mediastinal widening or pleural effusions
   - Contrast-enhanced CT is the most useful imaging modality; can define level and extent of venous obstruction as well as reveal presence of collaterals
   - MRI venography can be used in patients with contrast dye allergy
   - Doppler ultrasound

5. **What is the treatment for SVC syndrome?**
   - Management goals include symptomatic alleviation as well as treatment of underlying disease

- If time permits, a histologic diagnosis should be obtained prior to initiation of treatment
- Emergent radiation reserved for respiratory compromise (stridor) or central nervous system (CNS) symptoms only
- Chemotherapy and/or radiation directed at underlying malignancy
- Endovascular stenting provides rapid symptom palliation; can be performed emergently and in setting of occlusion (with appropriate clot-directed intervention prior)
- Anticoagulation and removal of intravascular catheter indicated if SVC is due to intravascular thrombosis
- Glucocorticoids and diuretics may be used for symptomatic relief; however, steroids should be avoided prior to tissue biopsy and diuretics need to be used with caution due to their potential for causing dehydration and cardiovascular compromise
- Conservative management includes elevation of head of bed, bed rest, and supplemental O_2

CHEMOTHERAPY EXTRAVASATION

1. **What is extravasation of chemotherapy?**
   - Unintended leakage of chemotherapy drug into extravascular space
   - Vesicants cause tissue necrosis; irritants cause inflammation only

2. **What are the common vesicant and irritant chemotherapeutic drugs?**

Vesicant	Commonly Used Treatments
Anthracyclines	
• Daunorubicin, doxorubicin, epirubicin, idarubicin, mitomycin C	• Dexrazoxane • Topical DMSO • Topical cooling
Vinca alkaloids	
• Vincristine, vinblastine, vinorelbine	• Subcutaneous hyaluronidase • Topical warming

Irritant	Commonly Used Treatments
Taxanes*	• Topical cooling
• Docetaxel, paclitaxel	• Subcutaneous hyaluronidase
Platinums*	
• Carboplatin, cisplatin	
Epipodophyllotoxins	• Topical warming
• Etoposide, teniposide	
Topoisomerase I inhibitors	• Topical cooling
• Irinotecan, topotecan	

*May have vesicant properties at high volume/concentration, but generally act as irritants.

Supportive Care

CHEMOTHERAPY-INDUCED NAUSEA AND VOMITING

1. **What are the types of chemotherapy-induced nausea and vomiting (CINV)?**
   - **Acute:** up to 24 hours after chemotherapy, mediated by 5-HT3 release from enterochromaffin cells
   - **Delayed:** more than 24 hours after chemotherapy, mediated by NK_1 receptors
   - **Anticipatory:** occurs on the day of or some hours before the anticipated chemotherapy; typically triggered by taste, odor, sight, distressing thoughts, or anxiety

2. **What is the emetogenicity of various chemotherapeutic agents?**

	Risk of Emesis (Without Antiemetics)			
	High >90%	Moderate 31%–90%	Low 10%–30%	Minimal <10%
IV agents	Carmustine	Alemtuzumab	Bortezomib	2-chlorode-oxyadenosine
	Cisplatin	Azacitidine	Carfilzomib	Bevacizumab
	Cyclophosphamide ≥ 1,500 mg/m²	Bendamustine	Cytarabine ≤1,000 mg/m²	Bleomycin
		Cabazitaxel	Docetaxel	Busulfan
	Dacarbazine	Carboplatin	Eribulin	Cetuximab
	Dactinomycin	Clofarabine	Etoposide	Fludarabine
	Mechlorethamine	Cyclophosphamide ≤1,500 mg/m²	5-Fluorouracil	Rituximab
	Streptozotocin	Cytarabine >1,000 mg/m²	Gemcitabine	Vinblastine
		Daunorubicin*	Ixabepilone	Vincristine
		Denileukin diftitox	Methotrexate >1,000 mg/m²	Vinorelbine
		Doxorubicin*	Mitomycin	
		Epirubicin*	Mitoxantrone	
		Idarubicin*	Paclitaxel	
		Ifosfamide	Panitumumab	
		Irinotecan	PEG-liposomal doxorubicin	
		Melphalan		
		Oxaliplatin		

(continued)

(continued)

	Risk of Emesis (Without Antiemetics)			
	High >90%	Moderate 31%–90%	Low 10%–30%	Minimal <10%
PO agents	Hexamethyl-melamine Procarbazine	Pralatrexate Temozolomide Altretamine Busulfan Crizotinib Cyclophosphamide Imatinib Lomustine Temozolomide Tretinoin Vandetanib Vinorelbine	Pemetrexed Romidepsin Temsirolimus Topotecan Trastuzumab Vorinostat Axitinib Bexarotene Capecitabine Cetuximab Dasatinib Estramustine Etoposide Everolimus Fludarabine Lapatinib Lenalidomide Nilotinib Panitumumab Pazopanib Sunitinib Tegafur uracil Thalidomide Topotecan Vemurafenib Vorinostat	6-Thioguanine Chlorambucil Erlotinib Gefitinib Hydroxyurea Melphalan Methotrexate Regorafenib Sorafenib

*When combined with cyclophosphamide, these anthracyclines have high emetic risk.

3. What antiemetic agents are available?

- Serotonin (5-HT$_3$) receptor antagonists

- ○ First generation: dolasetron, granisetron (transdermal patch option), ondansetron (oral dissolving tablet option), tropisetron
- ○ Second generation: palonosetron (higher affinity for receptor and longer half-life)
- ○ Oral and IV forms are similarly effective
- ○ Side effects: headache, diarrhea, transient transaminitis and EKG changes; prolonged QT interval seen primarily with dolasetron. Constipation with the 5-HT3 receptor antagonists can be severe
- NK$_1$ receptor antagonists
  - ○ Aprepitant and its prodrug fosaprepitant
  - ○ Potential drug interactions: moderate inhibitor of CYP3A4
- Steroids
  - ○ Oral and parenteral dexamethasone and methylprednisolone are equally effective
  - ○ Side effects: insomnia, mood changes, irritability, and hyperglycemia
- Dopamine (D$_2$) receptor antagonists
  - ○ Prochlorperazine, promethazine, haloperidol, and metoclopramide
  - ○ Side effects: sedation, extrapyramidal reactions, anticholinergic effects, EKG changes (haloperidol, droperidol), hypotension with rapid IV administration (phenothiazines)
- Benzodiazepines
  - ○ Lorazepam and alprazolam
  - ○ Side effects: dose-related sedation and delirium (especially in elderly patients). Benzodiazepines can potentiate the sedating effects of opioids and should be used with caution in patients receiving concomitant opioids
- Cannabinoids
  - ○ Dronabinol and nabilone
  - ○ Side effects: sedation, confusion, dizziness, short-term memory loss, euphoria/dysphoria, ataxia, dry mouth, and orthostatic hypotension
- Antihistamines
  - ○ Diphenhydramine and hydroxyzine
  - ○ Are not useful for CINV, but helpful for motion sickness
  - ○ Side effects: sedation, dry mouth, visual changes, mydriasis, decreased GI motility, urinary changes, and increased heart rate
- Neuroleptics
  - ○ Olanzapine
  - ○ Useful for both acute and delayed CINV refractory to other treatments

4. How do you prevent nausea and vomiting?

Risk	High		Moderate		Low		Minimal	
			Prophylaxis Recommended					
Type	Acute	Delayed	Acute	Delayed	Acute	Delayed	Acute	Delayed
	5-HT3RA + dex + aprepitant ± lorazepam	Dex + aprepitant ± lorazepam	Anthracycline/ cyclophosphamide: 5-HT3RA + dex + aprepitant ± lorazepam Others: 5-HT3RA ± dex ± lorazepam	Aprepitant ± dex ± lorazepam	Dex ± lorazepam prochlorperazine ± lorazepam Metoclopramide ± lorazepam	None	None	None

5-HT3RA, serotonin receptor antagonist; dex, dexamethasone.

5. **How do you treat breakthrough and refractory CINV?**
   - Avoid repeated dosing of agents that were given for prophylaxis and already failed
   - Consider adding prochlorperazine, metoclopramide, a benzodiazepine, or a neuroleptic (ie, olanzapine)

6. **What are nonpharmacologic measures for antiemetic prophylaxis?**
   - Ginger capsules or chews (prior to and during treatment cycle)
   - Cognitive distraction (ie, playing video games during treatment)
   - Systematic desensitization (visualization and learned relaxation techniques)
   - Hypnosis
   - Acupuncture
   - Transcutaneous electrical nerve stimulation
   - Mindfulness through guided meditation

GROWTH FACTORS

1. **What are the indications for the prophylactic use of granulocyte colony-stimulating factor (G-CSF)?**
   - Risk of febrile neutropenia is >20%
   - Consider use if the risk of neutropenia is between 10% and 20% based on patient risk factors
     - Prior chemotherapy or radiation therapy
     - Persistent neutropenia
     - Bone marrow involvement by malignancy
     - Renal or liver dysfunction
     - Age >65 and receiving full dose chemotherapy
   - Not indicated if the risk of febrile neutropenia is <10%

2. **When should you use G-CSF for the treatment of febrile neutropenia?**
   - Continue if the patient is currently receiving prophylactic filgrastim, filgrastim-sndz, or tbo-filgrastim
   - *Do not use* if the patient has already received prophylactic pegfilgrastim
   - Consider use if the patient has risk factors for infection-associated complications
     - Sepsis syndrome
     - Age >65 years
     - ANC <100/uL
     - Duration of neutropenia expected to be >10 days
     - Invasive fungal infection
     - Hospitalization at the time of fever
     - Prior episode of febrile neutropenia
     - Presence of pneumonia or other clinically documented infections

CANCER-ASSOCIATED VENOUS THROMBOEMBOLIC DISEASE

1. **What are the risk factors for venous thrombotic events (VTEs)?**
   - General patient-associated risk factors
     - Active cancer
     - Advanced stage of cancer
     - Higher risk cancer types: brain, pancreas, stomach, bladder, gynecologic, lung, lymphoma, myeloproliferative neoplasms, kidney
     - Bulky regional lymphadenopathy with extrinsic vascular compression
     - Inherited and/or acquired hypercoagulable states
     - Medical comorbidities: infection, renal failure, pulmonary disease, heart failure
     - Poor performance status
     - Older age
   - Treatment-associated risk factors
     - Major surgery
     - Central venous catheter
     - Certain chemotherapies (ie, thalidomide/lenalidomide/pomalidomide and high-dose dexamethasone)
     - Exogenous hormonal therapy (ie, oral contraceptives and tamoxifen/raloxifene)
   - Modifiable risk factors
     - Tobacco smoking
     - Obesity
     - Decreased activity/exercise

Khorana Predictive Model for Chemotherapy-Associated VTE

Patient Characteristic	Risk Score
• Site of primary cancer	
○ Very high risk (stomach, pancreas)	2
○ High risk (lung, lymphoma, gynecologic, bladder, testicular)	1
• Prechemotherapy platelet count ≥350 K/uL	1
• Hemoglobin <10 g/dL or use of ESA	1
• Prechemotherapy leukocyte count >11 K/uL	1
• BMI >35	1

BMI, body mass index; ESA, erythropoiesis-stimulating agents; VTE, venous thrombotic event.

Total Score	Risk Category	Risk of Symptomatic VTE
0	Low	0.8%–3%
1,2	Intermediate	1.8%–8.4%
3 or higher	High	7.1%–41%

2. When is outpatient VTE prophylaxis indicated?

- Surgical oncology patients: VTE recommended for up to 4 weeks postoperation, especially in high-risk abdominal or pelvic cancer surgery patients
- Patients with multiple myeloma receiving either thalidomide or one of its derivatives (lenalidomide, pomalidomide)
  - High risk: VTE prophylaxis with either low molecular weight heparin (LMWH) or warfarin
  - Low risk: aspirin 81 mg to 325 mg

3. When is inpatient pharmacologic VTE prophylaxis contraindicated?

- Absolute contraindications
  - Recent CNS bleed
  - Intracranial or spinal lesion at high risk for bleeding
  - Major active bleeding, defined as, >2U PRBC transfused in the past 24 hours
- Relative contraindications
  - Thrombocytopenia (<50 K/uL)
  - Severe platelet dysfunction
  - Recent major surgery at high risk for bleeding
  - Coagulopathy

PAIN MANAGEMENT

1. What are the critical features of a comprehensive pain assessment?

- Interview the patient to characterize the position, quality, severity, and timing of the pain. Rule out radiation or referred pain. Identify factors that provoke or palliate pain. Patients can have multiple sources of pain; each should be characterized separately.
- Identify psychosocial factors that may interfere with treatment of pain:
  - Concurrent mood disorders
  - Fear of addiction or death
  - Social, financial, and spiritual stressors
  - Prior history of substance abuse, tobacco, or chronic opioid use
- Inspect and palpate the site of pain, looking for associated physical signs. Rule out neurologic deficits.
- Reassess the patient when there is any change in quality or severity of pain or the consumption of pain killers
- Severe, uncontrollable pain is a medical emergency that may require IV therapy and/or hospitalization

2. What is an appropriate approach to cancer pain management?

- Determine the likely mechanism of the pain. Many patients with cancer have pain that is not cancer-related and should *not* be treated with opioids.
- Determine if the patient is a good candidate for opioids. Patients should be able to take the medication responsibly. Patients with prior history of polysubstance abuse should be provided opioids in smaller quantities (1–2 weeks at a time) and given additional supervision by staff.

		Immediate Prognosis	
		Good	Poor
Severity of Cancer Pain	Mild	NSAID and/or acetaminophen PRN	Dose find with strong, short-acting opioid PRN; rotate to long-acting opioid
	Moderate–Severe	Strong, short-acting opioid PRN only	Strong, short-acting PRN + long-acting opioid over time

NSAID, nonsteroidal anti-inflammatory drug.

3. What are opioid equivalences as compared with single dose morphine?

Drug	Parenteral Dose (mg)	Oral Dose (mg)	Factor (IV to PO)	Peak	Duration of Action (hours)	Starting IV Dose	Starting PO Dose
Morphine*	10	30	3	PO: 1.5–2 hr IV: 20 min	3–4	2–4 mg q2–4 hr	15 mg immediate release q4 hr
Hydro-morphone	1.5	7.5	5	PO and IV: 1 hr	2–3	0.2–2 mg q2 hr	2–4 mg q4–6 hr
Fentanyl	100 mcg	–	–	IV: 1–5 min Transdermal: 24 hr	1–3	0.25–1 mcg/kg prn	Transdermal: 12–25 mcg/hr q72 hr
Levorphanol	2	4	2	PO: 1 hr IV: 20 min	3–6	1 mg q3–6 hr	2 mg q6–8 hr
Oxycodone	–	15–20	–	1–2 hr	3–5	–	5–10 mg q4–6 hr
Hydrocodone	–	30–45	–	2 hr	3–5	–	5–10 mg q4–6 hr
Oxymorphone	1	10	10	PO: 1 hr	3–6	0.5 mg q4 hr	5–10 mg immediate release q4 hr
Codeine	–	200	–	1.5 hr	3–4	–	30–60 mg q4 hr
Tramadol	–	50–100	–		3–7	–	50–100 mg q4–6 hr

*Methadone's conversion ratio to oral morphine equivalents is dose-dependent.

4. What opioid do you choose?

- Short-acting opioids are indicated for intermittent or breakthrough pain.
- Long-acting opioids are indicated when patients are taking short-acting opioids round the clock.
- Compounded opioids should be avoided in patients whose pain condition is likely to worsen over time as there is a ceiling level, preventing upward titration.
- Choice of opioid depends upon the severity of the pain as well as the patient's past trials of opioids.
- First line:
  - Mild pain: hydrocodone
  - Moderate to severe pain: oxycodone or morphine
- Some situations merit specific opioids:
  - Poor compliance or mild cognitive impairment: transdermal fentanyl
  - Intractable constipation: transdermal fentanyl
  - Neurotoxicity: hydromorphone, oxycodone, or methadone
  - Renal impairment: buprenorphine, fentanyl, and methadone (if patient is not on dialysis)
  - Liver impairment: oxycodone
  - Opioid tolerance: hydromorphone
  - Complex pain (with heavy neuropathic component): methadone

5. How do you initiate short-acting opioids?

- For patients who are opioid-naïve, begin opioids at the lowest recommended dose (see the previous table); consider even lower doses for older patients or patients with renal or liver disease.
  - Effectiveness of a given dose can be gauged within 1 hour of taking an oral opioid and 15 minutes of taking an IV opioid
- For ambulatory patients with pain but not in crisis, start opioids as given in the preceding, have them keep a diary and follow up within a week. When pain control is not achieved, increase dose in increments by 30% to 50%.
- For ambulatory patients in a pain crisis, start opioids as recommended in the preceding, have them keep a diary, and reassess within 24 hours. When pain is not controlled, increase dose by 100% and reassess again within 24 hours.
- Patients in crisis whose pain cannot be controlled at home with oral opioids should be admitted to the hospital for IV treatment. IV is preferred for patients who have malabsorption or intractable vomiting.

6. How do you initiate long-acting opioids?

- Patients should not be started on a long-acting opioid without "dose finding" with a short-acting opioid first to determine the total daily dose (TDD)
- Once the TDD is known, divide the TDD by the number of times the patient will be taking the long-acting opioid per day. For example, for BID long-acting morphine, 50% of the TDD should be given in the morning and 50% of the TDD should be given in the evening.

- Try to use the short- and long-acting forms of the same opioid. Rarely is a combination of different opioids helpful.
- When converting a patient from one opioid to another (eg, morphine to oxycodone), calculate the TDD of the initial opioid and convert to the equivalent TDD of the replacement opioid using the equianalgesic doses (see the previous table). Account for incomplete cross-tolerance by decreasing the TDD of the new opioid by 25% to 50%. Then convert into long- and short-acting forms.

7. What is appropriate dosing for breakthrough pain medication?

- Once patients are on a long-acting opioid, the short-acting breakthrough opioid should be dosed at 10% to 20% of the TDD.
  - For example, if a patient is taking 40 mg long-acting oxycodone twice daily, then an appropriate dose of breakthrough medication would be 5 to 10 mg oxycodone every 4 hours as needed.
- Oral opioids may be safely dosed as often as every 1 to 2 hours during a pain crisis.
  - Short-acting opioids given orally reach peak effect at 1 hour and last no more than 4 hours.

8. What are common side effects of opioids?

- All patients on opioids get constipation.
- Other common side effects include delirium, myoclonus, urinary retention, sedation, nausea and vomiting, pruritus, and respiratory depression. Tolerance develops over time for all these effects **except delirium, myoclonus, and urinary retention**; these side effects and hypersensitivity reactions require switching to a different opioid.
- Prevent constipation in patients on opioids by administering a motility agent (bisacodyl or senna) daily.
  - Titrate the dose every 2 to 3 days for a bowel movement at least once every 48 hours.
  - Avoid constipating agents (eg, fiber, anticholinergics, haloperidol, calcium channel blockers, iron, anticonvulsants, ondansetron).

9. What are risks of long-term opioid use?

- Addiction: malingering for opioids is rare in patients with active cancer, but can be seen among patients whose cancers are in remission, especially those with a preceding history of polysubstance abuse. Every effort should be made to titrate patients entirely off opioids once their cancer is in remission.
- Dependence: manifests as withdrawal symptoms (nausea, chills, sweats) at cessation or dose reduction.
- Tolerance: all patients taking opioids regularly develop tolerance; providers should expect that TDD will go up over time, even when disease is stable.
- Hyperalgesia: increased pain sensitivity that develops with regular, long-term opioid use; precise mechanism is poorly understood; escalating the opioid dose may paradoxically increase the level of pain.

10. **How does one terminate opioid therapy?**
    - Decrease TDD by 10% to 20% daily or more slowly if withdrawal develops.
    - Treat withdrawal: loperamide (for diarrhea), prochlorperazine (for nausea/vomiting), clonidine (for sweats).

11. **What are examples of adjuvant analgesics?**
    - Anticonvulsant medications
      - Gabapentin, pregabalin, lamotrigine, topiramate, carbamazepine, valproic acid, and phenytoin
    - Antidepressants
      - Serotonin and norepinephrine reuptake inhibitors (SNRIs), selective serotonin reuptake inhibitors (SSRIs), and tricyclic antidepressants (TCAs)
      - Useful as single agents in patients without cancer
      - For patients with cancer, they should be added once opioids have been initiated. Patients should be monitored for anticholinergic side effects. Avoid TCA use in the elderly.
    - Bisphosphonates
      - Pamidronate, ibandronate, and zoledronate
      - Effective for treating bone pain related to metastases
    - Local anesthetics (ie, lidocaine patch)
      - Effective for treating localized, superficial neuropathic and somatic pain syndromes
    - Corticosteroids
      - Effective for pain and weakness associated with nerve impingement or bone metastases
    - Antispasmodics (ie, dicyclomine)
      - Effective for visceral pain
    - Interventional pain clinic
      - Referral for nerve/plexus blocks, infusion pumps, stimulation units, kyphoplasty/vertebroplasty

12. **What are examples of nonpharmacologic pain therapy?**
    - Acupuncture
    - Relaxation/biofeedback
    - Recreation/art/music therapy
    - Transcutaneous electrical nerve stimulation
    - Myofascial trigger release
    - Massage, healing touch
    - Behavioral counseling

CONSTIPATION

1. **What should an assessment of constipation entail?**
   - Assess cause and severity of constipation:
     - Goal: one bowel movement every 24 to 48 hours

- Rule out and treat other causes such as:
  - Impaction
  - Obstruction
  - Malignant neurogenic involvement
  - Medication-induced (5-HT3 antagonists, opioids)
  - Electrolyte imbalances

2. **What are preventive measures for constipation?**
   - Ensure adequate fluid intake
   - Encourage physical activity
   - Patients taking opioids should be instructed to stop fiber supplementation
   - Initiate a bowel regimen at the same time as initiation of opioids. Instruct patients that "every day you take a pain pill is a day you take a laxative."

3. **How do you manage constipation?**
   - Ask patients to keep a log of their bowel movements.
   - When an opiate is prescribed, prescribe senna (with or without docusate; 2 tablets BID).
     - Adjust the dose every 2 to 3 days according to results.
   - If the patient goes more than 3 days without a bowel movement, first prescribe either a bisacodyl or glycerin suppository. If ineffective, recommend a phosphate enema daily until a good bowel movement is achieved.
     - Note: do *not* use rectal approaches if patient is neutropenic or coagulopathic
   - When senna daily is ineffective, add lactulose or polyethylene glycol

CANCER CACHEXIA

1. **What is cancer cachexia?**
   - Characterized by loss of appetite, chronic nausea, fatigue, and weight loss ($\geq$6% decrease over 6 months). Thought to be secondary to:
     - Proinflammatory cytokines (TNF, IL-1, IL-6, IFN), which lead to hypermetabolism and anorexia (from changes in ghrelin, leptin, and serotonin production)
     - Tumor production of proteolysis-inducing factor and lipid-mobilizing factor causes fat and muscle loss
     - Inefficient energy metabolism and insulin resistance leads to further lean body mass depletion
   - Cancer cachexia is an independent predictor of early mortality
   - Overfeeding may lead to further metabolic derangement without resultant weight gain

2. **What are appropriate interventions for anorexia/cachexia?**
   - Treat reversible causes: for example, nausea and vomiting, xerostomia, mucositis, dental issues, dysgeusia, dysphagia, early satiety, bowel obstruction, constipation, pain, and depression.
     - Rule out endocrine abnormalities

- Review and eliminate medications that interfere with appetite
- Rule out social and economic factors
- Nutrition consultation to help identify barriers to increased intake or recommend dietary modifications
- Caloric supplementation:
  - Increased intake does not result in improved survival or tumor response
  - Enteral feeding is preferred (less infection risk, decreased catabolic hormones, improved wound healing, shorter hospital stays, and maintenance of gut integrity)
  - Parenteral nutrition (rarely indicated unless patient is NPO)
- Pharmacologic interventions:
  - Metoclopramide helps treat nausea as well as delayed gastric emptying in patients who complain of early satiety. Watch for extrapyramidal symptoms (EPS)
  - Glucocorticoids help to increase appetite, but should be used for short periods of time due to the long-term effects
  - Megestrol works like steroids and is rarely effective if the patient has not responded to steroids in the past. Do not give megestrol concurrently with steroids. Note: megestrol can increase risk for thromboembolic events
  - Mirtazapine
  - Dronabinol is not effective for increasing appetite in cancer patients

DYSPNEA

1. What is an appropriate approach to the management of dyspnea?
- Assess and identify the causes of the dyspnea
- Treat reversible causes:
  - Infection: antibiotics as indicated
  - Anemia: transfuse as needed
  - Bronchospasm
  - Pneumothorax
  - Pulmonary embolus: anticoagulation if possible
  - Airway mechanical obstruction (eg, mass)
  - Effusions (pleural and pericardial): thoracentesis and pleurodesis, respectively
  - Airway obstruction: bronchoscopic interventions and/or radiation
    - Comorbid chronic obstructive pulmonary disease (COPD): inhaled corticosteroids and bronchodilators
- Relieve symptoms
  - Nonpharmacologic
    - Fans (for patients without COPD or coronary artery disease [CAD]), cooler temperatures, stress management, and relaxation therapy
    - Supplemental oxygen for hypoxia (SaO_2 <90%) or subjective relief
    - Emotional, psychosocial, and educational support

- Pharmacologic
  - Low-dose opioids (ie, 2.5–5 mg morphine q2–4 hr) to reduce air hunger
  - Anxiolytics to reduce the anxiety that coexists with dyspnea (use with caution in patients who are taking concomitant opioids)
  - Expectorants (ie, guaifenesin) to thin secretions
  - Antitussives (ie, dextromethorphan, codeine, and hydrocodone) to reduce frequency of cough
  - Anticholinergics (ie, atropine and hyoscine) to control secretions
- Noninvasive positive pressure ventilation (CPAP and BiPAP)

PSYCHIATRIC SYNDROMES

1. **What are common psychiatric syndromes seen in cancer patients?**
   - Adjustment disorder
   - Major depression
   - Anxiety
   - Delirium

2. **What is adjustment disorder?**
   - Time-limited, maladaptive reaction to a specific stressor (eg, cancer diagnosis and treatment)
   - Onset within 3 months of stressor, duration <6 months
   - Lack neurovegetative signs and suicidal ideation
   - Treatment directed at crisis intervention, brief psychotherapy, and symptom management

3. **What are the diagnostic criteria for major depressive disorder (MDD)?**
   - Persistently low mood or anhedonia plus five of the following for at least 2 weeks:
     - Sleep disturbance
     - Loss of interest
     - Feelings of hopelessness, helplessness, or guilt
     - Low energy
     - Poor concentration
     - Appetite disturbance
     - Psychomotor retardation/agitation
     - Suicidal or homicidal ideation
   - Screen using the PHQ-2, and assess using the PHQ-9
   - Rule out pseudodepression

4. **What are some causes of pseudodepression?**
   - Uncontrolled pain
   - Hypothyroidism
   - Medications (steroids, certain chemotherapies such as interferon)

- Metabolic abnormalities (electrolytes, B12, or folate deficiency)
- Organic brain disease (metastatic brain involvement, endocrinopathies, etc.)
- Dementia
- Substance abuse
- Adjustment disorder
- Fatigue
- Personality disorders

5. **What is the treatment of MDD?**
   - Psychotherapy
   - Pharmacotherapy
     - ○ SSRIs and SNRIs are especially useful in patients who also have neuropathic pain. Can take 4 to 8 weeks to see full benefit.
     - ○ Methylphenidate has a shorter duration of action, but should be avoided in anyone who has insomnia, agitation, active CAD, or anxiety
     - ○ TCAs should be avoided in patients over the age of 65
     - ○ Mirtazapine is a good option for patients with cancer anorexia and/or insomnia
     - ○ Antidepressants should be continued for 12 months from the point of remission if first episode of MDD

6. **What are commonly used antidepressants?**

Class	Name	Dose Range (mg)	Side Effects
SSRI	Fluoxetine	5–60	GI symptoms, weight changes, sleep disruption, sexual dysfunction, dry mouth, hyponatremia
	Paroxetine	10–60	
	Sertraline	12.5–200	
	Citalopram	10–60	
	Escitalopram	5–40	
Mixed agents	Venlafaxine	18.75–300	GI symptoms, sexual dysfunction, anticholinergic effects, hypertension with doses >225 mg, reduces hot flashes
	Bupropion	37.5–450	GI symptoms, tremor, lowers seizure threshold
	Duloxetine	20–60	GI symptoms, headache, dizziness; also indicated for neuropathic pain

(continued)

(continued)

Class	Name	Dose Range (mg)	Side Effects
	Mirtazapine	7.5–45	Sedation, dry mouth, increased appetite, and weight gain
	Trazodone	25–200	Sedation, orthostatic hypotension, priapism
TCAs	Amitriptyline	25–150	Dry mouth, sedation, weight gain, GI symptoms, EKG changes, orthostatic hypotension, anticholinergic effects
	Nortriptyline	25–150	
	Desipramine	25–150	
	Doxepin	10–150	
Psychostimulants	Methylphenidate	2.5–60*	Hypertension, tachycardia, anxiety
	Dextroamphetamine	10–60	

*For off-label use in depression, maximum dose is 20 mg and sustained release product is not recommended. For stimulant use, maximum daily dose is 60 mg.

GI, gastrointestinal; SSRI, selective serotonin reuptake inhibitor; TCA, tricyclic antidepressants.

7. What is the management of anxiety?

- Rule out reversible causes
  - Poorly controlled symptoms
  - Metabolic disturbances (eg, hypercalcemia, hypoglycemia, and carcinoid syndrome)
  - Medications (eg, thyroxine and phenothiazines)
- Nonpharmacologic treatment
  - Behavioral therapy and psychotherapy
- Pharmacologic treatment
  - Benzodiazepines (eg, lorazepam, alprazolam, and clonazepam)
  - Antidepressants (eg, SSRIs and mixed agents)
  - Neuroleptics (eg, haloperidol and atypical antipsychotics) for severe and persistent anxiety
  - Other drugs: buspirone, propranolol (for autonomic symptoms), sedative hypnotics (for insomnia)

8. What is delirium?

- Acute confusional state characterized by fluctuating course of cognitive impairment, perceptual disturbances, delusions, mood changes, and disruption of sleep–wake cycle
- May be hyperactive (agitated) or hypoactive (quiet)

9. What is the management of delirium?

- Identify and treat precipitating factors
  - Direct CNS causes
    - Brain tumor
    - Brain metastases
    - Seizures
  - Indirect causes
    - Metabolic encephalopathy
    - Electrolyte imbalance
    - Medications (steroids, narcotics, anticholinergics, antiemetics)
    - Infection
    - Hematologic abnormalities
    - Nutritional deficiencies
    - Paraneoplastic syndromes
- Pharmacologic treatment
  - Neuroleptics (eg, haloperidol)
    - Side effects: sedation, EPS, hypotension, QT prolongation
  - Atypical neuroleptics (eg, olanzapine, quetiapine, and risperidone)
    - Side effects: sedation, weight gain, metabolic syndrome, and QT prolongation
  - Benzodiazepines (eg, lorazepam, midazolam):
    - Should not be prescribed in patients with delirium
  - Palliative sedation (only for terminal delirium, with patient and/or surrogate consent)
    - Propofol 10–70 mcg/hr
- Environmental modification
  - Keep the environment calm and quiet with adequate, but soft, indirect light and limit noise levels.
  - Provide glasses and hearing aids to maximize sensory perception.
  - Consider the use of night lights to combat nighttime confusion.
  - Use music that has an individual significance to the confused and agitated client to prevent the increase in or decrease agitated behaviors.

QUESTIONS

1. A 70-year-old male with past medical history significant for coronary artery disease status pacemaker placement and degenerative joint disease status post left hip replacement was recently diagnosed with Stage IV non–small cell lung cancer (NSCLC) to the bones. He is scheduled to undergo palliative chemotherapy with carboplatin and pemetrexed and presents to your office for a prechemotherapy visit. On your interview, he states that he has been experiencing acute

worsening of his chronic low back pain and also has had difficulty with walking. On neurologic exam, you note decreased strength of 4/5 in bilateral lower extremities. There is also decreased sphincter tone on rectal exam. What diagnostic imaging do you order emergently to make the diagnosis?
A. MRI of the spine
B. Bone scan
C. CT myelogram
D. PET scan

2. You are seeing a 56-year-old female with a history of metastatic breast cancer to the bone currently on palliative chemotherapy with palbociclib and fulvestrant and there is no evidence of progression on her most recent imaging. She is currently on oxycodone 5 mg as needed for pain control. She reports that she needs the oxycodone 6 times a day with improvement in her pain to a 3/10, which she states is tolerable. She is on an appropriate bowel regimen and is not having any constipation. She does not report any new pain. She is concerned about the frequency at which she needs to take the oxycodone, especially as she wakes up at night to take her medication, and is inquiring regarding long-acting pain medication. You recommend:
A. MS Contin 30 mg every 12 hours with 5 mg oxycodone PRN for breakthrough
B. Oxycontin 15 mg every 12 hours
C. Oxycontin 15 mg every 12 hours with 5 mg oxycodone PRN for breakthrough
D. Oxycontin 30 mg every 12 hours with 5 mg oxycodone PRN for breakthrough

3. You are on the inpatient hematology/oncology service and are taking care of a 34-year-old female with classical Hodgkin lymphoma status post two cycles of ABVD chemotherapy. She presented 4 days ago with fevers (T_{max} 101.2°F) and was found to be neutropenic with absolute neutrophil count (ANC) of 80/uL. She complained of general malaise and myalgias but did not have any localizing symptoms. Chest x-ray and urinalysis at the time of admission were unremarkable. After blood cultures were obtained, she was started on empiric therapy with piperacillin–tazobactam. Vancomycin was then added given that she does have a port in place. It is now day 5 and she is still persistently febrile with T_{max} of 100.9°F. Her vitals are otherwise stable and she continues to not have any localizing symptoms. Her cultures have thus far been negative. Her ANC is now 360/uL. What medication changes would you consider making next?
A. Discontinue piperacillin–tazobactam and start cefepime
B. Add tobramycin to the current regimen
C. Discontinue vancomycin and start daptomycin
D. Add fluconazole to current regimen

4. You are seeing a 28-year-old male in the outpatient oncology clinic. He was diagnosed with good risk advanced testicular germ-cell tumor about 6 weeks ago. He is currently receiving BEP chemotherapy and is tolerating it well. On your interview today, he appears to be more withdrawn than usual. He admits to occasionally feeling down and depressed when thinking about his cancer diagnosis. He also thinks that he has become more irritable with his family and friends. He continues to work full time and finds pleasure in golfing, which has been his favorite recreational activity. He denies any thoughts of harming himself. What is the most likely diagnosis?
   A. Adjustment disorder
   B. Major depressive disorder
   C. Anxiety
   D. Delirium

5. A 67-year-old male with past medical history of coronary artery disease (CAD) and chronic kidney disease (CKD) who was recently diagnosed with limited-stage small cell lung cancer (SCLC), not yet started on chemotherapy, was brought to the emergency department for a 3-day history of somnolence and confusion at home. His wife also noticed that he had become progressively weaker. Vital signs are stable. Physical exam reveals a mildly distended abdomen with diffuse tenderness to deep palpation. Bloodwork reveals a serum calcium of 10 mg/dL, creatinine of 3.5 mg/dL (at baseline), and albumin of 2.5 g/dL. In addition to starting intravenous (IV) fluids, what other medications do you want to consider prescribing?
   A. Pamidronate 30 mg IV
   B. Denosumab 120 mg SQ
   C. Zoledronic acid 4 mg IV
   D. Furosemide 40 mg IV

6. A 59-year-old male with a 100 pack smoking history presents to the emergency department with acute onset of shortness of breath. He states that this occurred suddenly 1 week ago and has become progressively worse. He does have a nonproductive cough, worse than his baseline. He states that he has tried over-the-counter remedies without any improvement in his symptoms. He notices that lying down makes his coughing worse. On physical exam, he is noted to be markedly dyspneic with respiratory rate in the 30s. He is also tachycardic. There is facial fullness. You order a CT of the chest with intravenous (IV) contrast, which preliminarily reveals a large mass in the right upper lobe but no evidence of any obvious thromboembolism; this has not been verified by radiology. As the patient is returning from CT, you notice that he is stridoring and developing worsening mentation. What is the next best step in management?
   A. Start empiric IV heparin therapy as you are still highly suspicious for pulmonary embolism
   B. Page radiation oncology for an emergent evaluation
   C. Page thoracic surgery to obtain a stat tissue biopsy of the mass
   D. Start glucocorticoid therapy

ANSWERS

1. **C. CT myelogram.** This patient's presentation is highly suspicious for cord compression from metastatic disease. While MRI of the spine is the preferred imaging modality, he has both a pacemaker and a prosthetic hip, both of which are contraindications to MRI. CT myelogram is therefore the next best option.

2. **C. Oxycontin 15 mg every 12 hours with 5 mg oxycodone PRN for breakthrough.** To convert from short-acting opioids to long-acting opioids, you calculate the total daily dose (TDD) and divide it by the frequency at which it will be taken. In the example of this patient, her TDD of oxycodone is 6 × 5 mg = 30 mg. Oxycontin is prescribed every 12 hours, so her a.m. and p.m. doses should be 15 mg. While BID Oxycontin may be sufficient for her pain control, breakthrough short-acting pain medications at 10% to 20% of her TDD are still recommended. Finally, if possible, the long-acting and short-acting formulation should be of the same opioid.

3. **D. Add fluconazole to current regimen.** The patient is persistently febrile despite being on appropriate broad-spectrum antibiotics for the past 5 days. It is appropriate to consider adding antifungal coverage in these patients.

4. **A. Adjustment disorder.** While the diagnosis of adjustment disorder and depression can be difficult to differentiate, the lack of neurovegetative signs and suicidal ideation suggests the diagnosis of adjustment disorder in this patient. He will need continued assessment as, by definition, the duration of adjustment disorder is less than 6 months.

5. **B. Denosumab 120 mg SQ.** The patient has hypercalcemia (remember to correct for albumin; can also check an ionized calcium to confirm) likely from paraneoplastic secretion of parathyroid-hormone-related protein (PTHrp), which is commonly seen in SCLC. His poor renal function precludes him from receiving bisphosphonates and loop diuretics and therefore he should receive denosumab.

6. **B. Page radiation oncology for an emergent evaluation.** The patient is presenting with signs and symptoms concerning for superior vena cava (SVC) syndrome. While it is preferable to obtain a histologic diagnosis prior to therapy, the patient is developing stridor and is at high risk for respiratory failure and death. This is the only situation where emergent radiation therapy and stent placement should be done prior to confirming a histologic diagnosis.

BONE MARROW
TRANSPLANTATION

XIV

39

Bone Marrow Transplant

Lyndsey N. Runaas and Mary Mansour Riwes

EPIDEMIOLOGY

1. **How many allogeneic stem cell transplants are performed in the United States each year?**
   - More than 8,000 per year

2. **How many autologous stem cell transplants are performed in the United States each year?**
   - Approximately 12,000 per year

CLASSIFICATION

1. **How can stem cell transplants be classified?**
   - Modality:
     - Autologous: patient's own stem cells transplanted
     - Allogeneic: stem cells from an human leukocyte antigen (HLA) matched donor transplanted
     - Syngeneic: stem cells from an HLA identical donor transplanted
   - Donor source: for allogeneic transplants:
     - Matched related: a related donor who is at least an 8/8 HLA match with the recipient (HLA-A, HLA-B, HLA-C, and HLA-DRB1 identical)
     - Matched unrelated: an unrelated donor who is at least an 8/8 HLA match with the recipient
     - Mismatched: a donor who is less than an 8/8 HLA match with the recipient
     - Haploidentical: a related donor who is mismatched at 3/6 HLA loci (HLA-A, HLA-B, and HLA-DR)
     - Umbilical cord blood: stem cells are collected from umbilical cord and placenta after a baby is born. Relative immaturity of the immune system of donors allows for level of HLA mismatch that would otherwise be prohibitive in other sources. Requires at least 4/6 HLA match at HLA-A, HLA-B, and HLA-DRB1. Adult recipients typically require two separate products.
   - Stem cell source:
     - Peripheral blood stem cell: stem cells are collected from donor with a peripheral blood pheresis procedure. Uses either chemotherapy-based or chemokine-based regimen to mobilize stem cells prior to collection.
     - Bone marrow: stem cells are collected directly from the bone marrow. Typically does not require any preprocedure mobilization medications.

- Preparative regimen:
  - Myeloablative: conditioning regimen that is expected to destroy hematopoietic stem cells with resulting long-lasting, usually irreversible, and often fatal pancytopenia unless patient is rescued with stem cell transplant. For example, total body irradiation (TBI) in doses ≥ 5 Gy in a single dose or busulfan >8 mg/kg.
  - Nonmyeloablative: conditioning regimen that causes less cytopenias but significant lymphopenia and would not require stem cell rescue. For example, fludarabine and cyclophosphamide, TBI ≤ 2 Gy.
  - Reduced intensity: intermediate between myeloablative and nonmyeloablative. For example, busulfan ≤ 8 mg/kg or melphalan at ≤ 140 mg/m^2.

2. **Why would you not prefer a syngeneic transplant for a malignant condition?**
   - Patients with an identical twin donor, while they are not at risk for developing graft-versus-host disease (GVHD), have a higher risk of relapse of any underlying malignant condition. This is due to lack of a graft-versus-tumor reaction.
   - The probability of relapse at 3 years with a syngeneic transplant versus an HLA-matched but nonidentical transplant is 52% versus 16% for acute myeloid leukemia (AML) and 40% versus 7% for chronic myelogenous leukemia (CML).

3. **What donor source is preferred for allogeneic stem cell transplants?**
   - When available, a matched related transplant is preferred due to both clinical (less GVHD) and logistical (speed and ease of finding donor) factors.
   - If a matched related donor is not available, it remains unknown which of several alternative donors is best—matched unrelated, haploidentical, or umbilical cord. Factors that are important in making a selection include the urgency of transplant and time needed to obtain a donor, the underlying disease process, and the familiarity of the transplant center with the transplant modality.

4. **What is the likelihood of finding a matched unrelated donor in the donor registry?**
   - The likelihood of finding an unrelated donor through the National Marrow Donor Program varies depending on race and ethnicity.
     - For White patients, the likelihood of a match is as high as 97%.
     - For American Indian and Alaskan Native patients, the likelihood is 90%.
     - For Asian or Pacific Islanders, the likelihood is 84%.
     - For Hispanic or Latino patients, the likelihood is 83%.
     - For African American patients, the likelihood is 76%.

5. **When would you favor bone marrow harvest over peripheral blood stem cell (PBSC) collection in the setting of an allogeneic stem cell transplant?**
   - Studies have generally confirmed slightly faster engraftment with infusion of PBSCs versus bone marrow. However, most studies have documented less chronic GVHD with bone marrow transplant over PBSC.

- Therefore, marrow is preferred in situations where the concern for chronic GVHD is higher (ie, matched unrelated transplants) or in nonmalignant conditions where there is no potential benefit of a graft-versus-tumor phenomenon.

6. **What are the risks to a stem cell donor?**

- The risks vary slightly depending on the source of the stem cells.
- For marrow donors, collection is typically done under regional or general anesthesia, with those inherent risks. Following the collection, some degree of back or hip pain, bruising at the incision sites, and fatigue are common. The donor's marrow is naturally repleted within 4 to 6 weeks.
- For peripheral blood stem cell donors, filgrastim is administered to the donor to mobilize stem cells. These shots are administered for several days prior to the apheresis procedure where the stem cells are collected. Side effects from filgrastim include headaches, muscle, and bone pain. Serious side effects occur in <1% of donors but can include splenic rupture. The apheresis procedure may require placement of a central line, with those inherent risks, as well as bruising at the needle site, lowering of the platelet count and mild muscle cramping or tingling around the mouth (due to calcium depletion from the citrate used during pheresis).

ELIGIBILITY

1. **What testing must be performed prior to transplant (autologous and allogeneic) in order to consider a patient eligible?**

- While specific guidelines vary among institutions, there are some basic tests that must be done for all patients due to the known and expected toxicities of the transplant process. Testing typically includes:
  - ○ Pulmonary function testing
  - ○ EKG and transthoracic echocardiography (TTE) or multigated acquisition scan (MUGA)
  - ○ Liver function tests
  - ○ Serum creatinine
  - ○ Infectious disease screening
  - ○ Assessment of performance status

INDICATIONS

1. **What are the common indications for autologous stem cell transplant?**

- Multiple myeloma: considered as part of initial therapy for most transplant-eligible patients with myeloma.
- High-grade lymphomas: considered as the standard of care for relapsed diffuse large B-cell lymphoma (DLBCL) and considered as up-front therapy for select groups of other high-grade lymphomas, such as mantle cell lymphoma (see Chapter 7).
- Acute promyelocytic leukemia: considered for either relapsed disease or molecular persistence.

- Germ-cell tumors: considered for refractory or relapsed cases.

2. **What are the common indications for allogeneic stem cell transplant?**
   - Acute myeloid leukemia: considered the standard of care for intermediate- or high-risk patients in first complete remission (CR1) as well as for all patients in subsequent complete remission.
   - Acute lymphoid leukemia, Philadelphia chromosome positive: recommended in CR1.
   - Acute lymphoid leukemia, Philadelphia chromosome negative: recommended in CR1 if other high-risk features.
   - Chronic myeloid leukemia: recommended for patients presenting in accelerated or blast phase or in patients initially diagnosed as chronic phase but for whom tyrosine kinase inhibitors are failing.
   - Myelodysplastic syndrome: considered for certain transplant-eligible patients depending on the status of their disease.
   - Myelofibrosis: considered for certain transplant-eligible patients depending on the status of their disease.
   - Chronic lymphocytic leukemia: Considered for transplant-eligible patients with poor risk disease.
   - Other nonmalignant conditions: aplastic anemia, sickle cell disease, and so on.

TOXICITY OF CONDITIONING REGIMENS

1. **What are common toxicities of all myeloablative preparative regimens?**
   - Mucositis, nausea, vomiting, alopecia, diarrhea, rash, peripheral neuropathies

2. **What are some busulfan-specific toxicities?**
   - Busulfan can cause interstitial lung disease, hepatic sinusoidal obstructive syndrome, and lowered seizure threshold. Prophylactic anticonvulsant therapy should be administered. Some institutions recommend monitoring busulfan pharmacokinetics to help reduce risk of these complications.

3. **What are some TBI specific complications?**
   - Asymptomatic alteration in pulmonary function, cataracts, sicca syndrome, hypothyroidism, and thyroiditis.

4. **What is hepatic sinusoidal obstruction syndrome (SOS)/hepatic veno-occlusive disease (VOD)?**
   - Hepatic SOS/hepatic VOD describes a nonthrombotic obliteration of the small intrahepatic veins. It is thought to be secondary to the conditioning regimen of stem cell transplant, though VOD has been reported after exposure to a wide variety of agents. Clinically, it is recognized by jaundice, tender hepatomegaly, weight gain, ascites, and platelet refractoriness.

COMPLICATIONS OF TRANSPLANT

1. **What is GVHD? How common is it?**
   - GVHD is an immunological phenomenon where donor lymphocytes respond to polymorphic HLAs present in host tissues, and mount an attack against

these tissues. The resulting clinical syndrome is best described as an inflammatory response predominantly involving the skin, intestine, and liver. The interactions between donor lymphocytes and polymorphic HLAs on host tissue are amplified by the significant tissue injury that occurs during the conditioning regimen.

- The risk of GVHD depends on many factors, including degree of HLA compatibility, stem cell source, and conditioning regimen. Acute GVHD can be estimated to occur in 40% to 50% of patients undergoing an HLA-matched related stem cell transplant and 50% to 70% of patients undergoing an unrelated donor stem cell transplant. Chronic GVHD occurs in more than 50% of all patients who undergo an allogeneic stem cell transplant and the majority of patients who develop acute GVHD.

2. What are the organs affected in acute GVHD?

- Acute GVHD classically affects the skin, gastrointestinal (GI) tract, and the liver.

  ○ Skin involvement is typically a maculopapular rash that may be painful or pruritic upon first development. In severe cases, rash may cover the whole body and be associated with bullae, vesicles, and desquamation.

  ○ Gut involvement can be either upper or lower GI involvement with symptoms most typically being diarrhea but can also include abdominal pain, nausea, vomiting, or ileus.

  ○ Liver involvement is typically recognized by hyperbilirubinemia.

3. How is acute GVHD quantified?

Stage	Skin	Liver (Bilirubin)	Gut (Stool Output/Day)
0	No GVHD rash	<2 mg/dL	<500 mL/day
1	Maculopapular rash <25% BSA	2–3 mg/dL	500–999 mL/day *or* Persistent nausea, vomiting, anorexia with a positive upper GI biopsy
2	Maculopapular rash 25%–50%	3.1–6 mg/dL	1,000–1,500 mL/day
3	Maculopapular rash >50%	6.1–15 mg/dL	>1,500 mL/day
4	Generalized erythroderma (>50% BSA) *plus* bullous formation and desquamation >5% BSA	>15 mg/dL	Severe abdominal pain with or without ileus, or grossly bloody stool (regardless of stool volume)

Overall clinical grade:

- Grade 0: no stage 1 to 4 of any organ
- Grade I: stage 1 to 2 rash and no liver or gut involvement
- Grade II: stage 3 rash, or stage 1 liver or stage 1 gut
- Grade III: stage 0 to 3 skin, with stage 2 to 3 liver or stage 2 to 3 gut
- Grade IV: stage 4 skin, liver, or GI involvement

4. **What is graft failure? How common is it?**
   - Graft failure is the term used when donor stem cells are not engrafted within the host marrow and are failing to produce the necessary hematopoietic elements. This may be demonstrated by either failure of the donor stem cells to ever engraft (primary graft rejection), or loss of donor cells after initial engraftment (secondary graft rejection).
   - The causes of graft failure may be rejection, an immunologic phenomenon, or other causes including infection and drugs.
   - The risk of graft rejection is related to degree of HLA incompatibility, stem cell source, and intensity of conditioning—with higher risk of rejection with increased HLA incompatibility, cord blood, and reduced intensity conditioning. Graft failure remains relatively rare, occurring in approximately 5% of transplants.

5. **What organs are typically affected in chronic GVHD?**
   - A multitude of organs can be affected by chronic GVHD. Typically, the following organs are considered:
     - Skin: variety of skin changes can be seen including atrophic changes, lichen sclerosis-like changes, sclerotic changes, hypo- or hyperpigmentation. Changes can include hair and nails.
     - Eyes/mouth: lichenoid changes of oropharynx, leukoplakia, xerostomia, dry eye, photophobia.
     - Liver: elevated bilirubin, alkaline phosphatase, or aminotransferases.
     - Lungs: may present with dyspnea or wheezing. PFTs demonstrate obstructive or restrictive changes. Lung biopsy can confirm bronchiolitis obliterans.
     - Musculoskeletal: fasciitis, joint stiffness, or contractures.

6. **How is chronic GVHD graded?**
   - Chronic GVHD is graded by the National Institutes of Health (NIH) grading system: each organ is given a score from 0 to 3. A score of 0 is no GVHD manifestations and a score of 3 is the most severe GVHD manifestations.
   - Mild disease involves only one or two organs or sites, with no lung involvement and a maximum score of 1 at each involved site.
   - Moderate disease involves at least one site with a maximum score of 2 or 3 or more organs with a score of 1. A lung score of 1 will also be considered moderate disease.
   - Severe disease is when any organ or site is scored as 3 or a lung score of 2 or greater.

7. **What measures are used to prevent GVHD?**
   - Nonpharmacologic preventive measures include use of properly matched donors, T-cell depletion, and minimizing pretransplant organ damage.
   - Medications used to prevent GVHD vary by transplant center, preparative regimen, and donor source but common agents include methotrexate, tacrolimus, mycophenolate, cyclosporine, and sirolimus.

8. **What medications are used to treat acute GVHD?**
   - First-line therapy for acute GVHD depends on the initial GVHD grade.
     - For grade 1(skin stage 1), topical steroids are recommended.
     - For grades II to IV, topical therapy in addition to high-dose intravenous (IV) steroids (methylprednisolone 2 mg/kg/day) is recommended.
   - If GVHD is progressing after 3 days of therapy, or if there is no response to treatment after 5 days of therapy, second-line therapies should be considered. There is no standard second-line therapy and decisions should be tailored to the patient and clinical scenario. Options include infliximab, etanercept, mycophenolate, antithymocyte globulin, sirolimus, alemtuzumab, and octreotide.

9. **What medications are used to treat chronic GVHD?**
   - First-line therapy for chronic GVHD typically consists of prednisone at a dose of 1 mg/kg/day for moderate or severe disease.
   - Second-line treatment should be considered if there is progression of chronic GVHD despite optimal first-line treatment for 2 weeks or if there is no improvement after 4 to 8 weeks of sustained therapy or if there is an inability to taper prednisone. Second-line therapies include phototherapy, tacrolimus, cyclosporine, mycophenolate, sirolimus, and rituximab.

10. **What are the infectious risks associated with stem cell transplant?**
    - Infectious risks are distinct depending on the phase of transplant.
    - *In the pre-engraftment period (approximately day 0 through day 30 posttransplant):* the major risk is related to neutropenia, altered barriers (mucositis and diarrhea), and vascular devices. Thus, bacterial organisms including skin, oral, and GI flora are the most common sources of infection. Invasive fungal infections and *herpes simplex virus* (HSV), typically reactivation, can be seen in this time period as well.
    - *In the postengraftment period (approximately day 30 through day 100 posttransplant):* severe neutropenia is resolved and barrier defenses are healing. However, patients remain immunosuppressed due to impaired cell mediated immunity, humoral immunity, and decreased phagocyte function. If acute GVHD has occurred, this can impair immune function and damage immune barriers, in addition to the immunosuppressive effects of the GVHD-directed therapies, thereby multiplying the immunocompromised state of patients. Overall, bacterial infections become less common during this period. Instead, viral infections are the most common infections encountered in this period of time. Specific pathogens of note include CMV, adenovirus, community acquired respiratory viruses, enterovirus, HHV-6, and BK virus. Invasive fungal infections can continue to occur, especially in those patients with GVHD.

In addition, parasitic infections with *Pneumocystis jirovecii* can occur in this time period, necessitating prophylaxis to prevent this infection.

- *In the late posttransplantation period (>100 days posttransplant):* cellular mediated immunity and humoral immunity recover. Immunosuppressive therapy is slowly withdrawn. Without GVHD, infection is unusual in this period. However, with chronic GVHD, there remain defects in both cellular and humoral immunity as well as deficits in the barrier function of the skin, oropharynx, and GI tract. Infections during this period tend to be localized to the skin and upper and lower respiratory tracts. Pathogens tend to be viral, especially VZV, followed by bacterial. Patients with chronic GVHD tend to have functional asplenia and therefore have increased susceptibility to encapsulated bacteria.

QUESTIONS

1. A 47-year-old man with a diagnosis of acute myeloid leukemia (AML) (normal cytogenetics, FLT3-ITD positive) in first complete remission presents to the transplant clinic to discuss proceeding with allogeneic stem cell transplant. He is otherwise fit with an Eastern Cooperative Oncology Group (ECOG) performance status of 0 and no other medical comorbidities. He is blood type O−. Which of the following would be an optimal donor?
   A. His identical twin brother
   B. Umbilical cord transplant
   C. His human leukocyte antigen (HLA) identical 50-year-old brother who is otherwise healthy and is blood type O+
   D. An HLA identical matched unrelated donor who is blood type O−

2. A 57-year-old woman is 145 days from a matched unrelated stem cell transplant for high-risk myelodysplastic syndrome. Her early transplant course was complicated by a severe viral pneumonia and gastrointestinal (GI) acute graft-versus-host disease (GVHD), which was treated with steroids with good improvement. She presents to clinic today complaining of progressive dry eyes and dry mouth as well as muscle and joint tightness. Her exam is notable for a mild weight loss of 2 kg, irritation of bilateral sclera, and an oropharynx that appears dry with lichenoid changes. She has limited range of motion of both her arms but no muscle tenderness on exam. She remains on tacrolimus for GVHD prophylaxis but this has been tapered. In addition, she continues to take acyclovir, fluconazole, and trimethoprim/sulfamethoxazole for infectious disease prophylaxis. What is the most likely diagnosis?
   A. Side effects from tacrolimus
   B. Chronic GVHD
   C. Infection with adenovirus
   D. Sjögren syndrome

3. A 37-year-old woman underwent a matched related full intensity conditioning stem cell transplant 42 days ago for Philadelphia chromosome positive acute lymphoblastic leukemia (ALL) in first complete remission. Her transplant course had been smooth and she was

discharged home on day 17. She remains on full dose tacrolimus for graft-versus-host disease (GVHD) prophylaxis and continues to take acyclovir, fluconazole, oral and intravenous (IV) magnesium, trimethoprim/sulfamethoxazole, and ursodiol. Her tacrolimus level is therapeutic. However, over the past 2 days she has had loss of appetite, mild epigastric pain, and 6 to 8 episodes of nonbloody diarrhea daily. She undergoes an upper and lower endoscopy and biopsies from both procedures confirm a diagnosis of GVHD. What is the most important first step in management?

A. Increase tacrolimus dose
B. Start mycophenolate mofetil
C. Start photopheresis
D. Start prednisone

4. A 58-year-old man with acute myeloid leukemia (AML) in first remission underwent a myeloablative transplantation conditioning regimen with busulfan and cyclophosphamide followed by infusion of matched unrelated peripheral blood stem cells 19 days ago. Graft-versus-host disease (GVHD) prophylaxis has consisted of tacrolimus and methotrexate. He now has had several days of significant nausea, vomiting, and anorexia but has been noted to gain 5 kilograms. He is noted to have dark urine, scleral icterus, and tender hepatomegaly. Laboratory testing is notable for a total bilirubin of 5.0 mg/dL and transaminases that are fourfold above baseline. Which is the most likely explanation for his current condition?

A. Hepatic sinusoidal obstruction syndrome (SOS)/hepatic veno-occlusive disease (VOD)
B. Engraftment syndrome
C. Methotrexate toxicity
D. Acalculous cholecystitis

5. A 27-year-old healthy man who is volunteering as a peripheral stem cell donor for his sister develops sudden onset of severe left upper quadrant pain on his third day of taking high-dose filgrastim for mobilization. He denies any fevers, nausea, or vomiting; no hematuria or dysuria; no dyspnea or pleuritic pain. What is the most likely cause of his abdominal pain?

A. Nephrolithiasis from a uric acid stone induced by mobilization
B. Rib pain from marrow expansion
C. Splenic rupture
D. Pulmonary embolism

6. A 60-year-old woman with Philadelphia chromosome negative acute lymphoblastic leukemia (ALL) underwent a matched unrelated transplant in CR2. Posttransplant course has been complicated by mild skin graft-versus-host disease (GVHD) and an admission for *Clostridium difficile*-associated diarrhea but has otherwise been unremarkable. At 3 months after transplant, she develops urinary urgency, suprapubic pain, and gross hematuria. Her laboratory work demonstrates only

mild anemia to 11.1 g/dL and no abnormalities in kidney or liver function. What is the most appropriate testing for further evaluation of the patient's symptoms?

A. CT of the abdomen and pelvis
B. Urine PCR for viral DNA
C. Urine cytology and cystoscopy
D. Coombs test and measurement of haptoglobin

ANSWERS

1. **C. His human leukocyte antigen (HLA) identical 50-year-old brother who is otherwise healthy and is blood type O+.** For hematologic malignancies, syngeneic transplant has proven to result in higher relapse rates and would not be the recommended donor source. While ABO compatibility is important to consider in deciding an optimal donor, this is only a minor ABO mismatch and related donor transplants remain preferred to unrelated donor transplants given lower rates of graft-versus-host disease (GVHD) with related transplants. There is no role for an umbilical cord transplant in a setting with available related donors.

2. **B. Chronic GVHD.** Her symptoms of dry eyes, dry mouth, and joint tightness are classic for symptoms of chronic GVHD, as is her exam demonstrating irritated sclera and lichenoid changes in her oropharynx. This is an appropriate time frame for chronic GVHD to begin and her history of prior acute GVHD as well as her unrelated donor transplant are both risk factors for development of chronic GVHD. While the symptoms of dry eyes and dry mouth in a patient who had not previously undergone allogeneic stem cell transplant may be suggestive of Sjögren syndrome, GVHD is a better explanation in this case. Viral etiologies can certainly have a protean presentation of symptoms, but viral ulcerations in the oral cavity tend to be painful and not lichenoid. Tacrolimus does not cause dry eyes, dry mouth, or arthralgias. More commonly, it results in renal wasting of magnesium and rarely microangiopathic hemolytic anemia, neurologic changes, or renal dysfunction. More importantly, the patient's tacrolimus is being tapered suggesting her symptoms are related to the withdrawal of this immunosuppressant (ie, GVHD) and are not a symptom of the medication itself.

3. **D. Start prednisone.** Optimal first line therapy for treating acute GVHD involving the gastrointestinal (GI) tract is steroids, typically prednisone with methylprednisolone reserved for patients who cannot tolerate oral therapy. It is critical to recognize and initiate therapy promptly. There is no role for increasing tacrolimus when levels are already therapeutic as there is significant risk for toxicity with limited increasing therapeutic effect. Photopheresis and mycophenolate can both be effective therapies for GVHD but are typically reserved for patients who are not responding to steroids.

4. **A. Hepatic sinusoidal obstruction syndrome (SOS)/hepatic veno-occlusive disease (VOD).** The patient's signs and symptoms are most suggestive of hepatic SOS/VOD as demonstrated by the rapid weight gain often associated with ascites and/or peripheral edema, tender hepatomegaly, and rapid rise in liver function tests (LFTs). The pathophysiology of this condition includes occlusion of the terminal hepatic venules and sinusoids, likely due to injury of the endothelium of hepatic venules. Most commonly, this condition is seen 3 to 30 days after transplant. Severe cases are almost universally fatal but most patients with mild to moder-

ate disease will recover with only supportive care. Engraftment syndrome more typically presents with fevers and a cytokine release syndrome. It would be unlikely to result in such significant LFT abnormalities. While methotrexate can cause LFT abnormalities, typically this is not associated with tender hepatomegaly. Acalculous cholecystitis, while possible in any critically ill patient, would not be expected to have tender hepatomegaly or weight gain. Instead, the patient may more likely be febrile and exhibiting signs or symptoms consistent with sepsis.

5. **C. Splenic rupture.** Splenic rupture is a potentially life-threatening complication of stem cell mobilization with the use of granulocyte colony-stimulating factors (G-CSFs), such as filgrastim. Luckily, it is an exceedingly rare complication but one that both providers and donors must be aware of. The patient's sudden onset of severe pain without any other significant symptoms is most suggestive of this diagnosis. Filgrastim is not known to cause uric acid stones and the lack of dysuria or hematuria argues against nephrolithiasis. While filgrastim can cause bony pain, this is more typically dull diffuse aches and not severe, sudden-onset focal pain. G-CSF is not known to induce pulmonary embolisms and a lack of pleuritic pain or dyspnea argues against this diagnosis.

6. **B. Urine PCR for viral DNA.** BK virus is a polyoma virus that can cause dysuria, hematuria, and suprapubic pain in posttransplant patients. It is best tested for with use of urine PCR test. With normal renal function and electrolytes, there is no indication for abdominal imaging at this time. While patients with previous chemotherapy exposure, such as this patient, may be at risk for a genitourinary malignancy, her current symptomatology is more consistent with BK infection and one would not consider screening for malignancy until infection is screened for and treated. While hemolytic anemia can result in dark-colored urine with mild dysuria, it would be unlikely to cause this degree of suprapubic pain, especially in light of a relatively stable hemoglobin.

XV

BIOSTATISTICS

Biostatistics

Alexander T. Pearson and Emily Bellile

BASIC CONCEPTS AND DEFINITIONS

1. What is a *P value* and what does it mean?

- The *P* value assumes a null hypothesis (often, the null hypothesis is that two measurements or datasets are equal) and describes the probability that an observed difference between them is due to chance or random variation alone. Generally, a *P* value $< .05$ (5%) is considered sufficient to indicate that the null hypothesis can be rejected because the difference between two datasets is not due to chance alone.

2. What do the terms *incidence* and *incidence proportion* mean?

- Incidence is the number of new cases that occur over a specific period of time.
- Incidence proportion refers to the total number of new cases in a population over a given time divided by the total number of people at risk initially.

3. What does the term *prevalence* mean?

- The total number of cases in a population at a given point in time

4. What is a *relative risk*?

- The probability (incidence proportion) of an event in patients exposed to a variable (treatment, exposure) divided by the probability (incidence proportion) of an event in patients not exposed to that variable. Also called "risk ratio." Often used in randomized controlled studies and cohort studies.

5. What is an *odds ratio*?

- The odds ($P/[1 - P]$, where P is the probability) of an event (condition/diagnosis) occurring in one group divided by the odds of the event (condition/diagnosis) occurring in another group. The odds ratio measures the strength of an association between a condition/diagnosis and other variables. Because of its connection with logistic regression analysis, it is used with multivariable analysis and case–control studies.

6. What is *absolute risk reduction*?

- Absolute risk reduction is the change in incidence attributable to an exposure or treatment. This rate is calculated by subtraction of the incidence proportion of a condition in an exposed group from the incidence proportion in a control population over a specific period of time.

7. **How is *number needed to treat* calculated?**
   - Number needed to treat is the number of patients needed to treat with a given intervention to prevent one event. It is calculated by: 1/(event rate in control group – event rate in intervention group).
   - Example: 50% – 30% = 20% or 0.2. 1/0.2 = 5. The number needed to treat is 5.

DIAGNOSTIC TESTS

1. **What is sensitivity?**
   - Sensitivity is the number of patients who have a positive test with the disease divided by the total number of patients with the disease, that is, what proportion of the total population with a disease is detected by the test.

   See Figure 40.1.

2. **What is specificity?**
   - Specificity is the number of patients who have a negative test and do not have the disease divided by the number of patients who do not have the disease.

   See Figure 40.1.

3. **What is positive predictive value (PPV)?**
   - PPV represents the likelihood that a patient with a positive test will actually have the disease. It incorporates the overall incidence of the disease.

   See Figure 40.1.

4. **What is the negative predictive value (NPV)?**
   - NPV represents the likelihood that a patient with a negative test does not actually have the disease. It incorporates the overall incidence of the disease in the population.

   See Figure 40.1.

5. **What is a likelihood ratio in diagnostic testing?**
   - Likelihood ratio is an aggregate of sensitivity and specificity for a given test and reflects whether a test result changes the probability that a condition exists. Positive likelihood ratio = sensitivity/(1 – specificity) is used for a positive test result. Negative likelihood ratio = (1 – sensitivity)/specificity is used for a negative test result.

	Condition or disease		
	Positive	Negative	
Test results — Positive	A	B	Positive predictive value = A/(A + B)
Test results — Negative	C	D	Negative predictive value = D/(C + D)
	Sensitivity = A/(A + C)	Specificity = D/(B + D)	

FIGURE 40.1 ■ Sensitivity and specificity calculations.

CLINICAL TRIALS

1. What is a confidence interval?

- A confidence interval refers to the range of values most likely to incorporate the true value in a population and is based on the concept of repeat sampling. This range incorporates the number of observations sampled and the variance within the sample dataset. The range will narrow as variability decreases and the number of observations increases.

2. What is a type 1 error (alpha)?

- A type 1 error is commonly referred to as the significance of a test and refers to the probability of rejecting the null hypothesis when the null hypothesis is true; that is, finding a significant difference when there is no difference but that from chance alone. The P value for any hypothesis test is the alpha level at which we are on the borderline of accepting or rejecting a null hypothesis. If a test between two groups in a dataset has a P value of .05, then there is a 5% chance that the difference found could occur by chance.

3. What is a type 2 error (beta)?

- Type 2 error refers to the probability that a study will not detect a true difference between two datasets when a difference truly exists. The power of a study is a function of the type 2 error.

4. What is the "power" of a study?

- Power refers to the probability that a given study will detect a difference between two populations if one actually exists. It is calculated by 1-beta. Power is influenced by the magnitude of the difference, the number of subjects included in the study, the population variance, and the significance level of the test desired.

5. What is multivariate analysis?

- Multivariate analysis (technically called multivariable analysis) is a statistical method of analysis to control for multiple variables that could contribute to an outcome.

6. What is a Kaplan–Meier survival analysis?

- This analysis generates predicted probabilities of survival by calculating the number of surviving patients divided by the number of patients at risk at each time point, allowing for varying follow-up times. When plotted over time, a characteristic survival curve is generated. A log-rank test is often used to test survival differences between two groups using the Kaplan–Meier estimates.

7. What is a Cox proportional hazards analysis?

- A Cox proportional hazards model is a way of analyzing survival or time-to-event data. Similar to multivariate analysis, this analysis can take multiple variables into account in predicting outcome. The models generate hazard ratios, which indicate the magnitude of increased risk of the event attributable to a given variable.

8. What is a cohort study?

- A form of longitudinal study where a group of patients is followed and associations between differential exposures and outcome can be compared. Study can be completed retrospectively or prospectively.

9. **What is a case–control study?**
   - A type of observational study where a group of patients with a disease is compared to a similar control group without the disease.

10. **What is a randomized controlled study?**
    - A type of experiment where subjects are randomly allocated to receive one or another treatment under study, and then followed in exactly the same way. The advantage of randomized studies is that it minimizes allocation bias and provides balance in the comparison groups on prognostic factors known and unknown that could influence outcome.

STUDY BIASES

1. **What is a reporting bias?**
   - Reporting bias is a shift in outcomes resulting from a selective inclusion or exclusion of results. A subtype of reporting bias is publication bias, wherein positive study results preferentially appear in the literature and negative studies are suppressed.

2. **What is lead time bias?**
   - Lead time bias is a false extension of the time length between disease diagnosis and time of death resulting from improvements in disease screening that do not impart an improvement in the length of life, but change the date of diagnosis.

3. **What is length time bias?**
   - Length time bias is an incorrect estimation of cancer mortality rate incurred when deaths are estimated from disease prevalence at a short time interval. Rapidly progressive cancers are less likely to be captured in a short time interval, and thus slowly progressive tumors are over-emphasized, thereby biasing the survival time estimates for slowly progressive diseases to appear longer incorrectly.

4. **What is centripetal bias?**
   - Centripetal bias is when a specific individual or institution draws a cohort of patients who are unlike the population at large, thereby changing the generalizability of outcome results produced from clinical studies. For example, patients who are fit enough to travel long distances to see an expert are more likely to live longer while participating in a clinical study, independent of the true effectiveness of the intervention.

QUESTIONS

1. **Which of the following quantities is not used when a power calculation is performed?**
   A. The magnitude of the expected difference between groups
   B. The number of subjects or events to be included in the study
   C. Statistical alpha
   D. The cost of the study
   E. The amount of statistical variance expected in the data

2. The Kaplan–Meier statistic requires which of the following quantities to calculate median cancer specific survival?
   A. Length of participating individuals' time in the study
   B. Number of participating individuals' deaths occurring during the study
   C. Participating individuals' date of cancer diagnosis
   D. A + B
   E. B + C

3. Which of the following combinations represents the best evidence for strong association?
   A. $r = -0.9, P = .001$
   B. $r = -0.09, P = .001$
   C. $r = 0.09, P = .009$
   D. $r = 0.9, P = .009$
   E. $r = 0.9, P = .9$

4. Which of the following statements regarding 95% confidence intervals is correct?
   A. The width of the confidence interval is dependent only on data variability
   B. The confidence interval does not necessarily contain the true value
   C. It is narrower than the 90% confidence interval holding other parameters equal
   D. If this experiment was repeated on 20 samples, 19 of these intervals would contain the true value

5. A new public health surveillance testing initiative is most likely to induce which of the following:
   A. Lead time bias
   B. Sampling bias
   C. Centripetal bias
   D. Bogus control bias

ANSWERS

1. **D. The cost of the study.** While the number of events and number of individuals in a study are important, the cost of the study is not required for a power calculation. In a power calculation, four of the following are held constant and the fifth is calculated for: statistical alpha, statistical beta, amount of variance, magnitude of expected variance, and number of subjects/events.

2. **D. A + B.** The Kaplan–Meier method can calculate the median survival for a clinical study that enrolls participants beginning at different time points, but will only require each participant's time on the study and their event class (eg, withdrawal from study, death).

3. **A. r = −0.9, P = .001.** For the correlation coefficient r, associations are measured between −1 and 1. Stronger associations are farther from 0, whether positive or negative. For P values, lower P values imply stronger evidence that associations are not due to random variation.

4. **B. The confidence interval does not necessarily contain the true value.** Confidence intervals are a mechanism for calculating the amount of variability around a point estimate of a parameter. The calculation is based on the quantity and variability of data used in calculation. Confidence intervals with higher degrees of confidence (such as 95% vs. 90%) must be wider to accommodate more variability. A confidence interval does not necessarily contain the true value being estimated, and when repeating the study there is no guarantee for the number of successful estimations.

5. **A. Lead time bias.** Lead time bias defines the time between when a disease is detected by preventive screening and when it would be detected by clinical symptoms. Sampling bias defines the deviations from reality induced when a sample is collected nonrepresentatively. Centripetal bias is the deviation from a representative population caused by a patient population seeking a particular type of medical institution (eg, a tertiary care center).

Index